eureka

Biochemistry & Metabolism

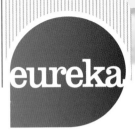

Biochemistry & Metabolism

Andrew Davison BSc (Hons) MSc CSci
EuSpLM FRCPath
Principal Clinical Biochemist and
Honorary Lecturer in Clinical
Biochemistry
Department of Clinical Biochemistry
Liverpool Clinical Laboratories
Royal Liverpool and Broadgreen
University Hospitals NHS Trust
Liverpool, UK

Anna Milan BSc (Hons) MSc PhD
FRCPath
Principal Clinical Biochemist and
Honorary Lecturer in Clinical
Biochemistry
Department of Clinical Biochemistry
Liverpool Clinical Laboratories
Royal Liverpool and Broadgreen
University Hospitals NHS Trust
Liverpool, UK

Suzannah Phillips BSc (Hons) MSc PhD
Principal Clinical Biochemist and
Honorary Lecturer in Clinical
Biochemistry
Department of Clinical Biochemistry
Liverpool Clinical Laboratories
Royal Liverpool and Broadgreen
University Hospitals NHS Trust
Liverpool, UK

Lakshminarayan Ranganath MD
MBBS MSc PhD CSci FRCP FRCPath
Professor and Consultant in Chemical
Pathology
Department of Clinical Biochemistry
Liverpool Clinical Laboratories
Royal Liverpool and Broadgreen
University Hospitals NHS Trust
Liverpool, UK

Series Editors

Janine Henderson MRCPsych
MClinEd
MB BS Programme Director
Hull York Medical School
York, UK

David Oliveira PhD FRCP
Professor of Renal Medicine
St George's, University of London
London, UK

Stephen Parker BSc MS DipMedEd
FRCS
Consultant Breast and General
Paediatric Surgeon
St Mary's Hospital
Newport, UK

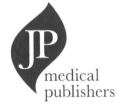

JP
medical
publishers

London · Philadelphia · New Delhi · Panama City

© 2015 JP Medical Ltd.

Published by JP Medical Ltd, 83 Victoria Street, London, SW1H 0HW, UK

Tel: +44 (0)20 3170 8910   Fax: +44 (0)20 3008 6180

Email: info@jpmedpub.com   Web: www.jpmedpub.com

ISBN: 978-1-907816-83-3

British Library Cataloguing in Publication Data
A catalogue record for this book is available from the British Library

Library of Congress Cataloging in Publication Data
A catalog record for this book is available from the Library of Congress

Publisher:	Richard Furn
Development Editors:	Thomas Fletcher, Paul Mayhew, Alison Whitehouse
Editorial Assistants:	Sophie Woolven, Katie Pattullo
Copy Editor:	Kim Howell
Graphic narratives;	James Pollitt
Cover design:	Forbes Design
Interior design:	Designers Collective Ltd

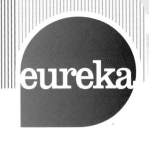

Series Editors' Foreword

Today's medical students need to know a great deal to be effective as tomorrow's doctors. This knowledge includes core science and clinical skills, from understanding biochemical pathways to communicating with patients. Modern medical school curricula integrate this teaching, thereby emphasising how learning in one area can support and reinforce another. At the same time students must acquire sound clinical reasoning skills, working with complex information to understand each individual's unique medical problems.

The *Eureka* series is designed to cover all aspects of today's medical curricula and reinforce this integrated approach. Each book can be used from first year through to qualification. Core biomedical principles are introduced but given relevant clinical context: the authors have always asked themselves, 'why does the aspiring clinician need to know this'?

Each clinical title in the series is grounded in the relevant core science, which is introduced at the start of each book. Each core science title integrates and emphasises clinical relevance throughout. Medical and surgical approaches are included to provide a complete and integrated view of the patient management options available to the clinician. Clinical insights highlight key facts and principles drawn from medical practice. Cases featuring unique graphic narratives are presented with clear explanations that show how experienced clinicians think, enabling students to develop their own clinical reasoning and decision making. Clinical SBAs help with exam revision while Starter questions are a unique learning tool designed to stimulate interest in the subject.

Having biomedical principles and clinical applications together in one book will make their connections more explicit and easier to remember. Alongside repeated exposure to patients and practice of clinical and communication skills, we hope *Eureka* will equip medical students for a lifetime of successful clinical practice.

Janine Henderson, David Oliveira, Stephen Parker

About the Series Editors

Janine Henderson is the MB BS undergraduate Programme Director at Hull York Medical School (HYMS). After medical school at the University of Oxford and clinical training in psychiatry, she combined her work as a consultant with postgraduate teaching roles, moving to the new Hull York Medical School in 2004. She has a particular interest in modern educational methods, curriculum design and clinical reasoning.

David Oliveira is Professor of Renal Medicine at St George's, University of London (SGUL), where he served as the MBBS Course Director between 2007 and 2013. Having trained at Cambridge University and the Westminster Hospital he obtained a PhD in cellular immunology and worked as a renal physician before being appointed as Foundation Chair of Renal Medicine at SGUL.

Stephen Parker is a Consultant Breast and General Paediatric Surgeon at St Mary's Hospital, Isle of Wight. He trained at St George's, University of London, and after service in the Royal Navy was appointed as Consultant Surgeon at University Hospital Coventry. He has a particular interest in e-learning and the use of multimedia platforms in medical education.

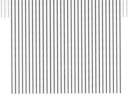

Preface

Knowledge of biochemistry is vital to the practise of clinical medicine, providing an understanding of disease processes at the molecular level. It is essential that clinicians and scientists have a firm grasp of the science that underpins disease, in order to select the appropriate treatment and investigations for their patients.

Eureka Biochemistry & Metabolism covers the fundamental building blocks of life, from basic metabolism to the investigation of disease. Chapter 1 provides an introduction to cellular structure and function, biochemical reactions and body fuels. Chapters 2-6 build on these themes and are enhanced by clinical cases; these highlight the importance of the core science and emphasise its relevance to real life and clinical medicine. Chapters 7 and 8 describe fluid and electrolyte balance and nutrition; like all the other chapters they include clinical insights to help clinicians make informed decisions around patient care. Lastly, chapter 9 provides an invaluable revision aid for undergraduate students in the form of clinical SBAs.

Throughout *Eureka Biochemistry & Metabolism*, we include diagrams and unique graphic narratives to help students understand key concepts. We have made every effort to carefully explain the knowledge you will need to succeed in your exams and become a successful doctor. We hope you enjoy the book and find it useful.

Andrew Davison, Anna Milan, Suzannah Phillips, Lakshminarayan Ranganath
April 2015

About the Authors

Andrew Davison is a Principal Clinical Biochemist with a special interest in phaeochromocytoma and one of the co-leads for the MSc course in Clinical Biochemistry at the University of Manchester. He has a keen interest in teaching undergraduate and postgraduate students about the science behind clinical medicine.

Anna Milan is a Principal Clinical Biochemist with a keen interest in bone markers, vitamins, mineralised tissue biochemistry and alkaptonuria. She is an Honorary Lecturer at the University of Liverpool and also lectures on the MSc course in Clinical Biochemistry at the University of Manchester. She has over 15 years' experience in teaching at all levels, in clinical and non-clinical settings, through lectures and problem-based learning examples.

Suzannah Phillips is a Principal Clinical Biochemist at the Royal Liverpool University Hospital. She has over 10 years' experience in teaching both undergraduate and postgraduate students and coordinates undergraduate medical teaching in clinical biochemistry. She also lectures on the MSc course in Clinical Biochemistry at the University of Manchester.

Lakshminarayan Ranganath is a Consultant Chemical Pathologist at the Royal Liverpool University Hospital and Clinical Director of the National Alkaptonuria Centre. He has extensive experience in teaching students, medical and non-medical trainees.

Contents

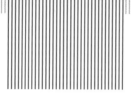

Glossary

A site	aminoacyl site		DNA	deoxyribonucleic acid
ABCA1	ATP-binding cassette transporter A1		dNTP	deoxyribonucleoside triphosphate
ABCG1	ATP-binding cassette transporter G1		dTMP	deoxythymidine monophosphate
ACE	angiotensin-converting enzyme		dTTP	deoxythymidine triphosphate
ADP	adenosine diphosphate		dUDP	deoxyuridine diphosphate
ADH	antidiuretic hormone		dUMP	deoxyuridine monophosphate
AMP	adenine monophosphate		dUTP	deoxyuridine triphosphate
ANP	atrial natriuretic peptide			
APRT	adenine phosphoribosyltransferase		E	enzyme
ATP	adenosine triphosphate		EDTA	ethylenediaminetetra-acetic acid
AVP	arginine vasopressin			
			F	ferroportin 1
BMD	bone mineral density		FAD^+	flavin adenine dinucleotide (oxidised form)
BNP	brain natriuretic peptide		$FADH_2$	flavin adenine dinucleotide (reduced form)
C:D	ratio of number of carbon atoms:double bonds		Fe^{2+}	oxidising iron
cAMP	cyclic adenosine monophosphate		Fe^{3+}	ferric iron
CDP	cytidine diphosphate		FMN	flavin mononucleotide (reduced form)
CE	cholesterol ester			
CHOL	cholesterol		G	Gibbs free energy
CMP	cytidine monophosphate		GDP	guanosine diphosphate
CoA	coenzyme A		GLUT	glucose transporter
CoASH	coenzyme A (reduced form)		GMP	guanine monophosphate
CTP	cytidine triphosphate		GP	general practitioner
cyt	cytochrome		G-protein	guanine nucleotide–binding protein
			GTP	guanosine triphosphate
dADP	deoxyadenosine diphosphate			
DAG	diacylglycerol		H	enthalpy
dATP	deoxyadenosine triphosphate		H	hephaestin
dCDP	deoxycytidine diphosphate		Hb	haemoglobin
dCTP	deoxycytidine triphosphate		HbA	adult haemoglobin
DEXA	dual-energy X-ray absorptiometry		HbA_2	haemoglobin A2
dGDP	deoxyguanosine diphosphate		HbC	haemoglobin C
dGTP	deoxyguanosine triphosphate		HbD	haemoglobin D
DHF	dihydrofolate		HbD_{punjab}	haemoglobin Punjab
DHFR	dihydrofolate reductase		HbF	fetal haemoglobin
DMT-1	divalent metal iron transporter-1		Hb_{lepore}	haemoglobin Lepore

HbM   haemoglobin M

HbS   sickle haemoglobin

HbSS   sickle cell anaemia

HDL   high-density lipoprotein

HGPRT   hypoxanthine–guanine phosphoribosyltransferase

HH   hereditary haemochromatosis

HMG CoA   3-hydroxy-3-methylglutaryl CoA

IDL   intermediate-density lipoprotein

IMP   inosine monophosphate

IP_3 inositol 1,4,5-triphosphate

Km Michaelis constant

LDL   low-density lipoprotein

Lp(a)   lipoprotein(a);

mRNA   messenger ribonucleic acid

MTHF   methylene tetrahydrofolate

MTHFR   methylenetetrahydrofolate reductase

NAD^+ nicotinamide adenine dinucleotide (oxidised form)

NADH   nicotinamide adenine dinucleotide (reduced form)

$NADP^+$ nicotinamide adenine dinucleotide phosphate (oxidised form)

NADPH   nicotinamide adenine dinucleotide phosphate (reduced form)

P site   peptidyl site

P   product

P_i inorganic phosphate

PIP_2 phosphatidylinositol 4,5-bisphosphate

PL   phospholipid

pre-mRNA   precursor messenger ribonucleic acid

pre-RNA   precursor ribonucleic acid

pre-rRNA   precursor ribosomal ribonucleic acid

pre-tRNA   precursor transfer ribonucleic acid

PRPP   5-phosphoribosyl 1-pyrophosphate

RANK   receptor-activated nuclear kappa

RANKL   receptor-activated nuclear kappa-B ligand

RNA   ribonucleic acid

rRNA   ribosomal ribonucleic acid

S entropy

S   substrate

T   temperature

TG   triglycerides

THF   tetrahydrofolate

TMP   thymidine monophosphate

TMPT   thiopurine methyltransferase

TPN   total parenteral nutrition

TPP   thiamine pyrophosphate

TRH   thyrotrophin-releasing hormone

tRNA   transfer ribonucleic acid

TSH   thyroid-stimulating hormone

UDP   uridine diphosphate

UMP   uridine monophosphate

UTP   uridine triphosphate

VLDL   very-low-density lipoprotein

V_{max} maximum rate (velocity) of reaction

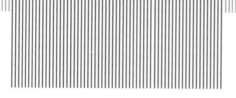

Acknowledgements

Thanks to the following medical students for their help reviewing chapters: Jessica Dunlop, Aliza Imam, Roxanne McVittie, Daniel Roberts and Joseph Suich.

Chapter 1
First principles

Introduction

Biochemistry is the study of all chemical and molecular processes occurring in the body, including:

- anabolism (building molecules)
- catabolism (breaking molecules down)
- molecular transport
- generation of energy

These reactions primarily use the key biological molecules carbohydrates, lipids, proteins and nucleic acids. Knowledge of how the body synthesises, uses and stores these molecules is fundamental to understanding normal body function and the mechanisms by which it goes wrong in disease states. In particular, an understanding of biochemical processes underlies many clinical investigations, diagnoses and treatments.

The cell is the basic unit of life, and the place in which and between which these processes occur. The body comprises about 100 trillion cells, each only 1–100 µm in diameter. All the cells in an individual person contain identical hereditary material for their design: the deoxyribonucleic acid (DNA) that encodes genes. Despite this, there are hundreds of different types of cell. Biochemistry is the story of how these living building blocks operate and communicate at the chemical level, and is key to understanding how and why they dysfunction.

Overview

Starter questions

Answers to the following questions are on page 39.

1. How many types of cell are there?
2. What is a stem cell?

Fundamental to biochemical processes are the molecular interactions between molecules, cells, tissues and organs. The body is composed of organs, which consist of tissues, which in turn are made of cells. Each cell contains organelles that have specific functions, and each cell is capable of numerous chemical reactions to provide usable energy. The energy provided is utilised to coordinate cellular activities and ultimately tissue and organ functions. This chapter focuses on the basic principles that govern these processes and functions.

Body systems

The average human contains over 10^{14} cells organised into tissues or organs, which form systems:

- the respiratory system to take up oxygen and remove carbon dioxide
- the gastrointestinal system to digest food and absorb nutrients
- the urinary system to remove waste products
- the cardiovascular system to transport oxygen and nutrients and to regulate temperature, blood pressure, electrolytes and water balance
- the reproductive system to enable procreation
- the nervous and endocrine systems to coordinate and integrate the functions of the other systems

Each system operates at a system, organ, tissue, cellular, organelle and molecular level to maintain its functions, and each is integrated in the whole organism through interorgan and intercellular communication, for example through chemical messengers called hormones.

Cells

Metabolic processes take place throughout the body and occur predominantly in cells. This compartmentalisation enables metabolites to be concentrated; their distribution regulated and also protects the body from harmful metabolites.

A cell is the fundamental unit of an organism. It is a microscopic membrane-bound sac of fluid and solid components, and its development and function depend on the controlled expression of the DNA it contains.

There are two main types of cell in organisms: prokaryotes (bacteria) and eukaryotes (animals, plants and micro-organisms). Eukaryotes have a nucleus, organelles and a compartmentalisation of materials, whereas prokaryotes do not. Both cell types have similar biochemical composition and share many metabolic pathways but are different in terms of structural elements and genetic processes (**Table 1.1**).

> The word 'cell' is derived from the Latin cella, which means small room.

An understanding of basic cell biology and the processes that occur in individual organelles is key to understanding cellular events at the molecular level. Organelles can be considered specialised subunits in a cell, much like organs are functional units in an organism.

Comparison of prokaryotic and eukaryotic cells		
Property	Prokaryotic	Eukaryotic
Size (µm)	0.2-2	10-100
Nucleus	Absent	Present
Organelles	Absent	Membrane bound organelles present
Cell division	By fission or budding	Mitosis or meiosis
Metabolism	Anaerobic and aerobic	Mostly aerobic
DNA	Single circular DNA	Linear DNA organised into chromosomes
Organisms	Bacteria	Fungi, protozoa, plants and animal

Table 1.1 Comparison of prokaryotic and eukaryotic cells

Cell structure

Starter questions

Answers to the following questions are on page 39.

3. Why are cell membranes both hydrophobic (water repelling) and hydrophilic (interact with water)?
4. How do cells die and how many die per day?

All eukaryotic cells have certain structures in common, such as a plasma membrane. However, specialised cells have additional features related to their function, such as the moving, high-surface area folds called villi in intestinal cells, which aid the absorption of intestinal contents. Cells are highly organised internally, with numerous organelles, each of which has a specific function (**Figure 1.1**).

Cell polarity

Cell polarity is the term for the asymmetrical organisation of cells, with differences in the properties of the cell surface, cell organelles and cytoskeleton at different ends. These differences reflect the function and location of the cells. For example, the epithelial cells of the intestine have two surfaces: the apical surface and the basolateral surface. Each is exposed to a different environment, and they differ both structurally and chemically.

The apical surface faces inwards towards the lumen, whereas the outer (basolateral) surface is exposed to extracellular fluids, facing outwards. The basolateral membrane is in contact with the basal lamina externally.

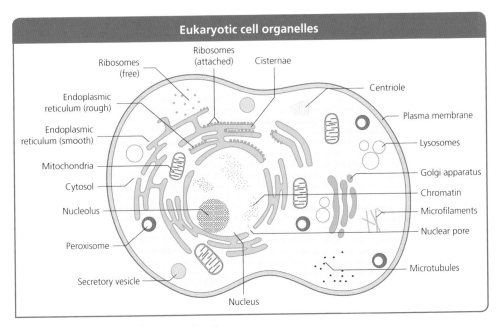

Figure 1.1 The organelles of a eukaryotic cell.

The two surfaces are evident in epithelial and endothelial cells. The basolateral membrane of a polarised cell is the surface of the plasma membrane that forms its basal and lateral surfaces. It faces outwards, away from the lumen. Thus the cell has apical–basal polarity that enables specialised diffusion and transport for ions and other macromolecules.

Cell membrane

Every cell is surrounded by a plasma membrane that separates the inside of the cell from the extracellular environment. It consists of lipids and proteins, which provide flexibility, motility and permeability.

Generally, biochemical processes occur more efficiently in an aqueous medium (a watery environment) because this facilitates movement of and interaction between substances. Therefore intracellular fluid, blood and other body fluids are aqueous environments.

To enable control of extracellular and intracellular environments, cells require a barrier through which water flow is controlled: the cell membrane. The cell membrane makes control possible because it is semipermeable: it selectively allows the passage of a limited number of substances. Membrane permeability is regulated by the lipid composition of the membrane and the proteins (ion channels and transport proteins) embedded in the lipid bilayer.

As well as isolating and controlling the intracellular environment, the cell membrane has other key roles, including:

- energy storage
- cell signalling
- cell adhesion
- anchoring of extracellular structures and the intracellular cytoskeleton
- ion conductivity
- membrane transport

The cell membrane protects the cytoplasm, also called cytosol, the large fluid-filled space inside the cell. In this fluid are all the organelles and the cytoskeleton.

Cytoplasm

The cytoplasm contains dissolved nutrients, helps break down waste products and moves material around the cell. It also contains salts, which make it a good conductor of electricity. Chemically the cytoplasm is 90% water and 10% proteins, carbohydrates, lipids and inorganic salts, providing a suitable environment for cellular function. The cytoplasm is predominantly fluid, and its flow is directed to transport molecules and organelles through cytoplasmic streaming.

> **Cytoplasmic streaming is like stirring the soup (the liquid cytosol) of the cell.** It allows organelles, metabolites, genetic material, nutrients and waste products to be circulated to where they are needed.

In the cytoplasm are the organelles, the most prominent of which is the nucleus.

The nucleus

The nucleus is the largest organelle, occupying up to half the cell volume. It is the operational centre of the cell because it contains DNA, the blueprint for the structure of the cell and the software for cell function.

The nucleus is separated from the cytoplasm by a protective double membrane called the nuclear envelope. This comprises two closely spaced membranes containing several hundred nuclear pore complexes. These pores allow macromolecules (larger molecules such as ribosomes, RNA and DNA polymerase enzyme) to move into and out of the nucleus. The nuclear envelope also protects the cell's DNA.

All cells have a nucleus except for red blood cells, which lose their nucleus on maturation. The lack of the nucleus enables the cell to develop the specific doughnut shape required to transport oxygen.

Chromosomes

The eukaryotic nucleus contains DNA organised into chromosomes. Each cell has the same DNA content (the genome) organised into the same number of chromosomes, unless there is a genetic abnormality.

Each chromosome consists of a single DNA molecule associated with numerous proteins. Humans have 46 chromosomes in 23 pairs, including one pair of sex chromosomes: XX in females and XY in males. The sex chromosomes carry information for sexual differentiation as well as other 'sex-linked' traits. The other 22 pairs, the autosomes, contain the rest of the genetic hereditary information.

Human cells are diploid, because each autosome is present in two copies. The cells of other organisms sometimes have more than two copies. This is especially common in plants, which can be hexaploid (e.g. in bread wheat) or tetraploid (e.g. durum wheat).

> **Chromosomal mutations are absent, damaged, swapped or extra chromosomes.** For example, Down's syndrome is usually caused by an extra copy of chromosome 21 (trisomy 21).

Ribosomes

Ribosomes are ribonucleoproteins; they consist of nucleic acid and protein. They are the machines that synthesise (or translate) proteins from messenger ribonucleic acid (mRNA), the messenger molecule that is transcribed from the DNA in the nucleus and then leaves through the nuclear pores (see Chapter 2).

Each ribosome comprises a large subunit and a small subunit. Each subunit is composed of proteins and one or more molecules of ribosomal RNA (rRNA). The small subunit reads the mRNA sequence, whereas the large subunit joins the amino acids encoded by the mRNA into a polypeptide chain.

The cell's ribosomes are either free in the cytoplasm or bound to another organelle called the endoplasmic reticulum. The bound ribosomes give the endoplasmic reticulum a rough appearance, hence the term rough endoplasmic reticulum.

Ribosomes have the same function whether free or bound. However, they synthesise different proteins, being controlled by signal sequences on the protein.

- Proteins synthesised by free ribosomes are released into the cytosol for use in the cell
- Proteins produced from bound ribosomes are usually used in the plasma membrane or are expelled from the cell through exocytosis (see page 13)

Endoplasmic reticulum

The endoplasmic reticulum is part of the cell's transport network for molecules, an interconnected network of membrane vesicles held together by the cytoskeleton. It has three forms:

- rough endoplasmic reticulum
- smooth endoplasmic reticulum
- sarcoplasmic reticulum

Rough endoplasmic reticulum has ribosomes on its surface and synthesises proteins for release, through the Golgi apparatus, to their destination.

Smooth endoplasmic reticulum does not have ribosomes. It has roles in lipid and carbohydrate metabolism, steroid metabolism, detoxification and calcium sequestration and release.

The functions of the endoplasmic reticulum vary depending on cell type, cell function and cell requirements. The cell can respond to changes in its metabolic needs, for example by adjusting the relative amounts of rough and smooth endoplasmic reticulum.

Sarcoplasmic reticulum is a type of smooth endoplasmic reticulum present in the myocytes (muscle cells) of smooth and striated muscle. It has a major role in excitation–contraction coupling, the molecular mechanism of muscular contraction. Its role is to collect and release calcium when the muscle cell is stimulated; the calcium ions are used to provoke muscular contraction. To carry out its functions, the sarcoplasmic reticulum has special membrane proteins not present in normal smooth endoplasmic reticulum.

The Golgi apparatus

The Golgi apparatus, also called the Golgi complex, is a folded membrane organelle that alters, sorts and packages newly made macromolecules such as proteins and lipids for secretion or for use in the cell. It also produces lysosomes, the small, membrane-bound vesicles (sacs) that contain digestive enzymes that break down unwanted molecules in the cytosol.

The Golgi apparatus consists of stacks of membrane cisternae: flat discs of folded membrane, with four to eight cisternae per stack and 40–100 stacks per cell. Each cisterna contains enzymes used to modify the proteins, which it then packs and transports.

Mitochondria

Mitochondria are self-replicating organelles that are present in various numbers, shapes and sizes in all eukaryotic cells. Their main role is to generate cellular energy by oxidative phosphorylation (see page 112). Oxidative phosphorylation is a chain reaction that occurs in the inner membrane of the mitochondria; oxygen is used to release energy from compounds, typically glucose, to generate adenosine triphosphate (ATP).

Other functions of mitochondria include regulation of programmed cell death (apoptosis), cell signalling, cellular differentiation and regulation of the membrane potential. The membrane potential is the difference in voltage inside and outside the cell; changes in membrane potential enable cells to send chemical and electrical messages around the body, and to and from the central nervous system. Different cells have different numbers of mitochondria. For example, erythrocytes are the only cells without them, and neurons and spermatozoa contain many.

> **Mitochondria are the power generators of cells.** They manufacture chemical energy in the form of ATP.

Mitochondria are sausage-shaped (**Figure 1.2**), 0.5–10 µm long and have five distinct features:

- an outer membrane
- an intermembrane space

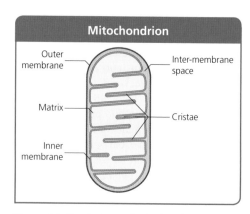

Figure 1.2 Key features of mitochondria.

- an inner membrane
- cristae, the folds of the inner membrane that contain the enzymes that catalyse oxidative phosphorylation
- a matrix, the central space, which contains mitochondrial DNA

> **Mitochondrial DNA replicates separately from the cell's DNA and is more prone to mutation.** The vulnerability to mutation is the result of mitochondria having no DNA repair system, like that of the nucleus. Mutations can cause mitochondrial diseases, a group of syndromes often featuring poor growth, loss of muscle coordination, visual and hearing problems, and neurological problems. The commonest parts of the body affected are the organs which have the highest energy requirements: the muscles, brain, liver, heart and kidneys.

The outer membrane

The mitochondrial outer membrane contains many integral porins. Porins are proteins that form channels for small molecules (≤ 5 kDa), thus making the membrane freely permeable to them. Because small molecules are able to diffuse freely across the outer membrane, the concentration of these molecules in the intermembrane space is equal to that in the cytosol.

Larger proteins are moved across the membrane by the translocase protein complex, which includes 19 proteins. This occurs by active transport, so energy is required in the form of ATP.

The intermembrane space

Cytochrome c is a protein in the intermembrane space with an essential role in the electron transport system, also known as the electron transport chain. This is the series of reduction–oxidation (redox) reactions between inner membrane proteins that produces most of the body's ATP. Cytochrome c also helps initiate apoptosis, the programmed cell death that ends the cell's life cycle and prevents disordered cell growth and behaviour.

The inner membrane

As well as being the fundamental site of the electron transport system, the inner membrane contains cardiolipin, a phospholipid (see page 9) also present in bacterial membranes. Cardiolipin contains four fatty acids instead of the two normally present on phospholipids; this property contributes to the impermeable nature of the inner membrane.

The inner membrane has no porins, so all ions and molecules require special membrane transport mechanisms to enter or exit the matrix. This property is central to the ability of the electron transport system to generate the concentration gradients that are exploited to generate ATP.

Cristae

Cristae are folds of inner membrane that provide an increased surface area for ATP production through the electron transport system. The number of folds varies according to the energy demand of the tissue or cell. For example, liver and muscle cells have many cristae, reflecting their higher energy demands.

Matrix

The mitochondrial matrix is the central space and contains two thirds of the total protein content of the mitochondria. It is the site of the citric acid cycle (also known as the tricarboxylic acid cycle or Krebs cycle), the oxidation of fatty acids and pyruvate, and all processes of ATP production.

> **Mitochondria look like bacteria because they probably evolved from endosymbiotic bacteria.** These bacteria formed a symbiotic relationship with the eukaryotic cells that engulfed them, becoming increasingly specialised to supply the cells with energy.

Lysosomes

Lysosomes are large, irregular vesicular structures in the cytoplasm. They break down old cell components and bacteria with degradative enzymes and acidic fluid bound by the lysosomal membrane. They engulf objects by endocytosis (cell takes up material; an energy dependent process) and phagocytosis (form of endocytosis whereby bacteria are internalised). They also help repair torn sections of plasma membrane by functioning as a 'patch'.

> **Lysosomal storage diseases result from mutations that inactivate a lysosomal enzyme, causing accumulation of the substrate that the enzyme would normally degrade.** These rare but serious diseases have variable clinical expression depending on age of onset, complexity of the storage product and tissue distribution. For example, in Tay–Sachs disease gangliosides accumulate in nerve cells to cause intellectual disability, blindness and death in childhood.

Peroxisomes

Peroxisomes are vesicular structures, 0.5 nm in diameter, required in synthetic (anabolic) and degradative (catabolic) processes. They contain more than 40 peroxisomal enzymes.

One major function of peroxisomes is the β-oxidation (i.e. breakdown) of very-long-chain fatty acids (with ≥ 22 carbons) to medium-chain fatty acids (6–10 carbons long). The shorter fatty acids are then transported to the mitochondria for further degradation. Peroxisomes are also the site of the breakdown of branched chain fatty acids, D-amino acids and polyamines.

Peroxisomes are also the site of anabolic activity.

- Synthesis of plasmalogen, the most abundant phospholipid in myelin, begins in peroxisomes, making peroxisomes essential for nerve cell myelination
- Peroxisomal β-oxidation of C_{27} bile acid intermediates forms C_{24} bile acids, which, when conjugated, are excreted into the bile. Bile acids are necessary for the absorption of fats and fat-soluble vitamins (vitamins A, D, E and K)
- Peroxisomes also contain 10% of the total activity of the two enzymes (see page 107) in the pentose phosphate pathway, producing the reduced form of nicotinamide adenine dinucleotide phosphate (NADPH, a key reducing agent used in biosynthesis) and 5-carbon sugars

In peroxisomal disorders, enzymatic mutations result in the accumulation of metabolites. These conditions usually present with neurological symptoms, because nerves are highly specialised and active cells with limited means of adapting to metabolite accumulation.

An example of a peroxisomal disorder is X-linked adrenoleukodystrophy, a disorder of peroxisomal fatty acid β-oxidation causing the accumulation of very-long-chain fatty acids. The central nervous system, adrenal cortex and Leydig cells of the testes are particularly affected.

Cell membranes and the transport of molecules and ions

Starter questions

Answers to the following questions are on page 39.

5. Why is sunflower oil liquid and animal fat solid?
6. What governs the shape of cells?
7. How can defects in water channel proteins in the kidney cause diabetes?

The cellular contents are surrounded by a phospholipid bilayer membrane composed primarily of phospholipids and proteins.

The **fluid mosaic model** of Singer and Nicolson describes biological membranes as 'two-dimensional liquids in which lipid and protein molecules diffuse more or less easily'.

The cell membrane

The phospholipid bilayer is 7.5 nm thick and consists of a thin layer of amphipathic phospholipids. They are 'amphipathic' because they have both polar hydrophilic (water-loving) and non-polar hydrophobic (fat-loving) domains.

The phospholipids are arranged with their hydrophilic head regions associating with the intracellular and extracellular surfaces of the bilayer, thus isolating the hydrophobic tail regions from the surrounding polar fluid inside and outside the cell (**Figure 1.3**).

The resultant lipid bilayer is impermeable to ions and polar molecules, but hydrophobic molecules are able to diffuse through it. This property enables the cell to control the movement of ions and polar molecules, regulating what the cell requires and transporting materials out of the cell. Hydrophilic molecules and ions are transported across the membrane through pores, channels and gates.

Cell membranes vary considerably in chemical structure and properties, depending on their location.

Lipids

Nearly half of the fatty acids in biomembranes are unsaturated, i.e. they contain one or more carbon–carbon double bond. Double bonds allow a molecule to exist in a *cis* or *trans* conformation; *cis* and *trans* molecules are stereoisomers that have the same molecular formula but a different geometric layout. Fatty acids, including those of phospholipids, are all in the *cis* conformation; this gives their structure a kink that prevents them from packing tightly together. This property enables the membrane to remain fluid-like at lower temperatures.

Phospholipids

These have an L–glycerol backbone with long-chain aliphatic fatty acids attached at the carbon–1 and carbon–2 positions in ester linkage (**Figure 1.4**). Phosphoric acid is linked as an ester at position carbon-3, and a polar head group, such as choline, is linked to the phosphate. Shorter fatty acid chains are less viscous, so their insertion into the membrane increases its fluidity.

Other lipids

Membranes contain other lipids besides phospholipids.

- Cholesterol is an essential component that strengthens the bilayer and makes it more flexible but also less fluid-like, especially at higher temperatures; cholesterol also

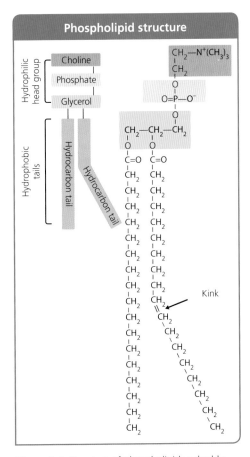

Figure 1.4 Structure of phospholipid: a double bond creates a kink in the hydrocarbon tail.

Figure 1.3 The lipid bilayer.

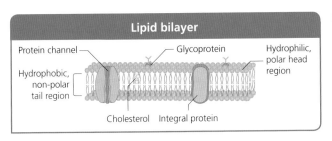

makes the membrane less permeable to water-soluble substances
- Glycosphingolipids are composed of a ceramide backbone and a carbohydrate moiety. These account for the majority of glycolipids in vertebrates and there are hundreds of structural variations
- Sphingomyelin constitute 10–20% of plasma membrane lipids. They are particularly abundant in myelin where they insulate nerve fibres. The hydrophobic chains are often mismatched in length and have a higher degree of saturation than other phospholipids

Carbohydrates

Carbohydrates are present in the plasma membrane predominantly as glycoproteins or glycolipids, which are mainly responsible for molecular recognition and cell-to-cell adhesion on the external side of the lipid bilayer.

Proteins

Proteins have specialised roles in transporting chemicals including ions, small molecules and other proteins, across the membrane. Membrane proteins are grouped as follows.

- Peripheral proteins on the intracellular or extracellular surface, which regulate cell signalling into multiprotein complexes
- Integral proteins are transmembranous and function as transporters, receptors and structural proteins; they also mediate cell adhesion
- Lipid-bound proteins are entirely within the lipid bilayer; these proteins are responsible for many membrane functions, including membrane transport

The ratio of protein to phospholipid varies between membranes and cell types. This ratio determines the fluidity and function of the membrane.

Transport across cell membranes

Cells need to take up nutrients and excrete waste, and the cell membrane regulates the transport of these substances (**Table 1.2**). Only water and gases are able to easily diffuse through the bilayer; the movement of almost all other chemicals through the membrane is tightly regulated. Transport occurs through various mechanisms, using both the biochemical properties of the membrane and the molecules to be transported.

Active versus passive transport

Mechanisms of transport are classified as either passive or active; passive movement does not require the input of cellular energy, whereas active transport does (**Figure 1.5**).

Chemicals are able to move down or up their concentration or electrochemical gradient.

- Movement down a concentration or electrochemical gradient means that the chemical is moving from an area of high concentration to an area of low

Relative permeability of the phospholipid bilayer		
Substance type	Example(s)	Permeability
Gases	Oxygen, carbon dioxide and nitrogen	Permeable
Small, uncharged polar molecules	Water, ethanol and urea	Totally or partially permeable
Large, uncharged polar molecules	Glucose	Not permeable
Charged polar molecules	Amino acids and adenosine triphosphate	Not permeable
Ions	Na^+, K^+, Cl^- and HCO_3^-	Not permeable

Table 1.2 Relative permeability of the phospholipid bilayer to different substances

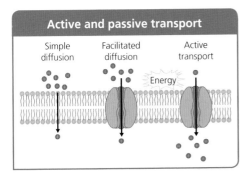

Figure 1.5 Active and passive transport across the cell membrane.

concentration (or from one electrical charge to the opposite electrical charge), therefore no energy is required
■ Conversely, a chemical moving against its gradient requires energy-dependent active transport; this can occur as a direct result of ATP hydrolysis, or by coupling the movement of one substance with that of another (a cotransporter)

Protein carriers

Most small molecules or ions require specific protein carriers to transport them across the membrane.

■ Ions and polar molecules are transported by ion channels
■ Water is transported by aquaporins
■ Carrier proteins are highly specific for the substance they transport, e.g. GLUT1 for glucose; cytochromes for electrons; cysteine carrier proteins in the kidneys for cysteine

> **Haemodialysis is a blood-filtering treatment for renal failure based on the principles of diffusion.** Mimicking renal filtration, blood flows on one side of a semipermeable membrane in one direction, and the dialysate flows on the opposite side in the other direction, creating a countercurrent. The countercurrent maximises the concentration gradient, enabling the efficient removal of waste products, including urea and creatinine, which are normally excreted in urine.

Transport mechanisms

Molecules are transported across membranes by:

■ passive diffusion
■ osmosis
■ facilitated diffusion
■ active transport
■ endocytosis and exocytosis

Passive diffusion

This is a spontaneous process in which small molecules or ions move across the plasma membrane by diffusion down a concentration gradient (see **Figure 1.5**). The diffusion velocity across the membrane depends on the gradient and the hydrophobicity, size and charge of the molecule.

Osmosis

This is similar to diffusion but refers specifically to movement of water; osmosis is the passive diffusion of water across a semipermeable membrane. The osmotic gradient is the movement of water from an area of low dissolved solute concentration to an area of high solute concentration, across a semipermeable membrane.

Facilitated diffusion

This is a passive transport process in which diffusion of a chemical down its gradient is aided by membrane channel proteins (see **Figure 1.5** and **Figure 1.8**). The cell membrane is impermeable to polar molecules and charged ions because of its hydrophobic nature. However, ion channel proteins and carrier proteins open or close to control the passage of molecules into the cells. This often involves conformational changes and specific binding of molecules to these proteins.

Channel proteins are very selective, and include ion channels, carrier proteins and aquaporins. Aquaporins specifically transport water.

> **Aquaporins are channel proteins that specifically facilitate the diffusion of water across membranes.** Aquaporins in the distal convoluted tubule of the kidney have a key role in regulating water reabsorption and excretion.

Active transport

This is the movement of a chemical against a concentration gradient (see **Figure 1.5**). Active transport requires ATP directly or secondarily. It occurs through transmembrane protein transporters.

Primary active transport

This process directly uses chemical energy such as ATP and redox energy (e.g. electron transport when NADH is used to move protons against a concentration gradient). The Na⁺–K⁺-ATPase pump is a primary active transport pump that maintains a steep concentration gradient of sodium and potassium across the cell membrane. Sodium concentration is high in the extracellular environment and low inside the cell; the concentration of potassium is the opposite.

This gradient represents a store of energy that is used by cells to transport other chemicals against their gradient.

The pump transports three sodium ions out of the cell in exchange for two potassium ions into the cell (**Figure 1.6**). It is powered by ATP, which phosphorylates the pump when sodium is bound to it. Phosphorylation induces a conformational change that opens the active site for potassium and releases sodium (**Figure 1.7**). The phosphate group is then released, which returns the protein to its original shape. This change in shape releases the potassium into the cytosol, enabling the cycle to start again.

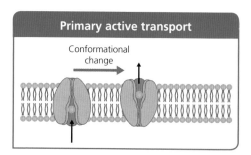

Figure 1.7 Movement across the cell membrane by primary active transport.

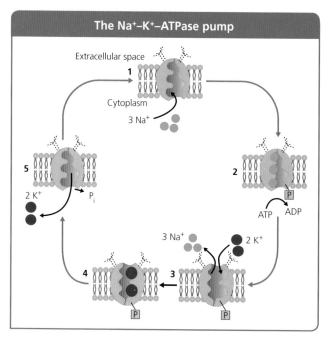

Figure 1.6 The Na⁺–K⁺-ATPase pump. ① Three cytoplasmic Na⁺ bind to the pump. ② Adenosine triphosphate (ATP) donates a phosphate group for energy. ③ The protein changes shape, expelling the Na⁺ into the extracellular space. ④ Two K⁺ bind to the pump. ⑤ The protein resumes its original shape, K⁺ is released and the pump relinquishes its phosphate. ADP, adenosine diphosphate; Pi, inorganic phosphate.

Secondary active transport

This process, also known as cotransport, uses energy to transport molecules. However, it does not use ATP directly; instead, it uses an electrochemical gradient to couple the movement of an ion down its gradient with that of another chemical up its gradient. Secondary active transport is analogous to a waterwheel harnessing the flow of water down a stream.

Cotransporters are symporters or antiporters, depending on the direction of movement (**Figure 1.8**).

Symporters move chemical species in the same direction across the membrane, but one is going down and the other up its concentration or electrochemical gradient. An example is the glucose symporter sodium–glucose transporter 1, which is responsible for glucose uptake in the intestine. This symporter transports one glucose molecule into the cell for every two sodium ions.

Antiporters move species in opposite directions across the cell membrane. One species moves with its electrochemical gradient (by facilitated diffusion), and this provides energy to drive the transport of another species in the opposite direction.

Integral transmembrane proteins maintain concentration gradients across membranes by tightly regulating concentrations of potassium ions (K⁺), sodium ions (Na⁺) and calcium ions (Ca²⁺). Intracellular concentrations of these are about 140 mM, 10 mM and 100 nM, respectively. In contrast, their extracellular concentrations are 5, 140 and 1 mM.

Endocytosis and exocytosis

These are reciprocal processes in which material is either brought into the cell (*endo-*) or secreted from the cell (*exo-*) in packages of plasma membrane (**Figure 1.9**). Endocytosis and exocytosis occur constantly, cell membrane lost by endocytosis is continually replaced by cell membrane gained by exocytosis.

Endocytosis

In this process, cells engulf molecules through invagination of the cell membrane (see **Figure 1.9a**); the membrane forms a small inward pouch, capturing the molecules to be transported. The pouch grows then separates from the membrane on the

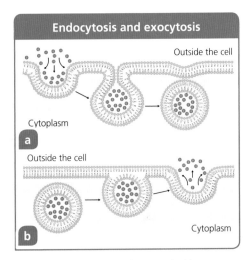

Figure 1.9 Endocytosis and exocytosis. (a) Endocytosis: a vesicle forms when a section of the cell membrane engulfs molecules that are otherwise unable to cross its lipid bilayer. (b) Exocytosis: a vesicle moves from within the cell to the cell membrane, with which it fuses to release its contents.

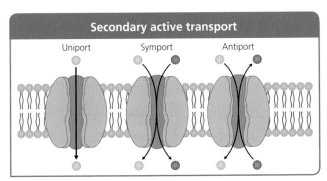

Figure 1.8 Movement across the cell membrane by secondary active transport using cotransporters. For comparison, uniport is equivalent to facilitated diffusion.

inside of the cell, creating a small vesicle containing the captured substance. This is an active process with three types:

- phagocytosis
- pinocytosis
- receptor-mediated endocytosis

Phagocytosis is the major mechanism for the removal of cell debris and pathogens. For example, a bacterium is endocytosed and digested, and the cell then reuses the products of its breakdown.

In pinocytosis, vesicles containing fluids with constituents are internalised and subsequently fuse with lysosomes. The lysosomes hydrolyse and break down the particles. Almost all cells perform pinocytosis whereas only specialised cells perform phagocytosis.

In receptor-mediated endocytosis, the molecule of interest binds to receptor complexes present in clatherin-coated pits on the cell surface membrane. They promote the formation of an endocytic pit. For example, LDL cholesterol binds to LDL receptor complexes and is then internalised, removing it from circulation. The clatherin pit then buds into the cell to form a coated vesicle. Thus a small area of cell membrane and a small volume of extracellular fluid are brought into the cell. Recycling of receptors via endocytosis enables the cycle to continue.

Exocytosis

This is the reverse of endocytosis. In exocytosis, packages of bilipid membrane originating within the cell fuse with the cell membrane to eject their contents (see **Figure 1.9b**). The process begins in the Golgi apparatus, which packages the molecules to be transported into vesicles. These vesicles migrate to the cell membrane. There, the cell membrane and the vesicular membrane fuse, enabling the contents of the vesicle to be released into the surrounding extracellular fluid. Exocytosis is used to transport hormones and enzymes out of cells.

Signalling pathways

Starter questions

Answers to the following questions are on page 40.

8. How do cells communicate?
9. Do all cells have the same response to a signalling molecule?

The survival of any multicellular organism depends on the ability of cells to communicate with each other. This communication is required to regulate cellular processes such as cell differentiation, cell growth and cell metabolism, and in this way ensures the coordinated function of the whole organism.

Such cell signalling occurs primarily through extracellular signalling molecules. These chemical messengers pass from one cell to another and alter cellular activity in the target cell. In a minority of cases, cells also communicate through electrical signals.

The cell signalling pathway has the following steps:

- synthesis and release of the signalling molecules
- transport of the signalling molecules to target cells
- detection of the signalling molecules by target cells, and changes to intracellular molecules in the target cell to produce a cellular response (signal transduction)
- removal of the signal

There are many different types of signalling molecules, but a much smaller number of signal transduction pathways through which they act. Typical cellular responses include enzyme activation or inhibition, stimulation of the synthesis of specific proteins, and increased cellular uptake of metabolites (**Figure 1.10**).

Signalling molecules

Signalling molecules include:

- amino acids and their derivatives
- protein molecules (peptides)
- cholesterol derivatives (steroids)
- fatty acid derivatives (eicosanoids)
- gases

They are broadly classified into six groups based on a combination of their chemical structure, mechanism of action and effects on cellular activity: pheromones, hormones, neurotransmitters, growth factors, eicosanoids and gases (**Table 1.3**).

> **Cortisol (and synthetic corticosteroids) can reduce inflammation by blocking the production of eicosanoid (oxidised 20-carbon fatty acid) signalling molecules.** This prevents the formation of arachidonic acid, a key intermediate in the generation of prostaglandins and leukotrienes, signalling molecules that mediate the inflammatory response. This is one of many anti-inflammatory mechanisms of cortisol.

Types of cell signalling

Signalling molecules reach their target cells by:

- direct transfer between cells
- diffusion through the interstitial space
- transport in the blood

Unstable signalling molecules are broken down rapidly, so they exert their effects on target cells only when close to them. In contrast, more stable signalling molecules survive long enough to be carried in the blood to more distant target cells. Cell signalling is classified into four types depending on the distance over which the signal acts (**Figure 1.11**):

- Direct cell-to-cell contact
- Autocrine signalling
- Paracrine signalling
- Endocrine signalling

Direct cell-to-cell contact

This occurs between adjacent cells, through either gap junctions (channels through the cell membrane) or binding of cell surface signalling molecules. This type of signalling is essential for the development and maintenance of tissues.

Autocrine signalling

This type of signalling occurs when cells respond to the signalling molecules they secrete themselves. Many growth factors act

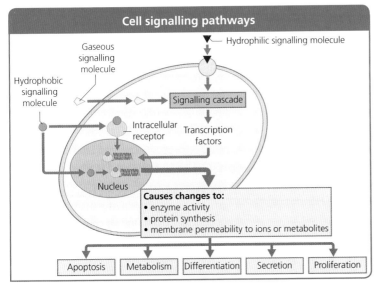

Figure 1.10 Overview of cell signalling pathways.

Cell signalling pathways

Hydrophilic signalling molecule

Gaseous signalling molecule

Hydrophobic signalling molecule

Signalling cascade

Intracellular receptor

Transcription factors

Nucleus

Causes changes to:
- enzyme activity
- protein synthesis
- membrane permeability to ions or metabolites

Apoptosis | Metabolism | Differentiation | Secretion | Proliferation

Signalling molecules					
Signalling molecule	Type of cell signalling	Chemical structure	Example(s)	Site(s) of receptors	Comment
Pheromones	Between organisms of the same species	Steroids Carbon chains	No known human pheromones	Nucleus Cell membrane	Influence behaviour of organism
Hormones	Endocrine	Steroids	Testosterone, oestrogen and cortisol	Nucleus	Regulate numerous bodily functions including: metabolism, growth, tissue function and reproduction
		Peptides	Insulin, glucagon, growth hormone and prolactin	Cell membrane	
		Amino acid derivatives	Thyroxine	Nucleus	
Neurotransmitters	Paracrine and endocrine	Amino acid derivatives	Adrenaline (epinephrine), dopamine and serotonin	Cell membrane	Signalling molecules in the nervous system
		Peptides (neuropeptides)	Endorphins	Cell membrane	
Growth factors	Autocrine and paracrine	Peptides	Cytokines and epidermal growth factor	Cell membrane	Control cell growth and differentiation
Eicosanoids	Autocrine and paracrine	Fatty acid derivatives	Prostaglandins and thromboxane	Cell membrane	Signalling molecules involved in the inflammatory and immune response
Gases	Paracrine		Nitric oxide and carbon monoxide	None (no receptors): they act directly to alter activity of intracellular target enzymes	Signalling molecule in nervous, immune and circulatory systems

Table 1.3 Summary of signalling molecules

through autocrine signalling. The uncontrolled, rapid growth of a tumour mass is often caused by oversecretion of growth factors by tumour cells.

Paracrine signalling

This refers to the communication between cells that are close to each other; the signalling molecules travel only short distances from one cell to the next. This type of signalling is used by neurotransmitters.

Endocrine signalling

This type of signalling occurs between cells that are some distance apart. Endocrine signalling is carried out only by hormones, which are carried in the blood to target cells.

Signal transduction

Once a signalling molecule reaches its target cell, it initiates a signal transduction cascade that results in a change in cellular activity.

Types of cell signalling

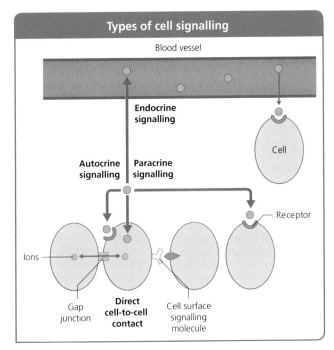

Figure 1.11 Direct cell-to-cell contact, autocrine signalling, paracrine signalling and endocrine cell signalling.

To alter cellular activity, the signalling molecule must be detected by the target cell and convey information to its interior. This process is called signal transduction. The signal transduction pathway begins with the detection of signalling molecules through specific receptors (proteins) on the cell membrane (membrane-bound receptors) or in the cytosol or nucleus of the target cell (intracellular receptors).

■ Small hydrophobic signalling molecules, such as steroids and some amino acid derivatives, are able to cross the plasma membrane of the target cell and bind to intracellular receptors
■ Hydrophilic signalling molecules, such as peptides and charged amino acids, are unable to cross the plasma membrane, so they must bind to membrane-bound receptors on the surface of the cell
■ Gaseous signalling molecules, such as nitric oxide, diffuse into the cell and directly influence enzyme activity

Hydrophilic signalling molecules bind to membrane receptors and tend to initiate a rapid cellular response (within seconds or minutes) by altering enzyme activity. Hydrophobic signalling molecules can cross membranes but induce a much slower and longer lasting cellular response by regulating gene expression.

Intracellular receptors

Intracellular receptors act as transcription factors: proteins that bind to specific regions of DNA to promote or inhibit transcription of a particular gene. They are located in the cytosol and the nucleus of the cell.

■ Receptors in the cytosol of the target cell undergo conformational change on binding a signalling molecule. They then diffuse to the nucleus, where they attach to DNA at the promoter regions of target genes. Steroid hormone receptors are an example of this intracellular cytosolic receptor.

- Receptors in the nucleus are converted by binding of a signalling molecule from a transcription inhibitor to a transcription activator. These receptors are bound to DNA at the promoter region of target genes. The thyroid hormone receptor is one example of this type of intracellular nuclear receptor.

Membrane-bound receptors

This type of receptor activates intracellular signalling cascades. This is done primarily by phosphorylation (addition of phosphate groups) to alter the activity of proteins. Protein phosphorylation is catalysed by a number of enzymes called protein kinases (see page 21).

Membrane-bound receptors all contain:

- an extracellular domain, which binds specifically to the signalling molecule

- a transmembrane domain, which crosses the cell membrane

Binding of the signalling molecule triggers a conformational change that activates the receptor and initiates an intracellular protein phosphorylation cascade through the activation of protein kinases. Some receptors have intrinsic protein kinase activity, whereas others act indirectly through the release of intracellular diffusible molecules (second messengers).

Membrane bound receptors are divided into three types (**Figure 1.12**):

- ion channels
- G-protein–coupled receptors
- enzyme-linked receptors

Ion channels

In this type of receptor, the transmembrane domain of the receptor acts as an ion-specific channel that allows certain ions to pass through the cell membrane. Binding of a sig-

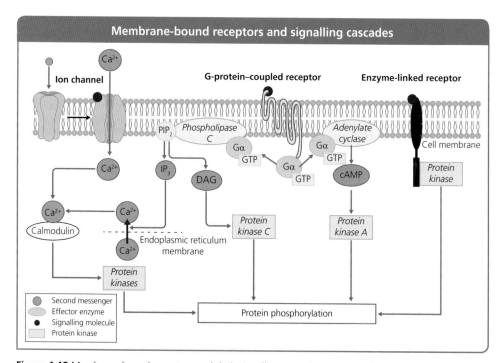

Figure 1.12 Membrane-bound receptors and their signalling cascades. cAMP, cyclic adenosine monophosphate; DAG, diacylglycerol; GTP, guanosine triphosphate; IP_3, inositol 1,4,5-triphosphate; PIP_2, phosphatidylinositol 4,5-bisphosphate.

nalling molecule induces conformational change in the receptor, and this change in shape opens the ion channel. Many neurotransmitter receptors are ion channels.

G-protein–coupled receptors

These receptors have seven transmembrane helical domains and an intracellular domain that bind to trimeric guanine nucleotide–binding proteins (G–proteins). The trimeric G-protein has three subunits: α, β and γ. The α subunit binds to guanosine diphosphate (GDP) or guanosine triphosphate (GTP).

- When its α subunit is bound to GDP, the receptor is inactive
- When the α subunit is bound to GTP, the receptor is active

Binding of the signalling molecule induces a conformational change that allows the receptor to interact with the intracellular G-proteins; this activates the receptor by causing the exchange of GDP for GTP. The α subunit can now dissociate from the receptor and bind to membrane-bound 'effector' enzymes that initiate further signalling through the release of second messengers.

Enzyme-linked receptors

These receptors have intrinsic enzyme activity in their intracellular domain, which is activated by a conformational change induced by binding of the signalling molecule. Examples of enzymes linked to receptors include tyrosine kinase, serine-threonine kinase, tyrosine phosphatase and guanylate cyclase.

In some cases, a single signalling molecule binds to two receptor molecules, causing them to come together (dimerise).The protein kinase activity on one receptor molecule can now phosphorylate the other receptor, and vice versa. This autophosphorylation reaction activates the receptors and initiates further signalling through the phosphorylation of other molecules.

> **Many diseases are caused by uncontrolled cell signalling.** For example, the cholera toxin inhibits the GTPase activity of the α subunit of trimeric G-proteins, so that the subunit remains bound to GTP and constitutively active. Constitutive activation of the α subunit causes continued activation of adenylate cyclase and the release of cyclic adenosine monophosphate (AMP). High cyclic AMP levels stimulate the active transport of ions from intestinal epithelial cells into the gut lumen, causing diarrhoea.

Second messengers

These are small molecules that are able to diffuse throughout the cytosol of the cell and propagate the signal transduction cascade. The main second messengers are cyclic AMP, calcium ions, inositol 1,4,5-triphosphate and diacylglycerol (**Table 1.4**). Second

Second messenger	Activation	Effects	Deactivation
Cyclic AMP	Produced from ATP by adenylate cyclase	Activates protein kinase A	Metabolised to 5'-AMP by cyclic AMP phosphodiesterase
Inositol 1,4,5-triphosphate	Produced from PIP_2 by the action of phospholipase C	Opens calcium ion channel on cell membrane to increase intracellular calcium	Converted to derivatives
Diacylglycerol	Produced from PIP_2 by the action of phospholipase C	Activates protein kinase C	Hydrolysed to glycerol and fatty acids
Calcium	Enters cell through open calcium ion channels	Activates calmodulin and changes cell membrane potential	Sequestered into intracellular stores or pumped out of the cell

AMP, adenosine monophosphate; ATP, adenosine triphosphate; PIP_2, phosphatidylinositol 4,5-bisphosphate.

Table 1.4 Common second messengers

messengers amplify the signal, because one signalling molecule generates many second messenger molecules.

Signal termination

For a cell to remain responsive to new signals, previous signalling pathways must be terminated. Controls to the signalling pathway are present at the receptor, signalling molecule and second messenger level.

Receptors can be inactivated through endocytosis of the activated receptor. The receptor is then degraded or recycled by the cell. In some cases, prolonged binding of the signalling molecule alters the conformation of the receptor so that the signalling molecule can no longer bind and thus the signal is terminated. Several mechanisms are used to deactivate second messengers (see **Table 1.4**). For example, phosphatases (enzymes that catalyse the removal of phosphate) are used to control phosphorylation cascades.

> **Graves' disease is excessive thyroid hormone production** caused by autoantibody stimulation of the thyroid-stimulating hormone receptor on the thyroid gland. Binding causes continuous activation of the receptors, resulting in oversecretion of thyroid hormone.

Enzymes and cofactors

Starter questions

Answers to the following questions are on page 40.

10. How are biochemical reactions regulated?

11. Why don't digestive enzymes degrade the cells of the gastrointestinal tract?

Biochemical reactions must be regulated to ensure efficient and effective cellular metabolism. This regulation is carried out through catalysts, the substances that increase the rate of reactions. Most biological catalysts are proteins called enzymes; however, RNA molecules called ribozymes also catalyse some reactions. Without enzymes, very few biochemical reactions would occur quickly enough to sustain metabolism.

Catalysts

All chemical reactions require the breakage of existing bonds and the formation of new ones. The energy required to break bonds in the reactant molecules and start the chemical reaction is called the activation energy. The higher the activation energy, the fewer molecules obtain enough energy for bonds to break and the slower the reaction rate.

The rate of a reaction can be increased in either of two ways:

- increasing the energy of the reactants, for example by increasing the temperature
- reducing the activation energy, for example by using a catalyst (**Figure 1.13**)

Catalysts are substances that lower the activation energy by stressing the bonds of the reactants so that they are easier to break. All catalysts:

- increase the rate of a reaction
- are not consumed or created during the reaction
- cannot cause a reaction to occur that is not energetically favourable

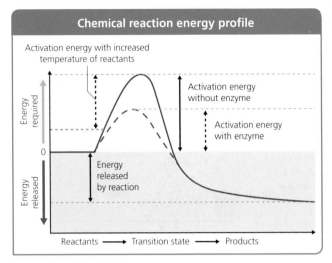

Chemical reaction energy profile

Activation energy with increased temperature of reactants

Activation energy without enzyme

Activation energy with enzyme

Energy released by reaction

Energy required

0

Energy released

Reactants ⟶ Transition state ⟶ Products

Figure 1.13 Energy profile of a chemical reaction.

■ have no effect on the equilibrium of a reaction, i.e. they do not alter the proportion of reactant molecules that are converted to product

Increasing the reaction rate by raising the temperature of the reactants (to make the particles move faster and thus more likely to collide) is not feasible, because many of the molecules would be degraded. Therefore organisms use enzymes to increase the reaction rate.

Enzymes

Almost every biochemical reaction is catalysed by an enzyme, and cellular metabolism is governed by the different enzymes expressed by each cell type. Hundreds of different enzymes have been identified, but they are generally classified into six groups according to the type of reaction they catalyse (**Table 1.5**).

The active site

Enzymes work by binding reactant molecules ('substrates') within a cleft on the enzyme surface called the active site. Enzymes are highly specific both for the type of reaction they catalyse and for their substrates. Substrate specificity is determined

Enzyme classification		
Enzyme class	Reaction catalysed	Examples
Oxidoreductases	Oxidation reactions (loss of an electron) and reduction reactions (gain of an electron)	Dehydrogenases and hydrolases, e.g. alcohol dehydrogenase
Transferases	Transfer of a chemical group from one molecule to another	Kinases and deaminases, e.g. hexokinase
Hydrolases	Breakage of bonds by addition of a water molecule (i.e. hydrolysis)	Proteases, lipases and nucleases, e.g. trypsin
Lyases	Formation of a double bond by addition or removal of chemical groups	Carboxylases, aldoases and dehydratasaes, e.g. pyruvate carboxylase
Isomerases	Rearrangement of chemical groups in a molecule to give a different isomer	Glucose-6-phosphate isomerase
Ligases	Formation of a bond by removal of a water molecule	DNA ligase

Table 1.5 Types of enzyme

by the precise shape, size, charge and amino acid sequence of the active site. The remainder of the enzyme molecule is important for maintaining this structure.

Substrate molecules interact with the active site in one of two ways.

- The substrate fits precisely into the active site; this is the lock-and-key model (**Figure 1.14a**)
- Once bound, the substrate distorts the shape of the active site to induce a precise fit; this is the induced fit model (**Figure 1.14b**)

Substrate binding lowers the activation energy of the reaction by inducing the transition state, the intermediate state between substrates and products. In the transition state, the chemical bonds of the substrate are strained and more easily broken. Once the bonds are broken and the products are formed, the product molecules dissoci-

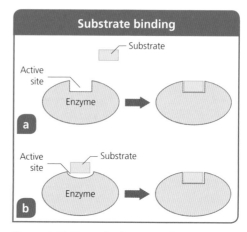

Figure 1.14 Types of substrate binding to an active site. (a) The lock-and-key model. (b) The induced fit model.

ate from the enzyme, leaving the active site available to bind other substrate molecules.

Enzyme cofactors			
Coenzyme(s)	Essential vitamin component	Reaction	Example
Thiamin pyrophosphate	Thiamin (vitamin B1)	Transferase	Pyruvate dehydrogenase
FAD	Riboflavin (vitamin B2)	Oxidoreductase	Succinate dehydrogenase
NAD⁺ and NADP⁺	Niacin (nicotinic acid) (vitamin B3)	Oxidoreductase	Alcohol dehydrogenase
Coenzyme A	Pantothenic acid (vitamin B5)	Transferase	Pyruvate dehydrogenase
Pyridoxal phosphate	Pyridoxine (vitamin B6)	Transferase	Alanine aminotransferase
Biotin	Biotin (vitamin B7)	Transferase	Alanine aminotransferase
Tetrahydrofolate and dihydrofolate	Folate (vitamin B9)	Transferase	Thymidylate synthase
Cobalamin	Cobalamin (vitamin B12)	Transferase	Methionine synthase
Zinc			Alcohol dehydrogenase
Magnesium			Glucose-6-phosphatase
Selenium			Gluathione peroxidase
Manganese			Arginase
Nickel			Urease

NAD⁺, nicotinamide adenine dinucleotide; NADP⁺, nicotinamide adenine dinucleotide phosphate; FAD, Flavin adenine dinucleotide.

Table 1.6 Enzyme cofactors

Some enzymes are able to bind more than one substrate and therefore catalyse more than one reaction. For example, alcohol dehydrogenase metabolises ethanol, methanol, and ethylene glycol. This is why methanol and ethylene glycol poisoning are treated by giving ethanol, which binds more readily and inhibits the metabolism of methanol and ethylene glycol to their toxic metabolites.

Cofactors

The activity of many enzymes depends on the presence of additional small 'helper' molecules called cofactors (**Table 1.6**). There are two groups of cofactor.

- Metal ions, including essential trace elements such as copper, zinc, magnesium and iron, work as cofactors by attracting the electrons in covalent bonds, thus promoting bond breakage
- Non-protein organic molecules called coenzymes, many of which are derived from the water-soluble B vitamins, act as either electron acceptors or electron donors in oxidation–reduction reactions. Some coenzymes are also able to transfer electrons from one enzyme to another in an electron transport chain, which drives ATP production.

Enzyme kinetics

Enzyme-catalysed reactions are a series of events in which the substrate (S) binds to the enzyme (E) and the product (P) is formed:

$$E + S \rightarrow ES \rightarrow E + P$$

The Michaelis–Menten equation

The kinetics of the above reaction, i.e. the rate at which it occurs, is characterised by the Michaelis–Menten equation. This describes how the rate (velocity) of the reaction (V) depends on the substrate concentration ([S]):

$$V = \frac{V_{max}\,[S]}{K_m + [S]}$$

Initially, the reaction rate increases as [S] increases. However, as the enzyme becomes saturated with substrate the rate becomes less able to increase, until finally it reaches its maximum (V_{max}) (**Figure 1.15a**).The Michaelis constant (K_m) is the substrate concentration at which the reaction rate is half V_{max}.

Graphical representations

The Michaelis–Menten equation can be represented graphically by the Lineweaver–Burk plot (**Figure 1.15b**) and the Eadie–Hofstee diagram (**Figure 1.15c**), which are useful for determining V_{max} and K_m from experimental

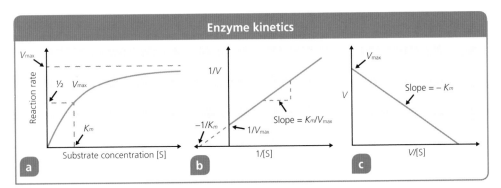

Enzyme kinetics

Figure 1.15 Enzyme kinetics. (a) The saturation curve. (b) The Lineweaver–Burk plot. (c) The Eadie–Hofstee diagram. V_{max}, maximum rate (velocity) of reaction; K_m, Michaelis constant; [S], substrate.

data. The Lineweaver–Burk plot is also useful in the analysis of enzyme inhibition (see page 25).

An understanding of enzyme kinetics, i.e. how quickly an enzyme becomes saturated with substrate and the maximum rate the reaction it catalyses can achieve, is useful when characterising enzymes and identifying altered enzymes that cause disease states. It is also useful when developing drugs that work by enzyme inhibition.

Substrate-binding affinity is a measure of how well a substrate binds to the active site of an enzyme. Substrates with high affinity bind readily to the active site, therefore the maximum rate of the reaction, V_{max}, is reached more quickly. High–affinity substrates also means a small K_m, i.e. a low substrate concentration at which half V_{max} is reached.

Enzyme regulation

Control of both the amount and the activity of an enzyme allows the cell to regulate its metabolism. Mechanisms of enzyme regulation are:

- regulation of gene expression, and thus how much enzyme is produced
- proteolytic enzyme activity, and thus how much enzyme is degraded
- covalent modification of enzymes for example by phosphorylation (addition of a phosphate group)
- allosteric regulation of enzyme activity; the binding of substances alters enzyme activity
- enzyme inhibition; the binding of substances stops enzyme activity

Enzyme activity is also affected by environmental factors such as temperature and pH, which alter the shape of the active site and its ability to bind a substrate.

Many enzymes are secreted as inactive precursors called zymogens or proenzymes, which become the active form once cleaved. This also adds a stage at which the timing and location of enzyme activity can be controlled. For example, blood clotting is mediated through the sequential cleavage of clotting factors in the clotting cascade of reactions.

Regulation of enzyme gene expression

The amount of an active enzyme can be altered by changing the expression of its gene. Cells use numerous signalling molecules that result in either the activation or the inhibition of transcription factors (see page 14). This allows the cell to change its expression of enzymes in response to metabolic demands, and provides a more long-term change in the levels of active enzyme. For example, the hormone insulin up-regulates transcription of the gene for the glycolytic enzyme glyceraldehyde 3-phosphate dehydrogenase.

Regulation of enzyme degradation

The amount of active enzyme can also be controlled by increasing its degradation when no longer required. Enzymes are broken down by proteases in lysosomes or by proteasomes in the cytosol. They are targeted for degradation by the addition of ubiquitin (a small, 72-amino acid peptide).

Covalent modification of enzymes

The activity of an enzyme can be modulated by various post-translational modifications (see page 83), which alter a protein's shape and hence its interactions with substrate.

These modifications can be either permanent or reversible. A common mechanism used by the cell is the reversible phosphorylation of enzymes through the action of kinases and dephosphorylation by phosphatases.

Allosteric regulation

Many enzymes can exist in an active or inactive state depending on the binding of an effector substance These allosteric molecules bind to specific allosteric sites on the enzyme, which differs from the active site. When bound, they cause a conformational change that either inhibits or activates the enzyme (**Figure 1.16**).

Enzyme inhibition

An enzyme inhibitor is any substance that binds to an enzyme and decreases its activity. This effect can be reversible, or if the inhibitor binds with covalent bonds, irreversible.

Enzyme inhibition can be competitive, non-competitive or uncompetitive (**Figure 1.17**). Each of these types of inhibition has distinct effects on enzyme kinetics (**Table 1.7**).

- In competitive inhibition, the inhibitor competes with the substrate for binding to the active site
- In non-competitive and uncompetitive inhibition, the inhibitor binds at a site different from the active site

Allosteric inhibitors are non-competitive inhibitors.

Negative feedback inhibition

Many biochemical reactions in a cell occur in sequences called biochemical pathways. In these pathways, the product of one reaction is the substrate for the next, and a different enzyme catalyses each step in the pathway.

Many biosynthetic pathways are regulated by feedback inhibition: the end product in the pathway is a non-competitive inhibitor for an enzyme further upstream in the pathway. This negative feedback prevents the cell wasting energy by making unneeded amounts of a product.

Effects of inhibition		
Type of inhibition	Mechanism of action	Kinetic effects
Competitive inhibition	Inhibitor binds to active site	$V_{max} \leftrightarrow$ $K_m \uparrow$
	Reversible	
Non-competitive	Binds enzyme at site other than active site	$V_{max} \downarrow$ $K_m \leftrightarrow$
	Irreversible by substrate	
Uncompetitive	Binds only to enzyme–substrate complex at site other than active site	$V_{max} \downarrow$ $K_m \uparrow$
	Prevents product formation	
	Irreversible by substrate	

Table 1.7 Effects of inhibitors on enzyme kinetics

Figure 1.16 Allosteric enzyme activation.

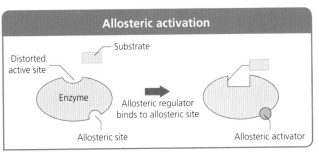

Allosteric activation

Substrate

Distorted active site

Enzyme

Allosteric regulator binds to allosteric site

Allosteric site

Allosteric activator

Enzyme inhibition

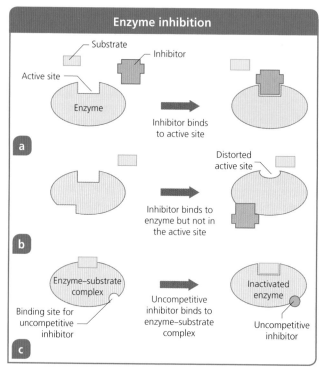

Figure 1.17 Enzyme inhibition. (a) Competitive inhibition. (b) Non-competitive inhibition. (c) Uncompetitive inhibition.

Many drugs are enzyme inhibitors that stop an unwanted reaction from occurring (or from occurring excessively). For example, penicillin is an irreversible inhibitor of the bacterial enzyme transpeptidase, which is required for bacterial cell wall synthesis and without which the bacteria are unable to survive.

Environmental factors

All enzymes have an optimal temperature and pH, at which their activity is greatest. At temperatures below the optimum, the enzyme is not flexible enough to permit binding of substrates, and at higher temperatures the enzyme is denatured, i.e. it loses its normal conformation. Unsurprisingly, normal body temperature 37°C, and a pH between 6 and 8 is the optimum for most enzymes. At lower or higher pH, the enzyme is denatured because its ionic bonds are disrupted.

Biochemical bonds and reactions

Starter questions

Answers to the following questions are on page 40.

12. What affects the rate at which a reaction occurs?
13. Why do some reactions require energy and others produce it?
14. Why does water form droplets?

In nature, atoms interact through chemical bonds. These are be divided into covalent and non-covalent bonds. The former define the structure of a molecule. They are of equal importance but non-covalent bonds are not as strong as covalent bonds.

Bonding

Bonding is the interaction between atoms that enables the formation of chemicals with two or more atoms. A bond is formed by electrostatic forces of attraction between opposite charges, which occurs between nuclei and electrons, or temporarily between structures with polarised bonds (the much weaker dipole attraction), such as the oxygen–hydrogen bond in water molecules. Bond strength varies considerably. For simplicity, bonding is divided into covalent and non-covalent.

Covalent bonds

Covalent bonds are the strongest type of bond. They form by the sharing of electrons between adjacent atoms; an example is the carbon–carbon (C–C) bond. More than one pair of electrons are shared between two atoms to form a double covalent bond, for example C=C. A simple example of covalent bonding is in the structure of methane (**Figure 1.18**).

Non-covalent bonds

Non-covalent bonds are reversible and vital molecular interactions. There are three types:

- electrostatic interactions
- hydrogen bonding
- van der Waals forces

Electrostatic interactions

Electrostatic interactions occur between positively and negatively charged atoms. They can be repulsive or attractive. The electric charge of an atom determines the extent of the electronic interaction between it and other atoms.

Hydrogen bonding

Hydrogen bonds are a form of electrostatic interaction and are considerably weaker than covalent bonds. They have a pivotal role in the structure and properties of many molecules. For example, in DNA, between nucleotide bases adenine–thymine and guanine–cytosine, there are two and three hydrogen bonds, respectively (**Figure 1.19**).

Van der Waals forces

These are weak non-covalent bonds (**Figure 1.20**). They are based on the distribution of charge around an atom and how this changes with time. At any time, the dispersion of charge is uneven, and as such it

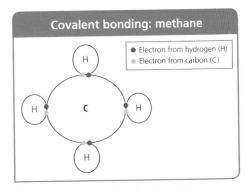

Covalent bonding: methane

- ● Electron from hydrogen (H)
- ● Electron from carbon (C)

Figure 1.18 Covalent bonding in methane.

Figure 1.19 Hydrogen bonding in deoxyribonucleic acid. Three hydrogen bonds exist between guanine and cytosine and two hydrogen bonds exist between adenine and thymine.

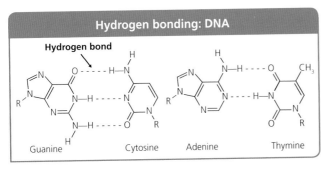

Hydrogen bonding: DNA

Hydrogen bond

Guanine   Cytosine   Adenine   Thymine

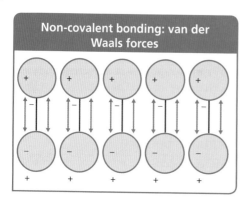

Non-covalent bonding: van der Waals forces

Figure 1.20 Non-covalent bonding: van der Waals forces are temporary interactions between atoms that are influenced by a differential electrostatic charge and intermolecular distance.

influences the distribution of charge around neighbouring atoms.

> **Chiral molecules have the same molecular formula but are mirror images of each other.** Optical isomers, like the left and right hand, cannot be superimposed on one another. The *dexter* (D, right)/*laevus* (L, left) system describes the chirality of sugars, fats and proteins. Many metabolites are chiral, with their isomers having different properties. Most amino acids are L and sugars are D.

Thermodynamics

Thermodynamics is the study of the relationship between temperature and energy. All biological activities involve changes in energy, and these are governed by two fundamental rules, the laws of thermodynamics.

First law of thermodynamics

The first law states that energy cannot be created or destroyed, but it can be transferred from one form to another (e.g. potential to kinetic energy). This means that the total energy in the universe stays the same. For example, when we eat food, we are acquiring energy, not creating or destroying it; the potential energy stored in food is transferred

into the energy that drives cellular processes, allowing us to sustain life.

When energy is transferred, there is always some lost as heat to the surroundings. The importance of this is addressed in the second law of thermodynamics.

Second law of thermodynamics

The second law is concerned with the transformation of potential energy to heat. When this happens, the disorder (entropy) in the universe increases. Chemical bonding increases order, and heat energy decreases order. An example of entropy in action is the changes in a bedroom; as time passes, the bedroom becomes more disorganised, thus the entropy in the room has increased. Energy is required to return it to a tidy, organised state, and entropy decreases.

This law is fundamental to all biochemical processes, because it determines whether biochemical reactions can happen in the body.

Free energy

To define the thermodynamic changes in a reaction, the free energy of a molecule must be considered. This is the energy available to break and form new chemical bonds, i.e. the energy available to do the work in a system such as a cell.

Free energy is closely related to the degree of disorder in a system. Under standard temperature and pressure conditions, it is defined by Gibbs free energy:

$$\Delta G = \Delta H - \Delta TS$$

In this equation, G is free energy, H is enthalpy, T is temperature, S is entropy and Δ is change.

Endergonic and exergonic

Chemical reactions in the body produce changes in free energy and are classified as endergonic or exergonic.

- Endergonic reactions require an input of energy, because the products of the reactants contain more free energy than the reactants do; an example is the stomach using acid to break down food

- Exergonic reactions produce energy, released as heat, because the products of the reactants contain less free energy than the reactants do; an example is respiration

Exothermic reactions transfer energy to the surroundings. Examples of exothermic reactions are combustion (burning), many oxidation reactions (e.g. rusting) and neutralisation reactions between acids and alkalis

Endothermic reactions take in energy from the surroundings. Examples of endothermic reactions are electrolysis, the reaction between ethanoic acid and sodium carbonate, and the thermal decomposition of calcium carbonate in a blast furnace

Reduction and oxidation (redox) reactions

During chemical reactions, energy stored in chemical bonds is used to make new bonds. In some reactions, electrons are passed from one atom or molecule to another (**Figure 1.21**).

- The atom or molecule that loses an electron is oxidised in the process of oxidation
- In contrast, an atom or molecule is reduced when it gains an electron in the process of reduction

This transfer of electrons results in a change in oxidation state.

Oxidation is loss, reduction is gain, hence the useful acronym OIL RIG. Oxidation is the loss of an electron from an ion, atom or molecule, and a gain in oxidation state. Reduction of a chemical species is the gain of an electron and thus a reduction of the oxidation state.

Redox reactions can be simple, for example when two substrates form one product. An example is the oxidation of carbon by oxygen to form carbon dioxide during cellular respiration.

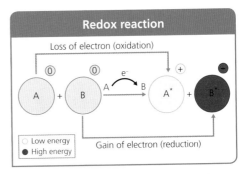

Figure 1.21 Reduction and oxidation (redox) reaction.

A more complex redox pathway is the citric acid cycle, in which energy is derived from the oxidation of a series of carbon-based compounds. It is summarised in two equations.

$$\text{succinate} + \text{FAD}^+ \rightleftharpoons \text{fumarate} + \text{FADH}_2$$

$$\text{malate} + \text{NAD}^+ \rightleftharpoons \text{oxaloacetate} + \text{NADH} + \text{H}^+$$

In equation 1, flavin adenine dinucleotide (FADH_2) carries the electrons, i.e. it is reduced. In contrast, equation 2 shows nicotinamide adenosine dinucleotide (NADH) carrying the electrons. FADH and NADH are coenzymes that are vital for numerous biochemical reactions as they donate electrons to reactions.

Types of biochemical reaction

Numerous biochemical reactions occur in the body. These are categorised as:

- reduction
- oxidation
- hydrolysis
- phosphorolysis
- decarboxylation
- deamination
- transamination

Hydrolysis

In hydrolysis, a molecule is cleaved into two parts by the addition of a molecule of water. One fragment of the molecule gains a hydrogen ion (H^+) from the additional water molecule. The other group gains the remaining hydroxyl group (OH^-). Hydrolysis reactions are important for the digestion of food.

ATP hydrolysis

Adenosine triphosphate is hydrolysed by the removal of a single phosphate residue to form adenosine diphosphate (ADP) and inorganic phosphate (P_i):

$$ATP + H_2O \rightarrow ADP + P_i$$

Alternatively, two phosphate groups (a diphosphate group) can be removed to form AMP and pyrophosphate.

$$ATP + H_2O \rightarrow AMP + PP_i$$

This fundamental reaction is used throughout the body to store and generate energy by forming and breaking the phosphate–phosphate bond.

Phosphorolysis

Phosphorolysis is similar to hydrolysis except that phosphate, not water, is used to cleave a molecule. Phosphorolysis reactions are used for glycolysis and glycogen breakdown in the body.

Glycogen (a carbohydrate energy store in liver and muscle) is broken down by the enzyme glycogen phosphorylase. This enzyme catalyses the reaction between inorganic phosphate and the terminal glycosyl residue of a glycogen molecule. If the glycogen chain has n glucose units, the products of a single phosphorolytic event are one molecule of glucose 1-phosphate and a glycogen chain of $n - 1$ remaining glucose units (**Figure 1.22**). The hormones glucagon and adrenaline (epinephrine) activate glycogen phosphorylase.

Sometimes, phosphorolysis occurs instead of hydrolysis, because reactions with glucose 1-phosphate yield more ATP than free glucose does when it is subsequently catabolised to pyruvate, the end product of glycolysis.

Decarboxylation

In decarboxylation, a carboxyl group (-COOH) is removed and carbon dioxide is released.

Decarboxylation is catalysed by decarboxylase enzymes and results in the removal of a carbon atom from a carbon chain. An example of this occurs when the ketone body acetoacetate is broken down by acetoacetate decarboylase.

Deamination

Deamination is the elimination of an amine group from a molecule. This is important for the removal of excess protein from the body and the recycling of carbon skeletons.

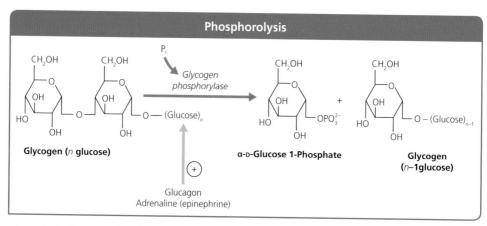

Figure 1.22 Glycogen phosphorylase acts by phosphorolytically removing a single glucose residue from α–(1,4)-linkages in the glycogen molecules. Glucose 1-phosphate is the production of this reaction.

This reaction is catalysed by deaminase enzymes. In humans, deamination takes place mainly in the liver. Deamination also occurs in the kidney, in which glutamate is converted to glutamine to facilitate the excretion of hydrogen ions. The amino group that is removed from the amino acid is converted to ammonia through the urea cycle.

Transamination

Transamination is the movement of an amine group between two molecules, and is catalysed by transaminase enzymes. These reactions are essential for the synthesis of non essential amino acids.

During transamination, an amine group on one acid is exchanged with the ketone group of another acid. An example is the formation of α–ketoglutarate, a citric acid cycle intermediate in transamination reactions.

Energy flow in cells

Cells need energy to survive. This energy comes from exergonic reactions in cells, which release free energy that is then used in endergonic reactions. An example of this is the oxidation of glucose, which releases energy then used to synthesise proteins (**Figure 1.23**). The most common energy coupler, i.e. transfer of energy from one process to another, in biochemical reactions is ATP.

Breakdown of food

The extraction of energy from the food we eat is divided into three stages (**Figure 1.24**).

1. Large macromolecules are broken down into smaller units
   - Proteins are hydrolysed to amino acids
   - Polysaccharides are hydrolysed to simple sugars
   - Fats are hydrolysed to glycerol and fatty acids
2. Most of the simple molecules produced in stage 1 are converted into the acyl unit of

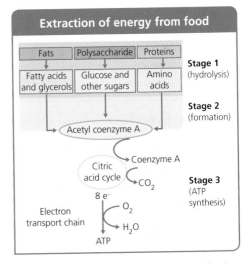

Figure 1.24 The extraction of energy from food: stage 1 (hydrolysis); stage 2 (formation of acetyl coenzyme A) and stage 3 (generation of ATP).

Figure 1.23 Energy transfer (exergenic and endogenic) between carbohydrates and proteins: the oxidation of glucose, which is coupled to the assembly of proteins in cells. ADP, adenosine diphosphate; ATP, adenosine triphosphate.

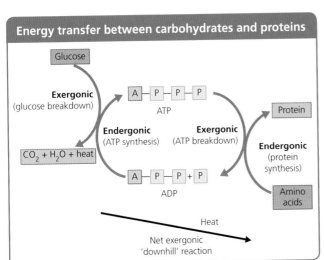

acetyl-coenzyme A, and a small amount of ATP is generated

3. Finally, ATP is generated from the complete oxidation of acetyl coenzyme A to carbon dioxide by the citric acid cycle and electron transport chain, in which four pairs of electrons are transferred (three to NAD^+ and one to FAD^+) for each acetyl group oxidised; the proton gradient across the inner membrane of mitochondria generated during this process is used to synthesise ATP

Adenosine triphosphate

Adenosine triphosphate is the fundamental currency of energy for cells, because it is needed for key processes such as the making of sugars, supplying activation energy to reactions, active transport across membranes and cellular growth. It is an essential portable source of on-demand energy for endergonic cellular processes.

The ATP molecule is composed of ribose (a 5-carbon sugar), adenosine (nucleoside) and a triphosphate group. The stores of energy are in the phosphate–phosphate bonds; hydrolysis of one of these bonds yields energy (delta G = –30.5 kJ/mol) (see **Figure 1.23**). ATP is synthesised when amino acids and sugars are broken down by coupling ADP and orthophosphate. Sugars are a more commonly utilised energy source, because they are more easily metabolised and stored. The direct synthesis of ATP occurs in glycolysis, a complex process in the cytosol that derives energy from glucose.

Body fuels

Starter questions

Answers to the following questions are on page 41.

15. Do biochemical reactions keep us warm?
16. Why is glucose the 'universal fuel' of all organisms?
17. Why can we digest starch but not cellulose?
18. Why are unsaturated fats good and saturated fats bad?

Sugars (carbohydrates), fatty acids and other lipids, amino acids and nucleotides are the key small molecules of biochemistry. They act primarily as sources of energy and as building blocks for larger macromolecules and other structures, such as membranes and tissues.

Carbohydrates

Carbohydrates are compounds that contain carbon, hydrogen and oxygen atoms. They typically have a carbon chain backbone and many hydroxyl groups, which confer the interactive properties of carbohydrates.

Carbohydrates are classified according to their number of carbon units:

- monosaccharides, such as glucose, have 1
- disaccharides, such as glycogen, have 2
- oligosaccharides have 2–10 monosaccharide units and are often the carbohydrate component of cell membrane glycoproteins or glycolipids
- polysaccharides, such as starch, typically have hundreds of monosaccharide units

In the polymers, monosacchride units are joined by glycosidic bonds (**Figure 1.25**). The glycosidic bond is a covalent bond between

Glycosidic bond: glucose and fructose

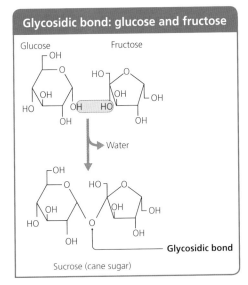

Figure 1.25 A glycosidic bond between glucose and fructose.

Table 1.8 Common carbohydrates in the body

No. of carbon atoms	Category	Examples
4	Tetrose	Erythrose
		Threose
5	Pentose	Ribose
		Ribulose
		Xylose
		Xylulose
6	Hexose	Glucose
		Fructose
		Galactose
		Mannose
7	Heptose	Sedoheptulose
		Mannoheptulose

the anomeric hydroxyl of a cyclic sugar and the hydroxyl of a second sugar.

> **Carbohydrate is the principal source of energy in most diets.** Starch usually accounts for two thirds of digestible dietary carbohydrate; the remainder is sucrose, lactose and their constituent monosaccharides.

Monosaccharides

Monosaccharides are classified by the number of carbon atoms in their carbon backbone; most, including glucose, have four, five or six (**Table 1.8**). Monosaccharides have a number of essential functions, including being an energy source within the cell.

Glucose is the key body fuel. It is one of the main products of plant photosynthesis and the main fuel for cellular respiration to produce ATP.

> **Glucose is an essential energy metabolite**, but its high energy content and potential reactivity can be pathological if blood levels are uncontrolled, as in cases of diabetes mellitus. Damage occurs through various mechanisms, including glucose forming permanent and disruptive glycation bonds with structural proteins, and the excessive production of free radicals during glucose breakdown.

Disaccharides

Disaccharides are produced by linking two monosaccharides with a glycosidic bond. During this reaction, water is eliminated (see **Figure 1.25**).

Examples of disaccharides are sucrose, lactose and maltose (e.g. lactose is galactose and glucose joined by a $\beta(1-4)$ link)

Disaccharides have one main function which is to provide a convertible source of monosaccharides.

Polysaccharides

The principle repeating monosaccharide unit present in polysaccharides is D–glucose.

- A homopolysaccharide is a polysaccharide made of only a single type of monosaccharide
- A heteropolysaccharide is a polysaccharide comprising more than one type of monosaccharide

Polysaccharides have essential functions, including the storage of energy (e.g. glycogen).

Glycogen, present in liver and muscle, is the main carbohydrate stored in humans. It is a homopolysaccharide composed of glucose. It has a compact branched structure, making it a physically efficient store of energy.

> **Glycogenesis is the formation of glycogen, which occurs when there is excess glucose and ATP in the presence of insulin and the enzyme glycogen synthetase.** In contrast, glycogenolysis, the breakdown of glycogen, occurs when blood sugar is low, is stimulated by glucagon hormone and catalysed by glycogen phosphorylase.

Glucose is also be produced from a non-carbohydrate source in a process called gluconeogenesis. Potential substrates for this process include lactic acid, some amino acids (e.g. alanine) from protein and glycerol from fat.

Amino acids and proteins

Amino acids have a common structure (**Figure 1.26**), with a central carbon atom, a basic amino group ($-NH_2$), an acidic carboxyl group ($-COOH$), a hydrogen atom($-H$) and a distinctive functional group ($-R$).

Proteins are made of a sequence of amino acids, which are the monomeric units that are linked together to form a polypeptide structure. The importance of amino acids and proteins is clear from the way DNA, the blueprint for all biological activity, is 'read

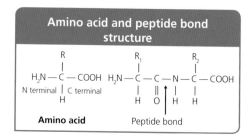

Figure 1.26 Structure of an amino acid and a peptide bond.

and translated' solely into sequences of amino acids that form functioning proteins, which oversee all cellular activity.

Amino acids

Plants and animals contain more than 300 amino acids; however, only 20 are coded by DNA (**Table 1.9**). In humans, only eight amino acids are essential, i.e. they cannot be synthesised by the body and so must be present in the diet.

Apart from glycine, all amino acids contain one asymmetrical carbon called an α carbon. This gives rise to two isomers called enantiomers, which have a D or an L configuration. All amino acids are present in the L configuration because proteins are synthesised by enzymes that insert the L form into the polypeptide structure.

The properties of an amino acid and therefore a protein depend on its functional group side chain ($-R$). This influences how the protein folds, its charge and its function. For example, proteins with many aromatic amino acids (e.g. phenylalanine) are relatively insoluble in water, whereas proteins rich in polar amino acids (e.g. lysine) are water-soluble.

Proteins

Proteins are the primary structural and functional polymers in all living organisms; all other polymers are made by proteins. For example, they:

- catalyse metabolic reactions
- build and repair tissues
- transport oxygen, vitamins and minerals
- form blood clots

Amino acids encoded by DNA

Amino acid	Three-letter code	One-letter code
Alanine	Ala	A
Arginine	Arg	R
Asparagine	Asn	N
Aspartic acid	Asp	D
Cysteine	Cys	C
Glutamic acid	Glu	E
Glutamate	Gln	Q
Glycine	Gly	G
Histidine*	His	H
Isoleucine*	Ile	I
Leucine*	Leu	L
Lysine*	Lys	K
Methionine*	Met	M
Phenylalanine*	Phe	F
Proline	Pro	P
Serine	Ser	S
Threonine*	Thr	T
Tryptophan*	Trp	W
Tyrosine	Tyr	Y
Valine*	Val	V

*Essential amino acids and can be obtained only from the diet.

Table 1.9 The 20 amino acids encoded by DNA

They are also central to hormone signalling.

Proteins must form a three-dimensional structure to function. This is described in terms of primary, secondary, tertiary and quaternary structure (**Figure 1.27**).

Primary structure

A protein's primary structure is the linear sequence of amino acids joined by peptide bonds. This bond is formed by linking the carbonyl group from one amino acid to the amino group of another amino acid, in a reaction that produces water (see **Figures 1.26** and **1.27a**). In the polypeptide chain:

■ the amino acid with a free amino group at the end is called the N-terminal amino acid

Protein structure hierarchy

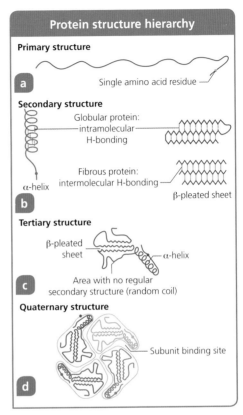

Figure 1.27 Hierarchy of protein structure. (a) Primary structure. (b) Secondary structure. (c) Tertiary structure. (d) Quaternary structure.

■ the amino acid with a free carboxyl group is the C-terminal amino acid

The peptide sequence of a polypeptide is represented by three and one letter codes, for example tyrosine is Tyr and Y (see **Table 1.9**).

Secondary structure

These structures are the result of how a polypeptide chain is influenced by hydrogen bonding between the carbonyl oxygen group of one peptide bond and the amide hydrogen of a neighbouring peptide bond. There are two types of secondary structures (**Figure 1.27b**): the α helix, a right-handed coil of amino acid residues on a polypeptide chain (typically 4-40 residues); and the β sheet, two segments of a polypeptide chain overlapping one another with a row of hydrogen bonds forming in between. This can be parallel or anti-parallel in arrangement.

Tertiary structure

The three dimensional, folded and biologically active structure is called the tertiary structure (**Figure 1.27c**). It is determined and stabilised by:

- side chain functional groups
- covalent disulphide bonds
- hydrogen bonds
- salt bridges
- hydrophobic interactions

Quaternary structure

This is the term for a complex or assembly of two or more peptide chains that are held together by either covalent or non-covalent interactions (**Figure 1.27d**). One of the best examples of this is haemoglobin, a tetrameric protein containing two α chains and two β chains and a haem prosthetic group (Figure 6.4).

> A triplet codon is the DNA code for a specific amino acid. The sequence of triplet codons in DNA determines the sequence of amino acids in a protein, which in turn determines the secondary and tertiary structures into which the chain of amino acids folds.

Lipids

Lipids are structurally and functionally diverse molecules consisting of carbon, hydrogen and oxygen atoms. Chemically, they contain principally non-polar carbon-hydrogen (C–H) bonds (**Figure 1.28**). They typically yield fatty acids, complex alcohols or both after hydrolysis. They are nearly insoluble in aqueous solutions, because of their hydrophobic hydrocarbon chain. However, they are soluble in organic solvents, because they have a non-polar hydrocarbon chain.

Some lipids also contain polar groups, such as sialic, phosphoryl, amino, sulfuryl and hydroxyl groups. These polar groups give them an affinity for water and organic solvents, making them amphipathic.

Lipids have four main roles. They are:

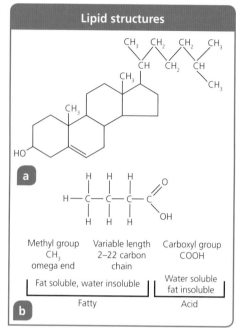

Figure 1.28 Basic lipid structures: (a) cholesterol and (b) butyric acid (fatty acid).

- structural components of biological membranes (see page 8)
- energy reserves, stored predominantly in the form of triglycerides (see page 129)
- biologically active molecules with a wide range of biological functions (e.g. hormones, and intracellular signalling molecules) (see page 16)
- lipophilic bile acids, which aid in lipid solubilisation, and absorption in the gut

Lipids can be broadly categorised into six main groups based on a combination of structure and function.

- Steroids such as cholesterol, which are essential for steroid hormone synthesis
- Fatty acids, including palmitic acid, which serve as an energy source
- Storage lipids (e.g. acylglycerols), which make up fat stores in adipose tissue
- Membrane lipids, e.g. glycerophospholipids and spingolipids
- Prostaglandins, such as prostacyclin, which are involved in inflammation and control of blood flow

- Terpenes, including squalene, which is the precursor of cholesterol

Steroids

Steroids are lipids that are composed of 17 carbon atoms arranged in a ring structure with a hydrocarbon chain, e.g. cholesterol (**Figure 1.28**). Cholesterol, a 27-carbon steroid alcohol present almost exclusively in animals, is a vital component of cell membranes and is often esterified with a fatty acid. Cholesterol forms the basis of various biological molecules, including vitamin D, steroid hormones and bile acids.

> **Bile acids are steroid lipids present in bile that form micelles, the small lipid bilayer globules that promote the digestion and absorption of dietary fat.** Once excreted in bile into the small intestine, they 'collect' dietary lipids, in effect making the lipid more soluble. This aids digestion by lipase enzymes and absorption by the intestinal epithelium.

Fatty acids

Fatty acids are hydrocarbon molecules with a carboxyl (-COOH) group at one end (see **Figure 1.28**). This makes them amphipathic.

Fatty acids are classified according to the length of their carbon chain (4–6 carbons, short chain; 6–10, medium chain; and 12–26 carbons, long chain) and their degree of saturation (**Table 1.10**):

- saturated (no double bonds)
- monounsaturated (one double bond)
- polyunsaturated (multiple double bonds)

The most important fatty acids in nutrition are long-chain fatty acids containing an even number of carbon atoms. In circulation, fatty acids are in a free form bound to albumin or in an esterified form (e.g. triglycerides).

Storage lipids

Storage lipids are the energy stores in adipose tissue. These are acylglycerols, also known as glycerol esters, that comprise a glycerol backbone with a fatty acid attached. This structure makes a good energy store because it is reduced and dehydrated, therefore providing a very concentrated energy source.

The class of acylglycerol is determined by the number of fatty acids attached. Thus monoacylglycerol has one and triacylglycerol (triglyceride) has three (**Figure 1.29**).

Triglycerides make up 95% of tissue storage fat in adipose tissue and are the main form of glycerol esters in plasma. Plant triglycerides tend to have more unsaturated fatty acids (such as linoleic acid) and are therefore liquid at room temperature. In contrast, animal triglycerides have more saturated acids and are solid at room temperature.

Common saturated and unsaturated fatty acids			
Unsaturated		Saturated	
Common name	C:D	Common name	C:D
Myristoleic acid	14:1	Caprylic acid	8:0
Palmitoleic acid	16:1	Capric acid	10:0
Oleic acid	18:1	Lauric acid	13:0
Linoleic acid	18:2	Myristic acid	14:0
Linoelaidic acid	18:2	Palmitic acid	16:0
α-Linolenic acid	18:3	Stearic acid	18:0
Arachidonic acid	20:4	Arachidic acid	20:0
Eicosapentaenoic acid	20:5	Behenic acid	22:0
Erucic acid	22:1	Lignoceric acid	24:0
Docosahexaenoic acid	22:6	Cerotic acid	26:0

C:D, ratio of number of carbon atoms:double bonds in the molecule.

Table 1.10 Common saturated and unsaturated fatty acids present in the body

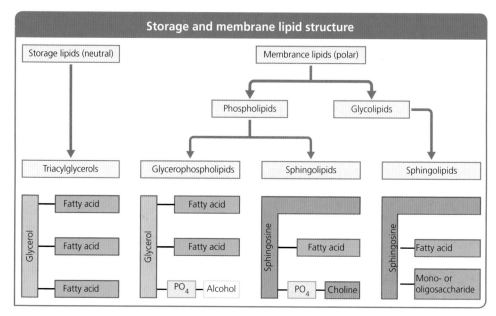

Figure 1.29 Basic structure of storage and membrane lipids.

Membrane lipids

Cell and organelle membranes (see **Figure 1.3**) consist predominantly of the phospholipids glycerophospholipids and sphingolipids (see **Figure 1.29**), which both usually have fatty acids with an even number of carbons, usually 14–24. In humans, the fatty acids are unbranched and can be saturated or unsaturated.

Glycerophospholipids

These are derived from phosphatidic acid. They have a glycerol backbone to which two fatty acids and a phosphoric acid are attached as esters. This basic structure is a phosphatidate, an intermediate in the synthesis of many glycerophospholipids, a major component of membranes. Glycerophospholipids are the most abundant lipid in cell membranes. They enable the formation of a lipid bilayer.

Plasmalogens are ether-linked glycerophospholipids in heart and brain membranes. Platelet-activating factor is an ether lipid with a signalling function in inflammation, platelet aggregation and vasoconstriction.

Sphingolipids

These are derived from sphingosine, an amino alcohol with an alcohol group at carbon-17. Sphingolipids give cell membranes their essential roles in signal transduction and cell recognition.

Ceramide is an intermediate for the synthesis of sphingomyelin, galactosylceramide and glycosylceramide. Ceramide is formed by attaching a fatty acid with 18 or more carbon atoms to the amino group of sphingosine through an amide linkage. Ceramide containing a sulphate group on the galactose residue form sulfatides; they have a major role in myelin stability and function.

Glycosylceramides also have additional monosaccharide groups such as N-acetylgalactosamine, to form globosides and gangliosides. The latter are abundant in the membranes of the grey matter of the brain, where they play a role in cell signaling and immune function.

Prostaglandins

Prostaglandins are derived from fatty acids, principally arachidonate. They all contain

20 carbon atoms, including a 5-carbon ring. Sixteen occur in nature, but only seven are regularly present in the body (see Table 5.6). These seven prostaglandins have several functions, including vasodilation and vaso-constriction. They also have other locally acting endocrine functions, such as those of local inflammation, as well as roles in fever and induction of labour.

Thromboxanes and leukotrienes are closely related to prostaglandins. The former have a role in blood clot formation and the latter in inflammation.

Terpenes

Terpenes are polymers of a 5-carbon iso-prene unit. Examples of terpenes include vitamins A, E and K, and dolichols.

Answers to starter questions

1. There are two main categories of cell – prokaryotes and eukaryotes. Eukaryotes have a nucleus, organelles and a compartmentalisation of materials, whereas prokaryotes don't. Bacteria are prokaryotes and plant, animal and other microorganisms are eukaryotes. Both cell types have similar biochemical composition and share many metabolic pathways but are different in terms of structural elements and genetic processes.

2. Stem cells are undifferentiated cells – effectively 'blank' unspecialised cells from which others can subsequently differentiate. They can renew themselves by dividing and under specific conditions can differentiate. There are two types, embryonic stem cells found in the inner cell mass of blastocysts and adult stem cells, generally isolated from bone marrow, adipose tissue or blood. Stem cells are used frequently in medical therapies and are one of the most expanding areas of medical research due to their potential to regenerate healthy cells, tissue or even organs.

3. Cells have a 'skin' of a lipid bilayer in which the hydrophobic tail regions of phospholipid molecules are repelled by the polar internal and external fluid. The hydrophilic heads are not repelled and form the surface layers inside and outside the cell. Some gasses and ions can diffuse passively across the bilayer, but proteins imbedded in the membrane selectively control the movement of other molecules. In this way, the membrane is responsible for maintaining both the intracellular and extracellular environment, by compartmentalising substances, and is essential for cellular and metabolic processes.

4. Cells can die either from a programmed/controlled suicide known as apoptosis, or by necrosis, where an external force such as a drug, poison, physical injury, overheating, or lack of oxygen results in uncontrolled cell death. Apoptosis is essential for normal health and development as it prevents damaged cells from persisting and allows for new cells to regenerate tissues. It involves many interlinking signals and pathways, but the end point is the organised degradation of the cellular organelles by proteolytic (i.e. protein-destroying) caspase proteins. Approximately 50-70 billion cells per day die via apoptosis in adults.

5. Both vegetable oil and animal fat are composed of triglycerides, however solid fats contain saturated fatty acids, i.e. they are fully saturated with hydrogen atoms and have no double bonds. Conversely, oils that are liquid at room temperature are unsaturated and have more double bonds that kink the triglyceride chain, preventing tight packing of the fatty acids thereby maintaining a liquid structure.

Answers *continued*

6. Cell shape is dictated by the environment of the cells, their function and the number of organelles. Cell structure is maintained by the three types of filaments that form the cytoskeleton. Microtubules give the cell its shape and organise the distribution and transport of the organelles. Microfilaments consist of actin and can contract the cell. Intermediate filaments resist tension placed upon the cell.

7. Aquaporins are cell membrane water-channel proteins that allow water to pass through the lipid bilayer quicker than diffusing through it. Aquaporin type 2 (AQP2) protein does this in the collecting duct of the kidney, to increase water reabsorption back into the blood in response to anti-diuretic hormone (ADH), to concentrate the urine and preserve water as needed. A disabling mutation of the AQP2 gene results in diabetes insipidus (DI) characterised by excessive thirst and excretion of large amounts of dilute urine. There are three types: cranial DI from lack of production of ADH. Nephrogenic caused by lack of aquaporin 2 response to ADH. Iatrogenic due to drugs and alcohol.

8. Cells communicate via signal molecules that are transferred directly between cells in a tissue or organ or they travel in the blood to cells of a different tissue. They are detected by the target cell via binding to receptors on or in the target cell. Once bound to their receptor they initiate a specific response in the target cells, such as the secretion of certain proteins, increased enzyme activity, cell division or cell death. Through this signalling, for example, one cell can tell another cell to alter its function, grow or even self-destruct.

9. The same signalling molecule can have different effects on different cells. A cell will only respond to it if they express the right receptor, and the extent of the response is related to the number and activity of receptors. The receptor response is also dependent on poorly understood and complex interactions between the different downstream effector molecules present in the cell.

10. Biochemical reactions are regulated by controlling the activity of the enzyme which catalyses the reaction via: control of enzyme gene expression, the presence of enzyme inhibitors or cofactors and enzyme activation through chemical modification or proteolytic cleavage.

11. Digestive enzymes are produced and stored in the pancreas as inactive zymogens – inert precursors. They are secreted in the pancreatic juice in response to a meal and are only activated in the gastrointestinal tract via proteolytic cleavage by the enzyme trypsin. Trypsin is itself secreted as the zymgen trypsinogen, which is in turn is activated by the enzyme enteropeptidase in the duodenum. The luminal cells of the GI tract are protected from digestive enzymes by a wall of mucus secreted by the goblet cells of the intestinal epithelium.

12. The rate of a reaction is affected by the: concentration of reactants, pressure of reacting gases, temperature, use of a catalyst, nature of reactants, orientation of reacting species, surface area of reacting solids, intensity of light and nature of solvent.

13. Reactions can be exothermic, where enthalpy is negative and energy is released, or endothermic, where heat is consumed from the environment. Typical examples of exothermic reactions are precipitation and crystallization, in which ordered solids are formed from disordered gaseous or liquid phases, i.e. they decrease entropy.

Answers *continued*

14. Water is polar in nature; there is a disproportion of electric charge between the oxygen and hydrogen atoms in the molecule. Oxygen has a higher electronegativity than hydrogen, the side of the molecule with the oxygen atom has a partial negative charge. This causes a difference in charge, a dipole that polarises water molecules. The relatively positive hydrogen atoms are attracted to the relatively negative oxygen atoms. This cohesion causes water to form droplets.

15. Thermogenesis is the production of heat; in organisms most heat is generated as a by-product of biochemical reactions, classified as non-shivering thermogenesis. This occurs only in brown adipose tissue (brown fat), which is very metabolically active. Brown fat cells contain a unique, uncoupling protein-1, which disrupts ATP synthesis so that the energy is released as heat. This process is controlled by thyroid hormone and the sympathetic nervous system.

16. All organisms use glucose as an energy store and energy source. There are two components: glucose must be suitable to its function and it must have evolved as suitable to its environment, i.e. in the context of evolution. Its successful properties are presumably – relative to other small molecules – that it is biochemically easy to make, contains a useful amount of energy, is relatively stable, and can be easily stored, converted and broken down. Its detailed evolutionary story is more difficult to untangle.

17. Starch and cellulose are both composed of D-glucose units. The difference is the linkage between the glucose molecules; starch consists of $\alpha(1–4)$–glycosidic bonds and cellulose $\beta(1–4)$ glycoside bonds. Humans do not have the cellulase enzymes to digest cellulose hence it contributes to the dietary fibre of the diet and helps maintain the smooth working of the intestinal tract. Ruminants such as cows, on the other hand, have symbiotic anaerobic bacteria in their intestines that have cellulase activity.

18. Saturated fats raise cholesterol levels whereas unsaturated, such as omega-3 essential fatty acids, can help lower cholesterol levels. Although the mechanism is not clear, it has been suggested that saturated fats activate liver metabolism, which results in an upsurge of very low-density lipoprotein (VLDL). These are the precursor of low-density lipoprotein (LDL), often known as 'bad' cholesterol due to its contribution to the formation of atheroma in arteries, the process that underlies coronary artery and cerebrovascular disease.

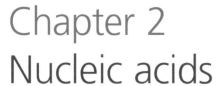

Chapter 2
Nucleic acids

Starter questions

Answers to the following questions are on page 67.

1. Why is DNA considered the 'blueprint' for life?
2. How is biological information passed from one generation to the next?
3. How does a species evolve?
4. Why do we age?
5. Why is DNA used as the genetic material of the cell and not RNA?

Introduction

The nucleic acids deoxyribonucleic acid (DNA) and ribonucleic acid (RNA) are long linear polymers of nucleotides. All biological information for an organism, from the receptors on a cell's membrane to how it develops, is encoded by the nucleotide sequence of DNA.

Nucleotides are small molecules containing:

- a five-carbon sugar
- a phosphate group
- a nitrogen base

As well as forming nucleic acids, nucleotides can function as essential providers of energy for many metabolic reactions. Adenosine triphosphate (ATP) is the best-known example of an energy transfer nucleotide.

Genes are sections of DNA that encode some or all of a protein; they control most cellular activity, metabolism and communication. The expression of genes to produce functioning proteins requires first transcription then translation:

1. Transcription: synthesis of an RNA template molecule
2. Translation: synthesis of a protein from the RNA template

The genome is the entire DNA content of an organism. The genome is present in every cell and must be replicated each time a cell divides. Therefore the processes of cell division and DNA replication are tightly coupled to ensure that replication is complete before division occurs.

Case 1 Pain and swelling in a big toe

Presentation

David Johnson, aged 58 years, presents to his general practitioner with severe pain in his left big toe. The pain had developed suddenly during the night.

On examination, the toe is red, swollen, warm and very tender to touch. David describes two previous similar attacks. Each attack lasted a few days and was successfully treated with non-steroidal anti-inflammatory drugs.

Analysis

A sudden, severe pain in the joint of the big toe, accompanied by redness and swelling, is the classic presentation of gout. This condition arises from the deposition of needle-shaped sodium urate crystals in the synovial fluid of joints.

Gout is associated with hyperuricaemia (high concentration of uric acid in the blood). Uric acid is produced by the breakdown of purine nucleotides, and hyperuricaemia is caused by:

- increased breakdown of nucleotides
- reduced uric acid excretion by the kidneys
- a combination of both

The condition can be primary but is usually secondary (Table 2.1). Hyperuricaemia is common in middle-aged and elderly patients, but not all develop gout.

Further case

David is overweight, and despite having reduced his alcohol intake, he admits to having drunk several pints the day before. He has hypertension.

Causes of hyperuricaemia		
Reason for increased uric acid levels	Primary	Secondary
Increased formation of uric acid	Lesch–Nyhan syndrome	Purine-rich foods
		Obesity
	Glucose 6-phosphate deficiency	Increased degradation of nucleic acids, for example because of malignancy, use of cytotoxic drugs, haemolysis, rhabdomyolysis and excessive alcohol consumption
Decreased excretion of uric acid	Idiopathic	Chronic renal failure
	Glucose 6-phosphate deficiency	Hypertension
		Acidosis, lactic acidosis and ketoacidosis
		Lead poisoning
		Salicylate (low dose) use
		Thiazide diuretic use
		Excessive alcohol consumption

Table 2.1 Primary and secondary causes of hyperuricaemia

Case 1 *continued*

This is the third attack of acute gouty arthritis in the past 10 months, and David's blood uric acid concentration is 620 µmol/L (reference range 200–430 µmol/L). Therefore the general practitioner prescribes allopurinol, a uric acid-lowering drug.

Allopurinol inhibits the enzyme xanthine oxidase, which catalyses uric acid production. Thus allopurinol prevents purine nucleotide degradation and the formation of uric acid.

Further analysis

Acute gouty arthritis is a complication of gout caused by an inflammatory response to uric acid crystals. The condition usually occurs in the toe, knee, elbow, wrist and ankle joints. One or two joints are affected once every couple of years, but the frequency of attacks and number of joints involved often increase as the disease progresses.

Acute attacks of gout are precipitated by certain risk factors for hyperuricaemia, such as excessive alcohol intake. Patients with frequent attacks and prolonged hyperuricaemia often develop tophi; these firm yellow nodules are caused by large accumulations of uric acid.

Tophi occur in the joints, bones and cartilage, as well as under the skin. They sometimes lead to bone erosion and joint deformity. Prolonged hyperuricaemia is also associated with the formation of uric acid stones in the kidney.

Gout: presentation and management

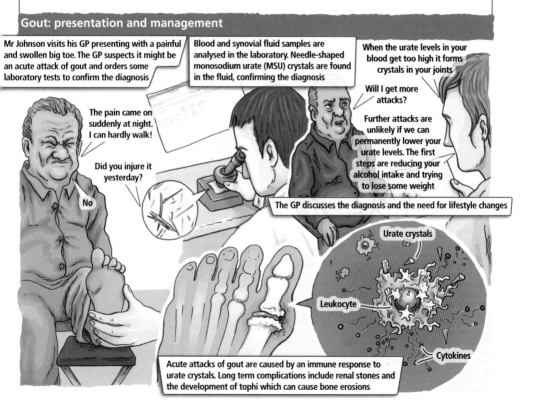

Mr Johnson visits his GP presenting with a painful and swollen big toe. The GP suspects it might be an acute attack of gout and orders some laboratory tests to confirm the diagnosis

The pain came on suddenly at night. I can hardly walk!

Did you injure it yesterday?

No

Blood and synovial fluid samples are analysed in the laboratory. Needle-shaped monosodium urate (MSU) crystals are found in the fluid, confirming the diagnosis

When the urate levels in your blood get too high it forms crystals in your joints

Will I get more attacks?

Further attacks are unlikely if we can permanently lower your urate levels. The first steps are reducing your alcohol intake and trying to lose some weight

The GP discusses the diagnosis and the need for lifestyle changes

Urate crystals

Leukocyte

Cytokines

Acute attacks of gout are caused by an immune response to urate crystals. Long term complications include renal stones and the development of tophi which can cause bone erosions

Case 6 *continued*

Gout progresses through four clinical stages. These are:

1. Asymptomatic hyperuricaemia
2. Acute attacks: sudden onset of intense pain and swelling in the affected joint
3. Intercritical gout: asymptomatic period between acute attacks
4. Advanced gout: development of tophi, chronic arthritis or both

Non-steroidal anti-inflammatory drugs or corticosteroids are used to treat acute attacks of gout by inhibiting the immune inflammatory response. Long-term treatment is based first on lifestyle changes to reduce blood uric acid levels (e.g. dietary improvements, exercise and weight loss); if required these are followed by the use of the drug allopurinol, which directly inhibits uric acid production.

Nucleotides

Nucleotides have essential and diverse roles in the body (**Table 2.2**):

- as precursors of nucleic acids
- in signal transduction
- in energy metabolism
- as components of coenzymes and other metabolites required for biosynthesis

They all share the same general structure (**Figure 2.1**) in that they have three components:

- a five-carbon sugar,
- a nitrogen-containing base and
- a phosphate group

Sugar group

The sugar component of a nucleotide is either ribose or deoxyribose (**Figure 2.2**). Nucleotides polymerise through linkage of the phosphate group of one molecule to the sugar group of an adjoining molecule in a phosphodiester bond (**Figure 2.3**). In this way, a nucleic acid is formed:

- Nucleotides containing ribose (ribonucleotides) polymerise to form RNA
- Nucleotides containing deoxyribose polymerise to form DNA

Nucleotide functions	
Function	Example(s)
Precursors of nucleic acids	RNA and DNA
Energy sources	ATP and GTP
Cellular signalling molecules and metabolic regulators	cAMP and cGMP
Components of coenzymes	NAD, NADP, FAD and coenzyme A (all derivatives of ADP)
Components of active metabolites	UDP–glucose (used in glycogen synthesis)
	CDP–choline (involved in phospholipid synthesis)

ADP, adenosine diphosphate; ATP, adenosine triphosphate; cAMP, cyclic adenosine monophosphate; CDP, cytidine diphosphate; cGMP, cyclic guanosine monophosphate; DNA, deoxyribonucleic acid; FAD, flavin–adenine dinucleotide; GTP, guanosine triphosphate; NAD, nicotinamide–adenine dinucleotide; NADP, nicotinamide–adenine dinucleotide phosphate; RNA, ribonucleic acid; UDP, uridine diphosphate.

Table 2.2 Cellular functions of nucleotides

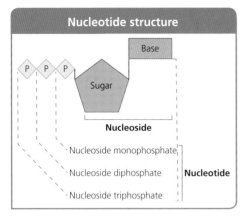

Figure 2.1 General structure of nucleotides.

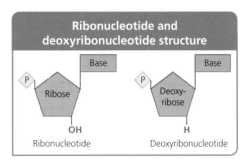

Figure 2.2 General structure of ribonucleotides and deoxyribonucleotides.

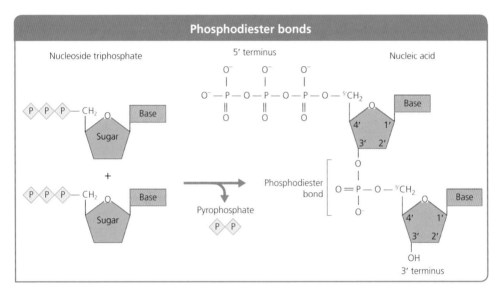

Figure 2.3 Formation of the phosphodiester bond.

Phosphate group

One, two or three phosphate units (mono, di- or triphosphate forms, respectively) attach to the 5' carbon of the sugar group (**Tables 2.3** and **2.4**). The breakage and formation of these phosphate bonds is the key way in which cells store and transfer energy. Base-specific phosphorylase and kinase enzymes catalyse the phosphorylation and dephosphorylation reactions.

Nucleosides are the forms with no phosphate; nucleotides are also known as nucleoside phosphates.

Nitrogenous base

Nucleotide bases are classified into two groups, purines and pyrimidines, which have different ring structures (**Figure 2.4**).

- Purines (adenine and guanine) have a double-ring structure
- Pyrimidines (thymine, uracil and cytosine) have a single ring

Adenine, guanine and cytosine are in both RNA and DNA. However, thymine occurs only in DNA and uracil only in RNA.

Base, nucleoside and nucleotide nomenclature: RNA				
Structure		**Purines**		**Pyrimidines**
Base	-	Adenine (A)	Guanine (G)	Uracil (U)	Cytosine (C)
Nucleoside:	Ribonucleoside	Adenosine	Guanosine	Uridine	Cytidine
Nucleotide:	Ribonucleotide	Adenylate	Guanylate	Uridylate	Cytidylate
	Ribonucleoside monophosphate	AMP	GMP	UMP	CMP
	Ribonucleoside diphosphate	ADP	GDP	UDP	CDP
	Ribonucleoside triphosphate	ATP	GTP	UTP	CTP

Table 2.3 Nomenclature for bases, nucleosides and nucleotides: ribonucleic acid (RNA)

Base, nucleoside and nucleotide nomenclature: DNA				
Structure		**Purines**		**Pyrimidines**
Base	-	Adenine (A)	Guanine (G)	Thymine (T)	Cytosine (C)
Nucleoside:	Deoxyribonucleoside	Deoxyadenosine	Deoxyguanosine	Thymidine	Deoxycytidine
Nucleotide:	Deoxyribonucleotide	Deoxyadenylate	Deoxyguanylate	Thymidylate	Deoxycytidylate
	Deoxyribonucleoside monophosphate	dAMP	dGMP	dTMP	dCMP
	Deoxyribonucleoside diphosphate	dADP	dGDP	dTDP	dCDP
	Deoxyribonucleoside triphosphate	dATP	dGTP	dTTP	dCTP

Table 2.4 Nomenclature for bases, nucleosides and nucleotides: deoxyribonucleic acid (DNA)

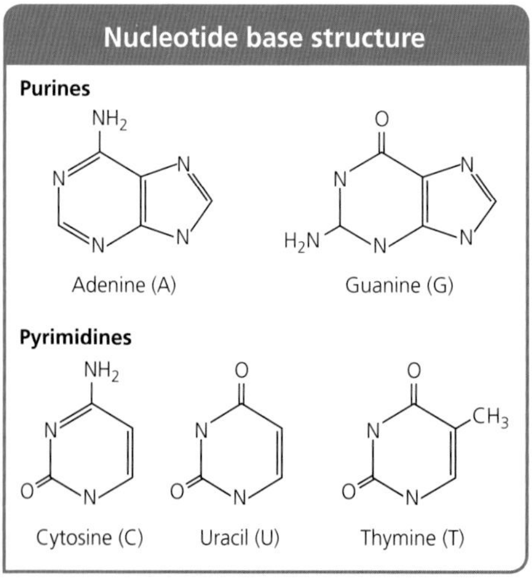

Figure 2.4 Structure of the nucleotide bases: purines and pyrimidines.

Nucleotide synthesis

All cells are able to synthesise purine and pyrimidine bases de novo from amino acids and other simple molecules to produce nucleotides. There are also salvage pathways, which use preformed purine and pyrimidine bases from the diet or recycled from nucleic acid breakdown to synthesise nucleotides. Most nucleotide synthesis is through salvage pathways.

Both de novo and salvage pathways produce monophosphate ribonucleotides. These molecules are then sequentially phosphorylated to give the diphosphate and finally the triphosphate forms (ribonucleoside triphosphates).

A key shared metabolite in all pathways is 5-phosphoribosyl 1-pyrophosphate (**PRPP**) (**Figure 2.5**). PRPP is a ribose derivative formed by the addition of pyrophosphate (diphosphate) to ribose 5-phosphate. This reaction is important, because it activates the molecule and allows the subsequent addition of a base.

Purine nucleotide de novo synthesis

The de novo synthesis of purine nucleotides starts with formation of inosine monophosphate (IMP) from the PRPP precursor (**Figure 2.6**). The conversion of PRPP to IMP is a complex pathway in which glycine, formate, ammonia, bicarbonate and aspartate are added to the molecule.

Inosine monophosphate is an intermediate purine nucleotide whose nitrogen base is hypoxanthine. IMP is a branch point in purine synthesis, because hypoxanthine is converted in one of two ways (see **Figure 2.6**):

- to adenine, to generate adenosine monophosphate (AMP)
- to guanine, to make guanosine monophosphate (GMP)

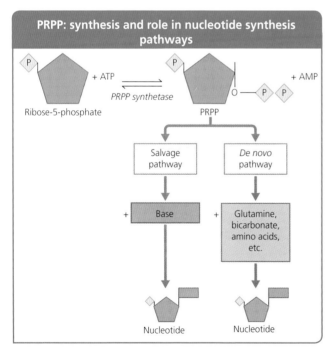

PRPP: synthesis and role in nucleotide synthesis pathways

Ribose-5-phosphate + ATP →(PRPP synthetase) PRPP + AMP

Salvage pathway → + Base → Nucleotide

De novo pathway → + Glutamine, bicarbonate, amino acids, etc. → Nucleotide

Figure 2.5 Synthesis of 5-phosphoribosyl 1-pyrophosphate (PRPP), and its central role in nucleotide de novo and salvage pathways. AMP, adenosine monophosphate; ATP, adenosine triphosphate.

Regulation of purine nucleotide synthesis

Purine synthesis is controlled by a negative feedback mechanism to avoid excessive production (see **Figure 2.6**).

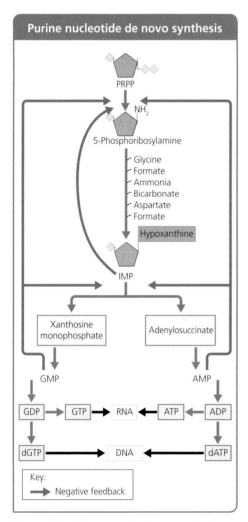

Purine nucleotide de novo synthesis

PRPP

NH$_2$

5-Phosphoribosylamine

Glycine
Formate
Ammonia
Bicarbonate
Aspartate
Formate

Hypoxanthine

IMP

Xanthosine monophosphate

Adenylosuccinate

GMP

AMP

GDP → GTP → RNA ← ATP ← ADP

dGTP → DNA ← dATP

Key:
→ Negative feedback

Figure 2.6 Purine nucleotide de novo synthesis and regulation of the pathway. ADP, adenosine diphosphate; AMP, adenosine monophosphate; ATP, adenosine triphosphate; dATP, deoxyadenosine triphosphate; dGTP, deoxyguanosine triphosphate; DNA, deoxyribonucleic acid; GDP, guanosine diphosphate; GMP, guanosine monophosphate; GTP, guanosine triphosphate; IMP, inosine monophosphate; PRPP, 5-phosphoribosyl 1-pyrophosphate; RNA, ribonucleic acid.

The first enzyme in the pathway is inhibited by the products IMP, AMP and GMP. AMP and GMP generation from IMP is also inhibited by AMP and GMP.

Additionally, the balance between AMP and GMP production from IMP is regulated by a reciprocal substrate mechanism. ATP is required for the conversion of IMP to GMP, and guanosine triphosphate (GTP) is required for the conversion to AMP. Therefore:

- excess ATP promotes GMP synthesis
- excess GTP promotes AMP synthesis

Pyrimidine nucleotide de novo synthesis

Pyrimidines have a less complex base ring structure than that of purines. Therefore pyrimidine synthesis is much simpler than purine synthesis.

Synthesis of pyrimidines involves the reaction of bicarbonate, glutamine and aspartate to form orotate. Orotate then couples with PRPP to produce orotidylate, an intermediate pyrimidine nucleotide.

In contrast to the pathway for purine synthesis, in pyrimidine synthesis the pyrimidine base is synthesised first and then attached to PRPP to form the nucleotide (**Figure 2.7**). The primary end product of the pathway is uridine monophosphate (UMP). UMP is then converted to the other pyrimidine nucleotides: cytidine triphosphate (CTP) and thymidine monophosphate (TMP).

Generation of CTP first requires phosphorylation of UMP to uridine triphosphate (UTP). UTP is then converted to CTP by CTP synthase. TMP production is slightly more complex and first requires formation of the deoxyribose form of UMP (dUMP).

Deoxyuridine monophosphate is then methylated to deoxythymidine monophosphate (dTMP) by thymidylate synthase. In this reaction, the methyl group is donated by methylene tetrahydrofolate, producing dihydrofolate. Methylene tetrahydrofolate is regenerated from dihydrofolate by the

Pyrimidine nucleotide de novo synthesis

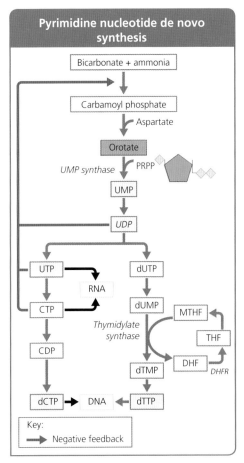

Figure 2.7 Pyrimidine nucleotide de novo synthesis and regulation of the pathway. CDP, cytidine diphosphate; CTP, cytidine triphosphate; dCTP, deoxycytidine triphosphate; DHF, dihydrofolate; DHFR, dihydrofolate reductase; DNA, deoxyribonucleic acid; dTMP, deoxythymidine monophosphate; dTTP, deoxythymidine triphosphate; dUMP, deoxyuridine monophosphate; dUTP, deoxyuridine triphosphate; MTHF, methylene tetrahydrofolate; PRPP, 5-phosphoribosyl 1-pyrophosphate; RNA, ribonucleic acid; THF, tetrahydrofolate; UDP, uridine diphosphate; UMP, uridine monophosphate; UTP, uridine triphosphate.

enzyme dihydrofolate reductase (see **Figure 2.7**). Cells that are unable to regenerate methylene tetrahydrofolate cannot synthesise sufficient deoxythymidine triphosphate (dTTP) for DNA synthesis, so they eventually die.

Folate (vitamin B9) is an essential component of methylene tetrahydrofolate, the methyl donor in de novo pyrimidine synthesis. Folate deficiency results in impaired nucleotide synthesis and prevents cell division. The production of red blood cells is particularly affected, leading to megaloblastic anaemia, a decreased number of red blood cells with an increased amount of abnormally large red cell precursors.

Regulation of pyrimidine nucleotide synthesis

As with purine synthesis, pyrimidine synthesis is regulated by negative feedback (see **Figure 2.7**). The downstream products uridine diphosphate (UDP), UTP and CTP all inhibit the first enzyme in the pathway, carbamoyl phosphate synthase II. CTP also inhibits CTP synthase. Additionally, because the purine nucleotides (ATP and GTP) are required for pyrimidine synthesis, this helps ensure that there is equal production of both pyrimidine and purine nucleotides.

- Excess ATP and GTP increase pyrimidine production
- Low ATP and GTP decrease pyrimidine production

Nucleotide salvage pathways

Salvage pathways produce up to 90% of the cell's nucleotides. These pathways reuse the nucleotide components released during nucleic acid and nucleotide breakdown, i.e. nucleosides and free purine or pyrimidine bases. Unlike de novo pathways, salvage pathways do not require energy.

Nucleosides are phosphorylated by kinase enzymes to generate the corresponding nucleotide. For example, thymidine kinase phosphorylates the thymidine nucleoside to first dTMP, then deoxythymidine diphosphate (dTDP), and then dTTP. Thymidine kinase is present in high concentrations in cells that are actively dividing.

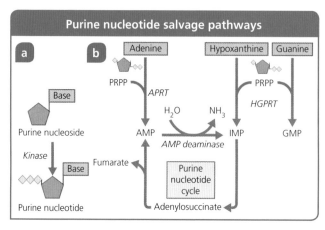

Figure 2.8 Purine nucleotide salvage pathways. (a) Pathway for nucleosides. (b) Pathway for free purine bases. AMP, adenosine monophosphate; APRT, adenine phosphoribosyltransferase; GMP, guanosine monophosphate; HGPRT, hypoxanthine–guanine phosphoribosyltransferase; IMP, inosine monophosphate; PRPP, 5-phosphoribosyl 1-pyrophosphate.

Purine salvage

The free purine bases adenine, guanine and hypoxanthine are salvaged by being added to PRPP by phosphoribosylation (**Figure 2.8**). This process involves two transferase enzymes:

- adenine phosphoribosyltransferase (APRT)
- hypoxanthine–guanine phosphoribosyltransferase (HGPRT)

A minor pathway for the salvage of IMP is through the purine nucleotide cycle (see **Figure 2.8b**). IMP salvage is particularly important in muscle cells during activity, because the fumarate generated is a substrate for the citric acid cycle (see page 110).

Severe combined immunodeficiency syndrome is an inherited disease commonly caused by a deficiency of adenosine deaminase. Adenosine deaminase is an enzyme in the purine salvage pathway and is required for the deamination of adenosine to inosine. Lack of the enzyme causes a build up of adenosine which is then converted to deoxyadenosine triphosphate (dATP).

Increased production of dATP in white blood cells inhibits the activity of ribonucleotide reductase, an enzyme required for deoxyribonucleoside triphosphate (dNTP) synthesis. Excess dATP impairs DNA replication and thus prevents lymphocyte proliferation and a sufficient immune response.

Lesch–Nyhan syndrome is an X-linked recessive disorder caused by a complete lack of the HGPRT enzyme. The absence of HGPRT results in:

- increased PRPP
- increased de novo synthesis of the purine nucleotides
- high concentrations of uric acid

Patients present with neurological symptoms, including intellectual disability, motor disorders, aggressive behaviour and compulsive self-mutilation (particularly chewing on their fingers and lips).

Pyrimidine salvage

The salvage of free pyrimidine bases (uracil and thymine) first involves generation of the corresponding nucleoside by their addition to ribose. This step is followed by phosphorylation to produce the nucleotide (**Figure 2.9**).

- uridine phosphorylase catalyses the addition of uracil to ribose 1-phosphate
- deoxythymidine phosphorylase adds thymine to deoxyribose 1-phosphate

Formation of deoxyribonucleotides

With the exception of TMP, both the de novo pathway and the salvage pathway for nucleotide synthesis form ribonucleoside triphosphates, which are the major nucleotides in all cells. Deoxyribonucleoside triphosphates (dNTPs) are required for DNA synthesis only; thus, the cellular requirement for these is generally small, because most cells are not actively dividing. However, during mito-sis an adequate supply of all four dNTPs is essential for DNA replication and cell division to proceed.

Deoxyribonucleotides are generated through reduction of their corresponding ribonucleotides by the enzyme ribonucleotide reductase (**Figure 2.10**). This process requires the reduced form of nicotinamide–adenine dinucleotide phosphate and the presence of a protein cofactor (thioredoxin or glutaredoxin).

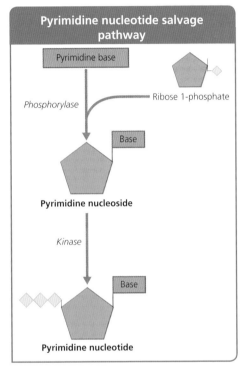

Figure 2.9 Pyrimidine nucleotide salvage pathway.

Regulation of deoxyribonucleotide formation

The activity of ribonucleotide reductase is tightly regulated to ensure that production of all four dNTPs is balanced to meet cellular requirements. The enzyme is stimulated or inhibited by the binding of nucleotides to two regulatory sites on the enzyme: the activity site and the specificity site.

The activity site of ribonucleotide reductase binds ATP and dATP:

■ binding of ATP increases its activity
■ binding of dATP decreases its activity

Thus production of dNTPs is increased when their concentration is low, and decreased when they are abundant.

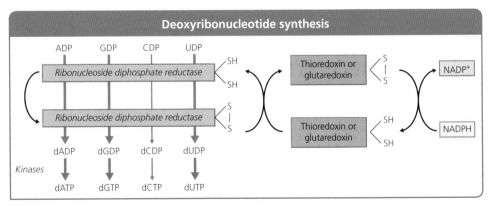

Figure 2.10 Synthesis of deoxyribonucleotides. ADP, adenosine diphosphate; CDP, cytidine diphosphate; dADP, deoxyadenosine diphosphate; dATP, deoxyadenosine triphosphate; dCDP, deoxycytidine diphosphate; dCTP, deoxycytidine triphosphate; dGDP, deoxyguanosine diphosphate; dGTP, deoxyguanosine triphosphate; dUDP, deoxyuridine diphosphate; dUTP, deoxyuridine triphosphate; GDP, guanosine diphosphate; UDP, uridine diphosphate.

The specificity site binds ATP, dATP, deoxyguanosine triphosphate (dGTP) and dTTP. Binding of the nucleotides to the specificity site alters the activity of ribonucleotide reductase towards its different substrates, so that nucleotides in scarce supply are preferentially selected. Thus the equal production of all four dNTPs is ensured.

Nucleotide degradation

Nucleotides are released by:

- intracellular breakdown of RNA or DNA
- extracellular hydrolysis of ingested nucleic acids

The released nucleotides are first degraded by phosphorylases to their nucleoside or free bases. Most of the products of nucleotide degradation are reused for nucleotide synthesis through salvage pathways. However, if demand for them is low, they are further degraded.

> Most animals, but not humans, have the enzyme uricase (uric acid oxidase), which degrades uric acid first to allantoin and then to urea. A recombinant form of uricase, rasburicase, is used to treat high uric acid levels in patients receiving chemotherapy.

Purine catabolism

In humans, breakdown of purine bases produces uric acid (**Figure 2.11**). Uric acid is insoluble, so it is excreted in the urine as its sodium salt, sodium urate.

Normally, the blood is close to saturated with uric acid. Therefore any slight impairment in purine catabolism often leads to hyperuricaemia (increased concentration of uric acid in the blood). The excess uric acid sometimes precipitates as crystals in the synovial fluid of joints, in a condition called gout (see page 45).

Purine breakdown products are insoluble. Therefore disruptions to purine catabolism cause a number of clinical disorders (**Table 2.5**).

Pyrimidine catabolism

Pyrimidine degradation leads to production of β-alanine from uracil and β–aminoisobutyrate from thymine (**Figure 2.12**). These metabolites are further converted to:

- malonyl coenzyme A, and thus diverted to fatty acid synthesis (see page 135)
- succinyl coenzyme A, which enters the citric acid cycle (see page 110)

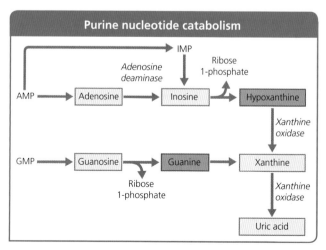

Figure 2.11 Purine nucleotide catabolism. AMP, adenosine monophosphate; GMP, guanosine monophosphate; IMP, inosine monophosphate.

Pyrimidine breakdown products are soluble and so easily excreted. Therefore disruption of the pyrimidine catabolism pathway has little clinical impact, and only a few effects are known (**Table 2.6**).

Primary disorders of purine metabolism		
Disorder	Enzyme or cofactor	Nature of defect
Gout	PRPP synthase	Increased activity
	HGPRT	Deficiency
	Glucose 6-phosphatase (Von Gierke's disease)	Deficiency
Lesch–Nyhan syndrome	HGPRT	Deficiency
Renal stones	Adenine phosphoribosyltransferase	Deficiency
Severe combined immunodeficiency syndrome	Adenosine deaminase	Deficiency
	Purine nucleoside phosphorylase	Deficiency
Exercise intolerance	Myoadenylate deaminase	Deficiency
Xanthinuria	Xanthine oxidase	Deficiency
	Molybdenum cofactor	Deficiency

HGPRT, hypoxanthine–guanine phosphoribosyltransferase; PRPP, 5-phosphoribosyl 1-pyrophosphate.

Table 2.5 Primary disorders of purine metabolism

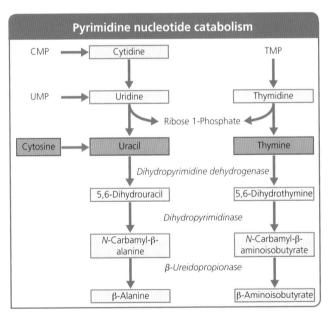

Figure 2.12 Pyrimidine nucleotide catabolism. CMP, cytidine monophosphate; TMP, thymidine monophosphate; UMP, uridine monophosphate.

Disorders of pyrimidine metabolism		
Disorder	Enzyme	Nature of defect
Orotic aciduria	Uridine monophosphate synthase	Deficiency
Neurological symptoms	Dihydropyrimidine dehydrogenase	Deficiency

Table 2.6 Primary disorders of pyrimidine metabolism

Drugs targeting nucleotide metabolism

Many chemotherapeutic and immunosuppressive drugs act by inhibiting nucleotide synthesis and thus reducing the production of dNTPs. This effect ultimately prevents DNA replication and cell division, causing cell death.

Such drugs target rapidly dividing cells with a high demand for dNTPs, including:

- cancer cells
- epithelial cells of the gastrointestinal tract
- hair follicles
- immune cells

Therefore nausea, hair loss and increased susceptibility to infections are some of the many common adverse effects of chemotherapy and immunosuppression.

These antimetabolites (drugs that inhibit the use of a metabolite in a pathway) are classified as:

- purine analogues, which disrupt purine nucleotide synthesis
- pyrimidine analogues, which disrupt pyrimidine synthesis
- antifolate drugs, which also disrupt pyrimidine synthesis

Purine analogues

Purine analogue drugs include the thiopurines:

- 6-mercaptopurine
- azathioprine, the precursor drug for 6-mercaptopurine

These drugs disrupt both the de novo and the salvage purine synthesis pathways.

6-Mercaptopurine disrupts the purine salvage pathway by competing for HGPRT. This drug is also converted to thioinosinic monophosphate (**Figure 2.13**), which inhibits several reactions involving IMP and de novo purine synthesis.

6-Mercaptopurine and azathioprine therapy are effective treatments for leukaemia and several autoimmune conditions, including psoriatic arthritis and inflammatory bowel disease (e.g. Crohn's disease).

> **Thiopurine methyltransferase activity is measured in patients due to start therapy with 6-mercaptopurine or azathioprine.** The results are used to determine the dose required.
>
> If normal drug doses are given to patients with low thiopurine methyltransferase activity, the risk of toxicity is high, because more 6-mercaptopurine is metabolised to the active thioguanine nucleotide analogue (see **Figure 2.13**).

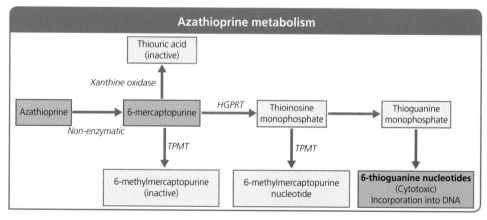

Figure 2.13 Azathioprine metabolism. DNA, deoxyribonucleic acid; HGPRT, hypoxanthine–guanine phosphoribosyltransferase; TPMT, thiopurine methyltransferase.

Pyrimidine analogues and antifolates

Pyrimidine analogues prevent dTTP production by directly inhibiting thymidylate synthase (see page 51). For example, the drug fluorouracil is converted in vivo to a dUMP analogue, which is a substrate for thymidylate synthase. However, once bound it irreversibly inhibits the enzyme.

Antifolate drugs, such as methotrexate (a dihydrofolate analogue), also prevent the synthesis of dTTP, in this case by inhibiting dihydrofolate reductase.

Nucleic acid structure

Most of the nucleotides within a cell are involved in the formation of the nucleic acids: DNA and RNA. These polynucleotide macromolecules are long chains of nucleotides linked together by their sugar and phosphate groups in a phosphodiester bond (**Figure 2.3**). This produces a repetitive 'sugar-phosphate backbone' which is common to all DNA and RNA molecules (**Figure 2.14**).

Variability between different DNA and RNA molecules is determined by the order of the bases in the polynucleotide chain – the primary structure. The secondary structure of the nucleic acids describes the three-dimensional shape of the molecules and is governed primarily by base-pairing (formation of hydrogen bonds between bases). Some nucleic acid molecules also undergo further, higher order folding, which is termed the tertiary structure.

Phosphodiester bonds

The phosphodiester bond forms between the phosphate group attached to the 5' carbon on one nucleotide and the hydroxyl group attached to the 3' carbon on the adjacent nucleotide (see **Figure 2.3**). Therefore the two ends of a nucleic acid molecule are different:

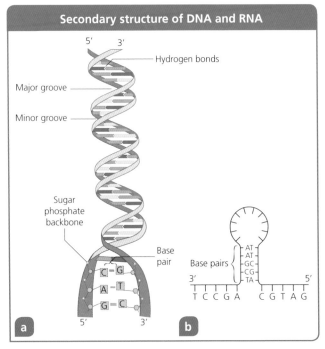

Secondary structure of DNA and RNA

Major groove

Minor groove

Hydrogen bonds

5'   3'

Sugar phosphate backbone

Base pair

C — G
A — T
G — C

5'   3'

a

Base pairs

AT
AT
GC
CG
TA

3'   5'

T C C G A   C G T A G

b

Figure 2.14 Secondary structure of DNA and RNA. (a) The deoxyribonucleic acid double helix. (b) The stem loop motif commonly present in ribonucleic acid.

- the 5' terminus has a free 5' carbon phosphate, which is not involved in the phosphodiester bond
- the 3' terminus has a free 3' carbon hydroxyl group

This means that the primary structure of a nucleic acid has a direction; 5' to 3'.

The energy required for the formation of the phosphodiester bond is provided by the cleavage of pyrophosphate (two phosphates) during the bond formation. Therefore, it requires the free nucleotides to be in the triphosphate form. The resulting phosphate group, involved in the phosphodiester link, is a strong acid and carries a negative charge at physiological pH. This is why DNA and RNA are known as nucleic acids.

Base pairing

The bases in nucleotides are not involved in the phosphodiester bond and are free to form hydrogen bonds with bases on other nucleic acids. These base pairs are between specific purine and pyrimidine bases (**Table 2.7**) and occur between complementary nucleotide sequences to give the secondary structure of a nucleic acid. Base pairing is also the fundamental mechanism for the synthesis of new nucleic acid molecules from a template molecule.

> Ultraviolet B rays in sunlight directly damage DNA in skin cells by disrupting base pairing and causing adjacent pyrimidine bases in a DNA sequence to bond together. These pyrimidine dimers are skipped in DNA replication and transcription, resulting in mutations and an increased risk of skin cancer. DNA repair mechanisms recognise and excise mutations but can be overwhelmed if there are too many.

Primary structure

The sequence of the bases (nucleotide sequence) in DNA and RNA molecules is

Base pairing		
Nucleic acid	Complementary bases	
Deoxyribonucleic acid	C	G
	A	T
Ribonucleic acid	C	G
	A	U

Table 2.7 Base pairing. Pairing occurs only between complementary bases, e.g. C and G can pair with each other but not with other bases.

called the primary structure; it is always written as the nucleotide base sequence, using the single letter abbreviation, in the 5' to 3' direction. This sequence encodes the genetic information required by the cell for protein synthesis. The bases can be joined together in any order providing an almost infinite number of possible sequences in a nucleic acid molecule. For example, a DNA molecule containing only ten nucleotides can have over one million (4^{10}) possible nucleotide sequences. This variability allows the cell to store massive amounts of information in its DNA using only four different nucleotides.

Secondary structure

DNA primarily forms a double helix (see **Figure 2.14**), whereas most RNA exists as a single-stranded molecule.

The double helix is created by base pairing between two DNA molecules (strands) with complementary base sequences. The two strands, running in opposite directions, twist around each other to form a right-handed helix (the B form). Double-stranded RNA molecules and DNA–RNA hybrid molecules form a right-handed helix (the A form), which is more compact. A small amount of DNA exists as a double-stranded left-handed helix (the Z form).

The polymerase chain reaction is one of the foundations of the molecular biology revolution of the late 20th century. In this technique, a short chain of known nucleotides (primers), a heat-resistant DNA polymerase enzyme originally found in an organism from a thermal deep sea vent, and a cycle of heating and cooling are used to generate many copies of a targeted sequence between the two primers. The primers bond by base pairing to a complementary sequence of nucleotides. Thus the DNA polymerase copies the nucleotide sequence between the primers. Many genetic diseases are detected this way.

Most single-stranded nucleic acid molecules have no defined secondary structure. However, base pairing often occurs between complementary sequences in regions of the molecule, causing them to fold back on themselves and form helices. The most common secondary structure in single stranded molecules is the simple stem loop motif (**Figure 2.14**).

Tertiary structure

Tertiary structure is the further higher-order folding of the nucleic acid molecules. Most DNA exists as a long linear double helix and has no tertiary structure. Sometimes however, the double helix twists around itself to form a more compact supercoiled tertiary structure.

Many RNA molecules also form more complex structures necessary for their function, by the folding together of helical regions.

Cellular organisation of DNA

In eukaryotic cells, DNA is found within the nucleus (nuclear genome) and within the mitochondrial matrix (mitochondrial genome). The nuclear genome, the chromosomal DNA, varies in size between different organisms, but the DNA always exists as double stranded linear molecules packaged into chromosomes. The mitochondrial genome is much smaller than the nuclear genome and the DNA usually exists as doubled stranded circular molecules.

Chromosomal DNA

DNA is packaged into chromosomes in a highly organised fashion, consisting of a repeating structure called a nucleosome (**Figure 2.15**). Each nucleosome contains a core, barrel-shaped protein complex, comprising a group of proteins called histones. Two tight turns of DNA are wrapped around each histone complex to form the nucleosome. The nucleosomes occur at regular intervals along the DNA molecule to give a 'beads-on-a-string' appearance. This structure is further folded to produce a more compact, 30 nm fibre, which is looped tightly into the chromosomes. This mechanism allows

Figure 2.15 Structure of chromosomes.

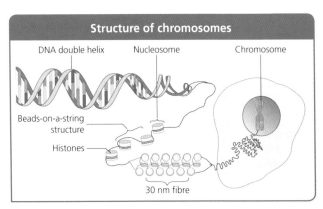

Structure of chromosomes

DNA double helix   Nucleosome   Chromosome

Beads-on-a-string structure

Histones

30 nm fibre

large amounts of genetic information to be contained within the cells. For example the human nuclear genome has a total length of approximately one metre, which is packaged into chromosomes with a total length of about 5 cm.

Mitochondrial DNA

The mitochondrial genome contains only a few genes, which encode for RNA and some of the proteins required for function of the mitochondria. The copy number of mitochondrial DNA varies between species, but in humans each mitochondria contains 10 identical mitochondrial DNA molecules. Since there are about 800 mitochondria per cell, this means every cell has approximately 8000 copies of mitochondrial DNA. A number of mitochondrial disorders, such as mitochondrial encephalomyopathy with lactic acidosis and stroke-like episodes (MELAS), are caused by mutations in mitochondrial DNA. Whether mitochondrial DNA mutations present clinically is very complex and depends on the number of the mitochondrial DNA molecules affected within the cell.

Nucleic acid synthesis

Nucleic acids are synthesised by the step-by-step addition of nucleotides to a polynucleotide chain:

- Replication is the term for synthesis of new DNA molecules
- Transcription is the term for synthesis of new RNA molecules

DNA molecules are several million nucleotides long. RNA molecules, in contrast, are usually no more than a few hundred nucleotides. Small polynucleotides with only a few nucleotides are called oligonucleotides.

Synthesis of a new DNA or RNA molecule occurs directly on a pre-existing DNA molecule, which acts as a template. The template determines the order in which the different nucleotides are join together during synthesis.

- In DNA replication, the whole DNA template molecule is copied to produce a new DNA molecule
- In transcription, only individual genes
- are copied; these are small segments of DNA up to a few hundred nuclotides in length

Although DNA and RNA are composed of a slightly differing set of nucleotides (see Table 2.7), the basic mechanisms of DNA replication and transcription to RNA are similar.

DNA replication

Synthesis of new DNA molecules involves separating the two DNA strands. Each strand then acts as a template for the synthesis of a complementary strand (**Figure 2.16**). Replication is semiconservative, so each daughter cell contains one DNA strand derived from the original cell and one newly synthesised strand. During replication, both DNA strands in the double helix act simultaneously as template strands for the synthesis of new molecules.

- The template DNA is read in the 3' to 5' direction
- Nucleotides are added to the new DNA strand in the 5' to 3' direction

Thus a new double helix forms comprising each template strand and a newly synthesised strand.

Replication of DNA is highly ordered. It has three distinct phases.

1. **Initiation**: recognition and start of replication
2. **Elongation**: synthesis of the new DNA molecule
3. **Termination**: cessation of replication

Each phase involves several enzymes and other proteins, each of which carries out a specific function.

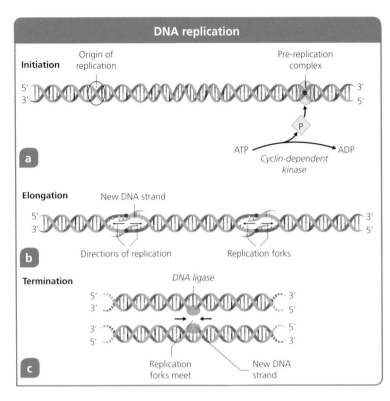

Figure 2.16
Replication of deoxyribonucleic acid (DNA). (a) Initiation. (b) Elongation. (c) Termination. ADP, adenosine diphosphate; ATP, adenosine triphosphate.

Initiation of DNA replication

Replication of DNA starts at several specific points along the DNA molecule: these are called origins of replication. The process begins with the formation of prereplication complexes. These protein complexes are activated by phosphorylation to recruit the enzymes and proteins required for DNA synthesis.

DNA replication is tightly coordinated with the cell division cycle and cell division does not occur before the genome of the cell has been completely replicated. This coordination is achieved by a number of proteins called cyclins, which are released at various stages of the cell cycle. Some cyclins bind to, and activate, cyclin-dependent kinases, which initiate replication by phosphorylation of the prereplication complex.

Other cyclins prevent reassembly of prereplication complexes after replication is complete. This action prevents the cell producing multiple copies of its genome before cell division.

Elongation

Once replication has been initiated, the enzymes helicase and DNA topoisomerase unwind the DNA double helix so that the base sequence is accessible.

- Helicase breaks the base pairs between the two DNA strands
- DNA topoisomerases remove the twists between the strands by breaking one of the strands, passing the intact strand through the gap, and then rejoining the strand

Single-strand binding protein then binds to the separated DNA strands to prevent reformation of the base pairs.

Replication fork

The region of the DNA where replication is occurring is the replication fork (**Figure 2.17**). As the enzymes move along the double helix, they unwind the strands so that the replication fork can proceed along the molecule. Replication occurs in both directions along the DNA molecule from

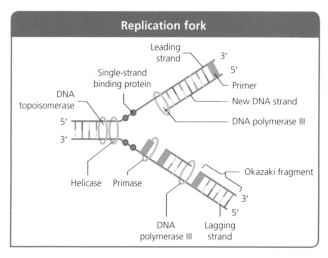

Figure 2.17 The replication fork, where deoxyribonucleic acid (DNA) is replicated.

the origin of replication, and new DNA molecules are synthesised simultaneously on both strands of the double helix.

Primers and polymerisation

Once the strands are separated, a primer (a short RNA oligonucleotide) is attached to the template strand by the enzyme primase. The primer provides a starting point for DNA synthesis. One by one, complementary free nucleotides bind to the DNA template by base pairing. Next, phosphodiester bonds are formed with the previous adjacent nucleotide by DNA polymerase III.

Synthesis always occurs in the 5′ to 3′ direction, so that replication of one DNA strand, i.e. the leading strand, occurs continuously in the 5′ to 3′ direction. In contrast, the other strand (the lagging strand) is formed in short sections called Okazaki fragments. The RNA primers are then removed by DNA polymerase I, and the Okazaki fragments are joined together by DNA ligase.

Acyclovir is a guanosine analogue used as an antiviral drug. It is phosphorylated by viral thymidine kinase to acyclo-GTP and incorporated into DNA. In DNA, acyclovir blocks DNA chain elongation, because it cannot form further phosphodiester bonds. With a greater affinity for viral DNA polymerase than for cellular, it preferentially inhibits viral DNA replication.

Termination

Replication continues until two replication forks meet. Synthesis then terminates when the two ends are ligated (joined) by DNA ligase, and the replication enzymes and proteins dissociate from the DNA strands. The precise mechanisms of this process are poorly understood.

Transcription

The biological information contained in the genome of a cell is divided into discrete units called genes. Each gene encodes a specific RNA molecule.

Gene expression is the synthesis of the functional end gene product. This process is regulated primarily by controlling transcription, although some RNA processing events also play a role.

Types of RNA

There are several types of RNA.

- Messenger RNA (mRNA) is coding RNA as it encodes the amino acid sequence required for protein synthesis (see page 79)
- Ribosomal RNA (rRNA) is non-coding RNA and so is not translated into a protein; instead, it has its own function in the cell: rRNAs are components of ribosomes and are the major type of RNA in a cell

- Transfer RNA (tRNA) is a non-coding RNA required for protein synthesis
- Small RNA molecules are a diverse group of non-coding RNA molecules with various functions including processing other RNA molecules (e.g. small nuclear RNAs)

> About 98% of DNA does not code for protein sequences and was previously considered 'junk DNA'. However, an increasing number of other functions are being discovered, including regulation of gene expression and organisation of chromosomal structure.

All RNA is synthesised from genes by transcription which generates an RNA copy of the gene (**Figure 2.18**). Transcription occurs in three steps.

1. Initiation
2. RNA synthesis
3. RNA processing

Initiation of transcription

Synthesis of RNA is catalysed by three different types of RNA polymerase (**Table 2.8**).

Promoter region

Transcription begins when RNA polymerase binds to a specific DNA sequence called the core promoter region. This region is usually upstream of the gene to be transcribed on the DNA template strand.

Through the actions of DNA-binding proteins, RNA polymerase binds directly or indirectly to core promoter regions. Different

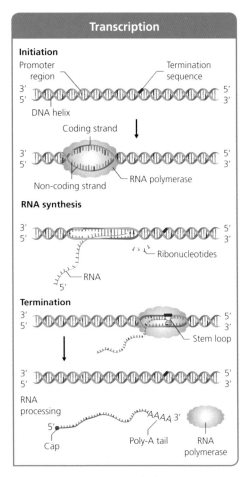

Figure 2.18 Transcription, which generates an RNA copy of a gene. DNA, deoxyribonucleic acid; RNA, ribonucleic acid.

RNA polymerases recognise different core promoter regions. For example, RNA polymerase II promoters are typically 40–50 nucleotides long and 25 nucleotides upstream of the start of the gene.

RNA polymerases in eukaryotes		
RNA polymerase	Type of RNA synthesised	Core promoter region
RNA polymerase I	Ribosomal RNA	Spans the transcription starting point
RNA polymerase II	Messenger RNA and small nuclear RNA	TATA box 25 bases upstream of the transcription starting point
RNA polymerase III	Transfer RNA and short RNA molecules	Usually two core promoter regions in the gene to be transcribed

Table 2.8 Different types of ribonucleic acid (RNA) polymerases in eukaryotic cells

Transcription factors

The recruitment and binding of RNA polymerases to their core promoters is regulated by transcription factors. These proteins bind to specific DNA sequences upstream of the core promoter.

- Transcription factors that promote RNA polymerase binding enhance transcription
- Factors that suppress RNA polymerase binding inhibit transcription

Gene expression is largely controlled by regulation of the synthesis of transcription factors and their transfer into the nucleus. Many transcription factors are receptors for cell signalling molecules such as steroid hormone receptors (see page 17) and thus provide a mechanism for external cell signalling molecules to influence gene expression in the cell.

Gilbert's syndrome is a common benign disorder of bilirubin metabolism. It is caused by an increase in the number of TA repeats in the promoter region of the UDP–glucuronosyltransferase gene. This decreases the affinity between DNA-binding proteins and RNA polymerase, and thus reduces gene transcription. The reduced UDP–glucuronosyltransferase activity in hepatocytes leads to an increased concentration of unconjugated bilirubin in the blood.

RNA synthesis

Once transcription is initiated, RNA synthesis continues by the addition of ribonucleotides, similar to elongation of the DNA chain in DNA replication.

Open complex

Once RNA polymerase is bound to the DNA at the core promoter region, some of the base pairs in the DNA double helix molecule are broken to produce an open promoter complex. This complex is an unwound section of DNA of about 13 base pairs. Free ribonucleotides then bind, one by one, to the DNA template strand by base pairing. In this way, each ribonucleotide forms a phosphodiester link with the previous adjacent nucleotide.

Continuation

The RNA polymerase synthesises RNA in the 5' to 3' direction, reading the DNA template in the 3' to 5' direction. RNA synthesis occurs only on the template strand of the DNA helix. Therefore the RNA molecule has a complementary sequence to the DNA template strand and the same sequence as the non-template DNA strand.

Dissociation

The new RNA molecule is attached to the DNA template strand by only a few RNA-DNA base pairs. As RNA polymerase moves along the DNA, these base pairs disassociate to release the new RNA molecule and allow the DNA double helix to reform.

Termination

The process ends when the whole gene has been transcribed and RNA polymerase dissociates from the DNA molecule. The precise mechanism underlying termination of transcription is poorly understood. However, it may involve the formation of a hairpin loop structure in the newly synthesised RNA molecule. The hairpin loop disrupts the RNA-DNA base pairs and releases the RNA molecule from the DNA template.

A 42-year-old woman presents to the emergency department with vomiting, diarrhoea and severe abdominal pain. The results of routine biochemistry tests are unremarkable except for increased liver enzymes, therefore poisoning or drug misuse is suspected. The patient says she ate two wild mushrooms 6 h ago; these are later identified as death caps (Amanita phalloides).

The death cap mushroom is extremely toxic because it contains α-amanitin, an inhibitor of RNA polymerase II. Inhibition of this enzyme causes cell death by preventing DNA transcription, and this effect results in liver and kidney failure and often death.

RNA processing

The initial precursor RNA (pre-RNA) is altered, for example by changes to length and chemical modifications, to produce mature RNA (**Table 2.9**).

Some processing events play a role in regulating gene expression; for example, capping of mRNA is required for protein translation. However, the reasons for many other processing events are unknown.

Chemical modifications to RNA nucleotides, such as methylation, result in alterations to the sequence or nature of the bases. In the non-coding rRNA and tRNA, this affects only the secondary structure of the RNA molecule. However, chemical modifications to mRNA (RNA editing) often change the coding and subsequent amino acid sequence of the protein translated.

> **Processing of mRNA enables a single gene to encode multiple types of protein.** For example, the *apolipoprotein B* gene encodes apolipoprotein B100, a 4563–amino acid protein synthesised in the liver. However, in intestinal cells the mRNA is modified by deamination of a cytosine nucleotide to uracil. This change introduces a stop codon, so translation produce apolipoprotein B48, which comprises only 2153 amino acids.

RNA processing		
Processing event	Type of RNA	Description
End modification		
End capping	Pre-mRNA	Addition of a 7-methylguanosine nucleotide to the 5′ end of pre-mRNA
Polyadenylation	Pre-mRNA	Addition of up to 250 adenosine nucleotides to the 3′ end of pre-mRNA to form a poly(A) tail; this process is catalysed by poly(A) polymerase
Splicing	Pre-mRNA, pre-rRNA and pre-tRNA	Removal of introns (sections of non-coding segments) and ligation of exons (coding regions)
Cutting	Pre-rRNA and pre-tRNA	Cleavage of a large pre-RNA transcript containing multiple genes into individual mature RNAs
Chemical modification	*mRNA, rRNA and tRNA	Modification to one or more nucleotides, including: methylation deamination addition of sulphur conversion of a double bond to a single bond in the nucleotide replacement of one nucleotide with another

Pre-mRNA, precursor messenger RNA; pre-rRNA, precursor ribosomal RNA; pre-tRNA, precursor transfer RNA.

*Chemical modification of mRNA is called RNA editing.

Table 2.9 Types of ribonucleic acid (RNA) processing

Mutations

The human genome contains about 3 billion nucleotide base pairs. These must be accurately replicated at each cell division.

Mechanisms

Errors in the DNA nucleotide sequence (mutations) are introduced by three mechanisms:

- errors in the replication process
- recombination (exchange of DNA between chromosomes)
- the action of mutagens (chemical or environmental factors that alter the chemical structure of DNA)

Cells contain several DNA repair mechanisms to correct errors. However, some errors escape detection and are passed to subsequent daughter cells. The consequences for multicellular organisms are as follows.

- Any mutations that occur in germ cells (during formation of spermatocytes or oocytes) are passed to the next generation; this process is the basis of inherited disease but is also essential for evolution
- Mutations that occur in somatic cells are not passed down to subsequent generations and are expressed only in the individual organism

Functional effect

The effect of a mutation depends on where it occurs in the DNA.

Silent mutations

Silent mutations have no effect. They occur in regions of DNA that are not expressed, or they occur in coding regions of DNA but have no effect on protein activity.

Loss-of-function mutations

Loss-of-function mutations tend to occur in coding sequences. Therefore this type of mutation leads to reduction or absence of a protein's activity.

These mutations are usually recessive, so the individual organism must be homozygous (carry two mutated genes, one on each chromosome pair) for the effect to be expressed. The presence of an unmutated (wild type) protein expressed in a heterozygote (an individual organism with one mutated and one unmutated gene) compensates for the mutated protein.

For example, the disorder cystic fibrosis is caused by a loss of function mutation in the gene encoding for the protein cystic fibrosis transmembrane conductance receptor (CFTR). Loss of CFTR function causes abnormally thick mucus secretions which block the lungs and pancreatic ducts; leading to frequent lung infections and malabsorption.

Gain-of-function mutations

Gain-of-function mutations are rarer than loss-of-function mutations and tend to occur in regulatory sequences. If this type of mutation affects proteins controlling cell division, it often leads to uncontrolled cell proliferation and cancer.

Gain-of-function mutations tend to be dominant. Therefore only one mutated gene is required.

For example, the disorder hereditary pancreatitis is caused by gain of function mutations in the gene encoding the protein cationic trypsinogen. Trypsinogen is secreted by the pancreas and cleaved to produce trypsin, (a digestive enzyme) which is degraded when no longer required. In hereditary pancreatitis mutations prevent trypsin degradation, and the resulting elevated trypsin levels damage the pancreatic tissue causing inflammation.

A genetic disease may not always be expressed clinically (i.e. phenotypically) in everyone who has it. Therefore mutations in some people with the disease are not always clinically evident.

Variation in clinical expression is referred to as the penetrance of a disease in a population. Disease penetrance may depend, for example, on the presence or absence of compensatory pathways or proteins that not all people have.

Answers to starter questions

1. The sequence of nucleotides in DNA is considered the 'blueprint' for life. It encodes all the proteins involved in cell development and function. Each cell contains all the information required for all the cells of an organism to develop, specialise and function. In multicellular organisms this includes signalling molecules and receptors that control cell division and the coordinated organisation of cells into specialised cells, functioning tissues and organs during development.

2. Cells replicate their entire genome prior to cell division, so that it is inherited by both daughter cells. In germ cells, this division occurs to create the haploid gametes: spermatazoa and oocytes (eggs). Two gametes combine in fertilisation to form the diploid zygote, with DNA inherited from both parent germ cells. This new combination of genetic material retains its genome in all its subsequent daughter cells created in divisions as development occurs.

3. The evolution of a species is caused essentially by germ cell mutations, i.e. those that occur in DNA replication during gametogenesis, the formation of spermtazoa and oocytes. Mutations that confer an advantage over the unmutated form lead to more individuals with the mutation surviving to pass it on to subsequent generations. Over time, the mutation becomes prevalent within the population. The mutations might be a single base pair change, or a large rearrangement of a chromosome.

4. In one sense aging is the accumulation of mutations in cells due to errors in DNA replication and mutagenic agents such as free radicals and UV radiation, and the accumulation of damage to the (mostly protein) infrastructure of tissues and organs, such as degeneration of the cornea causing cataracts, or of arteries promoting loss of elasticity and atheroma formation. But implicit in this is the decline in the ability of the body to repair damage in DNA and proteins and regenerate cells, which may be more genetically determined. For example, every time a cell divides and replicates its DNA, some nucleotide sequences are lost from the ends of the DNA molecules causing it to gradually shorten. To prevent the loss of coding DNA all cells have large sequences of non-coding nucleotides here called telomeres, a buffer protecting the valuable coding regions. Telomeres get shorter with each cell division, until they eventually reach a critical length and the cell stops dividing. This cessation of cell division is one of the reasons we age.

5. The phosphodiester bonds in nucleic acids have a negative charge. This makes both RNA and DNA relatively resistant to breakdown by hydrolysis because the negative hydroxide ions required for hydrolysis are repelled by the negative charge. However, DNA is more stable then RNA due to the absence of the hydroxyl group on ribose. This greater stability is probably why DNA evolved as the hereditary material.

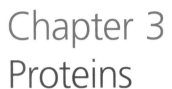
Chapter 3
Proteins

Starter questions

Answers to the following questions are on page 92.

1. Do changes in a gene's DNA sequence always lead to changes in protein function?
2. What determines the shape of a protein?
3. How do changes in protein structure lead to disease?
4. What stops water from leaking out of blood vessels?
5. Why is monosodium glutamate used as a food additive?

Introduction

Proteins are the most versatile compounds in living organisms. They are involved in virtually all cellular processes, and every cell contains thousands of different proteins, each with a specific function.

The proteome is the total amount of functioning protein in a cell. It changes constantly, according to cellular protein requirements. Therefore the proteome is a balance between the synthesis of new proteins and the degradation of proteins no longer required.

All proteins are polymers of small nitrogen-containing molecules called amino acids. Therefore an adequate cellular supply of amino acids is vital for protein synthesis and cellular function. Some amino acids can be synthesised de novo. Others, the essential amino acids, must be obtained from food.

Case 2 Seizure and lethargy in a baby

Presentation

A 5-day-old boy, Charlie Stillman, is admitted to the neonatal intensive care unit after having a seizure. He is lethargic, and his mother says that he has been increasingly irritable since birth and is reluctant to feed.

Initial laboratory tests show a marked increase in plasma ammonia concentration (hyperammonaemia), as well as respiratory alkalosis (increased blood pH). Due to the raised ammonia, a urea cycle disorder is suspected. The results of further investigations show increased plasma glutamine and alanine, as well as a high concentration of orotic acid in the urine. These findings suffice for ornithine transcarbamylase deficiency to be diagnosed.

Analysis

Ornithine transcarbamylase deficiency is one of several urea cycle disorders. Each of these disorders arises from a deficiency in one of the urea cycle enzymes (**Table 3.1**), which results in hyperammonaemia.

Urea cycle disorders present at any age, depending on the severity of the enzyme deficiency. The most acute neonatal presentations usually occur in boys with ornithine transcarbamylase deficiency, because the ornithine transcarbamylase gene is on the X chromosome (i.e. it is X-linked).

Symptoms of urea cycle disorders include:

- lethargy
- irritability
- vomiting
- hepatomegaly
- hypothermia
- delirium
- seizures
- poor feeding
- self-destructive behaviour (in children)

Coma and death occur if the condition is untreated.

Further case

Haemodialysis is started immediately, and sodium benzoate administered. Charlie is placed on a protein-restricted diet for 48 h and given intravenous dextrose. This treatment successfully reduces the level of ammonia in his body, and his condition steadily improves.

Further analysis

Hyperammonaemia is extremely toxic to brain cells. Therefore the aim of treat-

Urea cycle disorders		
Enzyme	Disorder	Mode of inheritance
N-acetyl glutamate synthetase	N-acetyl glutamate synthetase deficiency	Autosomal recessive
Carbamoyl-phosphate synthetase	Carbamoyl-phosphate synthetase I deficiency	Autosomal recessive
Ornithine transcarbamylase	Ornithine transcarbamylase deficiency	X-linked
Argininosuccinate synthase	Citrullinaemia	Autosomal recessive
Argininosuccinate lyase	Argininosuccinic aciduria (argininosuccinate lyase deficiency)	Autosomal recessive
Arginase	Arginase deficiency	Autosomal recessive

Table 3.1 Disorders of the urea cycle

Case 2 *continued*

Urea cycle defects: presentation, investigation and treatment

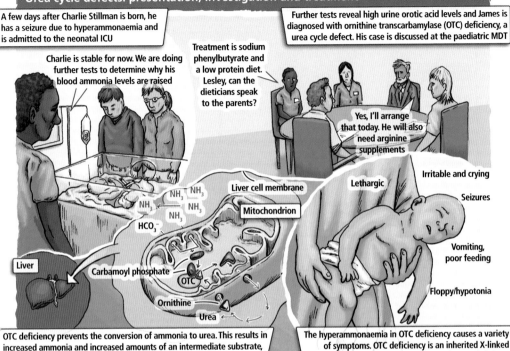

A few days after Charlie Stillman is born, he has a seizure due to hyperammonaemia and is admitted to the neonatal ICU

Further tests reveal high urine orotic acid levels and James is diagnosed with ornithine transcarbamylase (OTC) deficiency, a urea cycle defect. His case is discussed at the paediatric MDT

Charlie is stable for now. We are doing further tests to determine why his blood ammonia levels are raised

Treatment is sodium phenylbutyrate and a low protein diet. Lesley, can the dieticians speak to the parents?

Yes, I'll arrange that today. He will also need arginine supplements

Liver cell membrane

Mitochondrion

NH_3 NH_3 NH_3 NH_3 NH_3

HCO_3^-

Liver

Carbamoyl phosphate

OTC

Ornithine

Urea

Irritable and crying

Lethargic

Seizures

Vomiting, poor feeding

Floppy/hypotonia

OTC deficiency prevents the conversion of ammonia to urea. This results in increased ammonia and increased amounts of an intermediate substrate, ornithine, which is excreted in the urine as orotic acid

The hyperammonaemia in OTC deficiency causes a variety of symptoms. OTC deficiency is an inherited X-linked disorder and it classically presents acutely in male infants

ment is to reduce the ammonia and thus prevent neurological damage. Immediate treatment involves:

- stopping protein intake to prevent ammonia production
- removal of ammonia by haemodialysis and ammonia-scavenging drugs

Protein restriction should not exceed 48 h, otherwise the body will begin to break down endogenous proteins which will generate ammonia. Ammonia-scavenging drugs include sodium benzoate and phenyl acetate, as well as the latter's precursor drug, phenyl butyrate (**Figure 3.1**).

Long-term management includes use of a low-protein diet and an ammonia-

scavenging drug. Arginine is synthesised by the urea cycle, so patients with urea cycle disorders are usually arginine-deficient and require supplementation.

Carbamoyl phosphate is an intermediate in both the urea cycle in mitochondria and pyrimidine synthesis in the cytosol (see page 51). In ornithine transcarbamylase deficiency, excess carbamoyl phosphate enters the cytosol and stimulates pyrimidine synthesis, thus increasing orotic acid in the blood and urine.

Case 2 *continued*

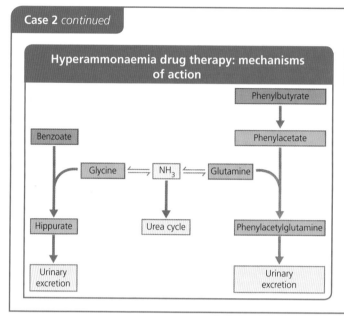

Figure 3.1 Mechanisms of action of drugs used to treat hyperammonaemia.

Amino acids

Amino acids are vital for life, not least because they function as building blocks for proteins. They also serve as precursors for other important compounds, such as nucleotides, porphyrins, neurotransmitters and hormones (**Table 3.2**).

The amino acids are a large and diverse group of molecules that contain:

- an amino group ($-NH_2$)
- a carboxyl group ($-COOH$)
- an organic side chain that is unique to each amino acid

Most of the biologically important amino acids are α-amino acids. In this type of amino acid, the amino group is attached to the α carbon (the carbon attached to the carboxyl group). Other types of amino acids are present in humans, for example the neurotransmitter γ-aminobutyric acid is a γ-amino acid, in which the amino group is attached to the γ carbon atom.

Amino acid precursors of biologically important compounds

Amino acid	Compound
Tryptophan	Serotonin
	Nicotinamide adenine dinucleotide and nicotinamide adenine dinucleotide phosphate
Tyrosine	Dopamine
	Adrenaline (epinephrine) and noradrenaline (norepinephrine)
	Melanin
	Thyroxine
Arginine	Nitric oxide
Histidine	Histamine
Serine	Choline
Glycine	Porphyrins
	Creatine
	Glutathione
	Bile salts
	Purines
Glutamate	γ-Aminobutyric acid

Table 3.2 Amino acid precursors of various physiologically important compounds

- the carboxyl group is deprotonated and has a negative charge

Therefore its overall net charge is zero.

R group side chains

The same 20 α-amino acids are present in the proteins of all organisms. They are classified by the chemical properties of their side chains (**Figure 3.3**) which differ in:

- size
- shape
- charge
- hydrophobicity
- chemical reactivity

This variation confers these amino acids, and the proteins they form, with different chemical properties.

With the exception of glycine all of the α-amino acids are chiral (exist in two different arrangements which are mirror images of each other). Only the L isomers are found in proteins.

Non-polar side chains: aliphatic

Amino acids with carbon and hydrogen (i.e. aliphatic) side chains are non-polar: glycine, alanine, valine, leucine and isoleucine (**Figure 3.3a**). Their non-polarity makes them hydrophobic; the longer the aliphatic chain, the more hydrophobic the amino acid.

> **Creatine is a nitrogenous compound synthesised from the amino acids arginine, glycine and methionine.** It is present in tissues with a high-energy requirement, such as the brain and skeletal muscle. In such tissues, creatine is phosphorylated by creatine kinase and acts as a store of phosphate for the generation of ATP.

Amino acid structure

The α-amino acids share a common basic structure (see **Figure 1.19**). They comprise a central α carbon atom, which is linked to an amino group, a carboxyl group, a hydrogen atom and a unique side chain (the R group).

Ionisation state

With both an amino group and a carboxyl group, amino acids can be either positively or negatively charged. Their ionisation state depends on the pH and whether or not the amino and carboxyl groups are protonated (have a hydrogen attached) (**Figure 3.2**).

At about neutral pH, amino acids exist predominantly as zwitterions. In a zwitterion:

- the amino group is protonated and has a positive charge

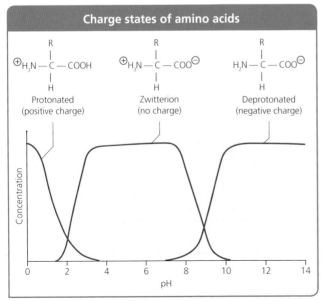

Figure 3.2 Different charge states of amino acids.

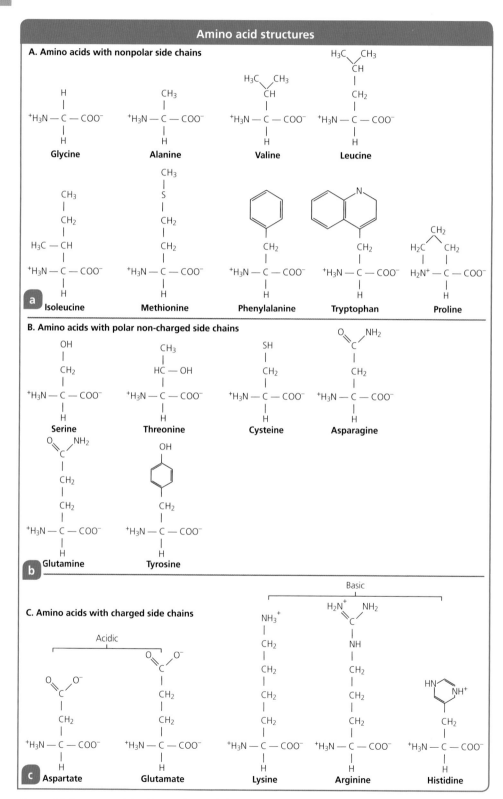

Figure 3.3 Structures of the 20 α-amino acids found in proteins. (a) Amino acids with non-polar side chains. (b) Amino acids with polar non-charged side chains. (c) Amino acids with charged side chains.

Non-polar side chains: aromatic

Other non-polar hydrophobic amino acids are the aromatic amino acids (phenylalanine and tryptophan) (**Figure 3.3a**). Aromatic amino acids have side chains containing an aromatic ring. This feature is a ring of carbon atoms stabilised by π bonds (covalent bonds formed by the sharing of electrons among all the carbons).

Hydrophobic amino acids influence the tertiary structure of proteins. This is because their hydrophobicity causes them to pack together in the centre of the protein to be shielded from water.

The amino acid proline contains an essentially cyclic aliphatic side chain and is also hydrophobic. The cyclic structure of the side chain is rigid compared with the other side chains. This makes proline less flexible than the other amino acids, and this property influences protein folding.

Polar non-charged side chains

The polar side chains are more hydrophilic than the non-polar side chains, and they contain hydroxyl (-OH), sulphur or amide ($CONH_2$) groups (**Figure 3.3b**). The amino acids with polar side chains are serine, threonine, cysteine, asparagine, glutamine and the aromatic amino acid tyrosine.

The thiol (-SH) groups of two cysteine molecules can oxidise to form disulphide bonds (**Figure 3.4**). These bonds stabilise protein structure.

Charged side chains

Three amino acids (lysine, arginine and histidine) contain positively charged side chains at neutral pH (**Figure 3.3c**). These amino acids are termed the basic amino acids, because they readily accept protons.

Conversely, the amino acids aspartate and glutamate contain negatively charged side chains at neutral pH. They are called the acidic amino acids, because they readily donate protons.

Both the basic and the acidic amino acids are very hydrophilic. Therefore they are often found on the external surfaces of proteins in contact with water.

The charged amino acids, along with tyrosine and cysteine, are readily ionised. They have an essential role in stabilising protein structure by forming ionic bonds.

Charged amino acids are also often present in the active site of enzymes (see page 21). Here, they promote biochemical reactions through the donation or acceptance of protons.

Other amino acids

As well as the 20 α-amino acids found in proteins, several other amino acids also have functional roles in nature. For example, some D isomers (e.g. D-alanine) are found in polypeptides in bacterial cell walls, and carnitine is used to transport fatty acids.

Additional amino acids are produced through chemical modification of one of the 20 α-amino acids after incorporation into proteins. For example, proline can be hydroxylated to hydroxyproline, which is a major component of the protein collagen. Other amino acids are intermediates in the synthesis or catabolism of the 20 α-amino acids, for example homocysteine.

Amino acid synthesis

Many organisms are able to make all 20 of the amino acids found in proteins. However, humans can synthesise only 11: the non-essential amino acids (**Table 3.3**).

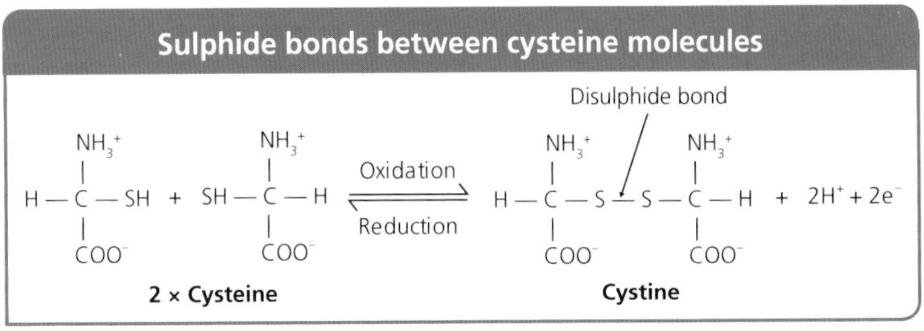

Sulphide bonds between cysteine molecules

Figure 3.4 Formation of sulphide bonds between two cysteine molecules.

α-Amino acids	
Non-essential	Essential
Alanine	Histidine
Arginine	Isoleucine
Asparagine	Leucine
Aspartate	Lysine
Cysteine	Methionine
Glutamate	Phenylalanine
Glutamine	Threonine
Glycine	Tryptophan
Proline	Valine
Serine	
Tyrosine	

Table 3.3 The essential and non-essential amino acids found in proteins

The nine essential amino acids cannot be synthesised by humans, because they lack the necessary enzymes. Instead, these amino acids must be obtained from the diet.

Arginine is also an essential amino acid in children, because the rate of its synthesis is too low to meet the requirements of growth.

The synthetic pathways for the non-essential amino acids are simple, with only a few steps. The process involves the addition of an amino group onto the carbon backbone. Intermediates in the glycolytic pathway, the citric acid cycle or the pentose phosphate pathway provide the carbon backbone, and ammonia provides the nitrogen component.

Utilisation of ammonia

Ammonia is the source of nitrogen for all nitrogenous compounds, for example nucleotides and amino acids. Ammonia is synthesised by only certain organisms, using one of two pathways:

- the reduction of atmospheric nitrogen gas (N_2) to ammonia (nitrogen fixation) in some species of bacteria
- the reduction of soil nitrate (NO_3^-) to ammonia in most plants, fungi and bacteria

Ammonia intake

Because ammonia cannot be synthesised by humans, it must be obtained from the breakdown of proteins and amino acids in their food. Once acquired, the first step in ammonia utilisation is the generation of either carbamoyl phosphate or the amino acids glutamate and glutamine. These three compounds are then used to synthesise all other nitrogen-containing compounds (**Figure 3.5**). Glutamate is the central compound used in the generation of the other amino acids.

Cachexia is the muscle wastage seen in malnourished patents. Muscle is broken down to obtain the nitrogen needed to synthesise more essential compounds, because unlike lipids and carbohydrates, the body has no mechanism for storing excess nitrogen.

Ammonia excretion

About 80% of the excess nitrogen in humans is excreted in the urine as urea (see page 89). The rest is excreted in the urine as uric acid (see page 54), creatinine or free ammonium ions.

Creatinine is produced from free creatine or phosphocreatine in muscle and is excreted in the urine. Measurement of the renal clearance of creatinine (creatinine

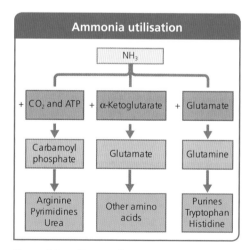

Figure 3.5 Utilisation of ammonia.

clearance) is a useful indicator of glomerular filtration rate.

Transamination

Transamination is the transfer of an amino group from one compound to another. This reaction has an essential role in amino acid synthesis. It is catalysed by aminotransferase enzymes, which require a vitamin B_6 derivative, pyridoxal phosphate, as a cofactor.

In amino acid synthesis, the amino group is transferred from glutamate to an α-ketoacid (a compound containing a carboxylic acid group and an adjacent ketone group). The ketoacids provide the carbon backbone of the resulting amino acid.

Generating glutamate from ammonia also involves a transamination reaction, in which ammonia is added to α-ketoglutarate, a ketoacid intermediate in the citric acid cycle. Three common α-ketoacids can be directly transaminated to their respective amino acids (**Figure 3.6**).

> **The enzymes alanine aminotransferase and aspartate aminotransferase have a key role in the assessment of liver disease.** Hepatocellular damage causes these aminotransferases to leak into the bloodstream. Therefore their increased concentration in the blood indicates damage to hepatocytes.

Synthesis of non-essential amino acids

All 11 non–essential amino acids are synthesised either from direct transamination of their respective α-ketoacids or from other amino acids (**Figure 3.7**).

Glutamate, glutamine, arginine and proline

Glutamate is synthesised directly from α-ketoglutarate and ammonia by glutamate dehydrogenase, an aminotransferase. This amino acid is the precursor for three other non-essential amino acids: glutamine, arginine and proline. Glutamine is synthesised by the addition of ammonia to glutamate by the enzyme glutamine synthetase, and arginine is synthesised from glutamate and carbamoyl phosphate in the urea cycle.

The conversion of glutamate to proline is slightly more complex, involving three enzymes and formation of the cyclic side chain.

Aspartate and asparagine

Aspartate is generated directly by the transamination of its ketoacid, oxaloacetate, an intermediate in the citric acid cycle. This amino acid is converted to asparagine by addition of ammonia.

Serine, glycine and cysteine

Serine is synthesised from 3-phosphoglycerate, an intermediate in the glycolytic pathway,

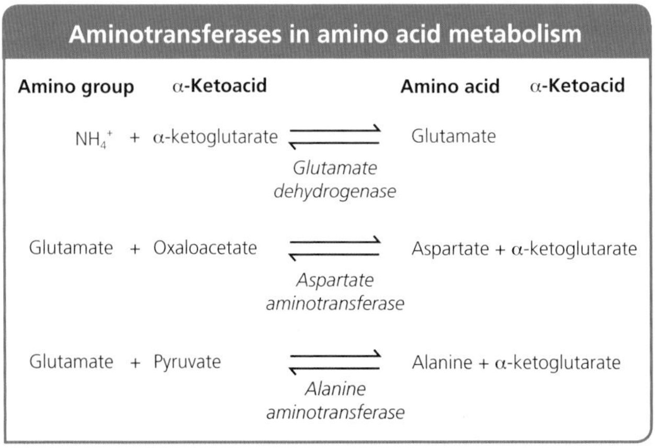

Aminotransferases in amino acid metabolism

Amino group	α-Ketoacid		Amino acid	α-Ketoacid
NH_4^+ + α-ketoglutarate		⇌ *Glutamate dehydrogenase*	Glutamate	
Glutamate + Oxaloacetate		⇌ *Aspartate aminotransferase*	Aspartate + α-ketoglutarate	
Glutamate + Pyruvate		⇌ *Alanine aminotransferase*	Alanine + α-ketoglutarate	

Figure 3.6 Common aminotransferases in amino acid metabolism.

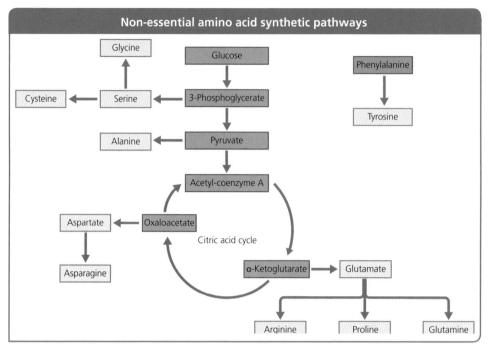

Figure 3.7 Synthetic pathways of the non-essential amino acids.

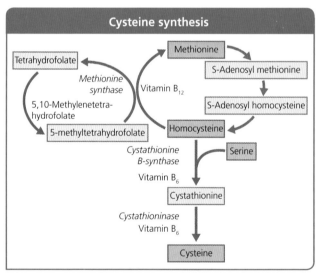

Figure 3.8 Cysteine synthesis. MTHFR, methylenetetrahydrofolate reductase.

through a transamination reaction. It is converted to glycine by the enzyme serine hydroxymethyltransferase. This reaction also requires tetrahydrofolate, which acts as a carrier of one-carbon groups.

Serine is also a precursor for the sulphur-containing amino acid cysteine. The sulphur group is provided by the essential amino acid methionine, which is first converted to homocysteine (**Figure 3.8**).

Homocystinuria is an inherited disorder caused by defects in the synthetic pathway for cysteine. It is characterised by an increased concentration of homocysteine in the blood and urine. Symptoms include a tall and thin build, lens dislocation in the eye, intellectual disability and vascular disease.

Alanine

Alanine is synthesised from pyruvate through a transamination reaction.

Tyrosine

Synthesis of tyrosine differs from that of the other non-essential amino acids, in that it is derived directly from an essential amino acid, phenylalanine. Therefore tyrosine also becomes an essential amino acid if phenylalanine is scarce.

Regulation of amino acid synthesis

The rate of amino acid synthesis depends on both the amount and the activity of the required enzymes. Enzyme activity is controlled by negative feedback. The amino acids act as allosteric inhibitors (see page 25) for their biosynthetic enzymes, so their synthesis is inhibited when there is a sufficient supply.

Cells require adequate amounts of all 20 α-amino acids for protein synthesis to occur.

Protein synthesis

Proteins are synthesised from a messenger ribonucleic acid (mRNA) template molecule through translation. Translation involves the stepwise addition of amino acids to linear polypeptide chains.

The final functional protein comprises one or more polypeptide chains linked by covalent interactions. Small singular polypeptide chains, containing up to about 70 amino acids, are called peptides.

Ribosomes

Translation occurs on ribosomes (see page 5) in the cytoplasm of the cell. Therefore in eukaryotic cells (cells with a nucleus) mRNA must be transported from the nucleus to the cytoplasm before translation begins.

Ribosomes coordinate and catalyse the polymerisation of amino acids to form polypeptide chains. Newly synthesised polypeptide chains then undergo post-translational modification (chemical modification, folding and cleavage) to produce the final functional protein (**Figure 3.9**).

Each cell contains tens of thousands of ribosomes, and each mRNA molecule is translated by more than one ribosome at a time. Thus multiple polypeptide chains are synthesised from one mRNA molecule.

Translation continues until the mRNA is degraded. The processes regulating the half-life of mRNA are poorly understood. However, degradation is triggered by removal of the poly(A) tail, a long repeat sequence of adenosine monophosphates.

Not all peptides are translated from mRNA. One example is glutathione, a tripeptide derived from the amino acids glutamate, glycine and cysteine. Its reduced form (γ-glutamylcysteinylglycine) is the most abundant peptide in cells and has a major antioxidant role; it protects the cell from oxidative damage by maintaining proteins in their reduced form and scavenging free radicals.

The genetic code

The sequence of amino acids in a protein is coded by the sequence of nucleotides in the mRNA molecule. The mRNA is a transcript of the DNA and therefore reflects the nucleotide sequence of the gene for that protein.

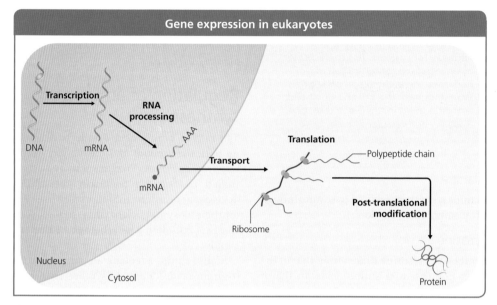

Figure 3.9 Gene expression in eukaryotic cells. DNA, deoxyribonucleic acid; mRNA, messenger ribonucleic acid; RNA, ribonucleic acid.

Each amino acid is encoded by a triplicate sequence of nucleotides called a codon. There are 64 possible codons, and most amino acids are encoded by more than one codon (**Table 3.4**). Some codons do not encode for amino acids but are used to signal the initiation or cessation of translation. They are the start and stop codons, respectively.

Transfer RNA

Transfer ribonucleic acids (tRNAs) are the pivotal link between the codons in a mRNA molecule and the amino acids they encode. These RNA strands, comprising 70–100 nucleotides, bring amino acids to the ribosomal translation machinery.

Structure of transfer RNA

Cells contain up to 50 types of tRNA. What these different transfer RNAs have in common is the same cloverleaf structure (**Figure 3.10**) and certain conserved nucleotide sequences required for the structure and function of tRNA.

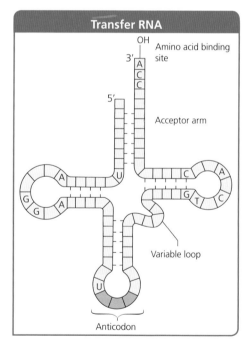

Figure 3.10 Secondary structure of transfer ribonucleic acid. Each square represents a codon. The CCA sequence at the 3' end is universal and is present in prokaryotic as well as eukaryotic tRNAs. The most highly-conserved bases in the arms and loops of the molecule are shown here.

The genetic code				
First position	Second position			Third position
	U	C	A	G
U	Phenylalanine	Serine	Tyrosine	Cysteine	U
	Phenylalanine	Serine	Tyrosine	Cysteine	C
	Leucine	Serine	Stop	Stop	A
	Leucine	Serine	Stop	Tryptophan	G
C	Leucine	Proline	Histidine	Arginine	U
	Leucine	Proline	Histidine	Arginine	C
	Leucine	Proline	Glutamine	Arginine	A
	Leucine	Proline	Glutamine	Arginine	G
A	Isoleucine	Threonine	Asparagine	Serine	U
	Isoleucine	Threonine	Asparagine	Serine	C
	Isoleucine	Threonine	Lysine	Arginine	A
	Methionine or start	Threonine	Lysine	Arginine	G
G	Valine	Alanine	Aspartate	Glycine	U
	Valine	Alanine	Aspartate	Glycine	C
	Valine	Alanine	Glutamate	Glycine	A
	Valine	Alanine	Glutamate	Glycine	G

A, adenine; C, cytosine; G, guanine; U, uracil.

Table 3.4 Codons and their respective amino acids

Each tRNA molecule contains an anticodon, a nucleotide sequence that is complementary to a specific mRNA codon. These complementary sequences enable tRNA to bind to mRNA by creating base pairs between codon and anticodon through the formation of hydrogen bonds (see page 58).

Binding of amino acids

Each tRNA binds to a specific amino acid to form an aminoacyl-tRNA. Binding occurs between the 3' terminal hydroxyl group of the tRNA and the carboxyl group of the amino acid. These reactions are catalysed by aminoacyl-tRNA synthetases.

For the genetic code to be preserved, each amino acid must be attached only to the tRNA containing its corresponding anticodon sequence. This is ensured by specificity of the aminoacyl-tRNA synthetase enzymes. Each of the 20 α-amino acids has its own aminoacyl-tRNA synthetase enzyme, which recognises only the correct tRNAs.

Translation

Translation occurs in three phases: initiation, elongation and termination (**Figure 3.11**). The site of translation is different for different types of protein.

■ Translation of secretory or membrane proteins occurs on ribosomes attached to the endoplasmic reticulum, which facilitates post-translational processing of the protein and targeting the protein for secretion via the Golgi apparatus (see page 5)
■ Translation of cytoplasmic proteins occurs on ribosomes free in the cytoplasm

Ribosomes consist of two subunits, large and small, which contain ribosomal ribonucleic acid and the numerous proteins required for

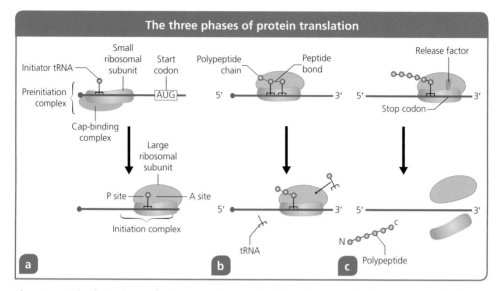

Figure 3.11 The three phases of protein translation. (a) Initiation. (b) Elongation. (c) Termination. A site, aminoacyl site; P site, peptidyl site; tRNA, transfer ribonucleic acid.

each phase of translation. These proteins are known as initiation factors, elongation factors and release factors.

When a ribosome is not actively participating in translation, its two subunits dissociate.

Initiation of translation

Translation is initiated as follows.

1. The small ribosomal subunit binds to an initiator tRNA to form the preinitiation complex
2. Initiation factors bind to the 5' cap of the mRNA to form the cap-binding complex
3. The preinitiation complex attaches to the mRNA by associating with the cap-binding complex; it then scans along the mRNA molecule until it reaches the start codon, which binds to the initiator tRNA
4. The large ribosomal subunit then attaches to form the initiation complex; the subunit contains two sites for tRNA binding: the peptidyl (P) site and the aminoacyl (A) site (in the initiation complex, the initiator tRNA occupies the P site and the next codon aligns with the A site)

The synthesis of some proteins is regulated by controlling their translation. For example, the mRNA for ferritin (an iron storage protein) contains sequences called iron response elements upstream of the translation start codon.

- In the absence of iron, proteins bind to iron responses elements to block the ribosome and thus inhibit ferritin synthesis
- In the presence of iron, the proteins dissociate from the mRNA to permit translation

Elongation of the polypeptide chain

Elongation begins when the correct aminoacyl-tRNA enters the A site. Peptidyltransferase then forms a peptide bond between the amino acid in the P site and the amino acid in the A site, and in so doing releases the former from its tRNA.

The ribosome moves along the mRNA molecule so that the next codon aligns with the A site. At the same time, the tRNA in the A site moves to the P site with the attached polypeptide chain, and the tRNA in the P site is released.

The next aminoacyl-tRNA enters the A site, and the process is repeated. Elongation continues until a stop codon is reached and translation is terminated.

Termination of translation

When the ribosome reaches a stop codon on the mRNA (a nucleotide triplet signalling to the ribosome to cease translation), a release factor enters the A site. The release factor prevents further elongation of the polypeptide chain, by preventing entry of aminoacyl-tRNA into the A site and releasing the polypeptide from the tRNA in the P site. The ribosomal subunits then dissociate and remain in the cytosol until required for another cycle of translation.

Post-translational modification

Newly translated polypeptide chains are inactive and must be processed to form the final functional protein. Three types of post-translational modification occur:

- Proteolytic cleavage
- Chemical modification
- Protein folding

In proteolytic cleavage, protease enzymes remove small fragments from one or both endsof the polypeptide molecule to produce a shortened active protein. This mechanism is often used to activate enzymes and peptide hormones. Alternatively, the polypeptide may be cleaved into two or more active proteins.

In chemical modification, the amino acid side chains of the polypeptide are chemically

altered by the addition of different compounds (**Table 3.5**).

All newly synthesised polypeptide chains must be folded to create their correct three-dimensional structure. Protein folding is facilitated by specific proteins called chaperones, which bind to hydrophobic regions and prevent protein aggregation.

> Heat shock proteins are a group of chaperones whose expression is induced when cells are exposed to high temperatures or other stress conditions, such as hypoxia or exposure to toxins. They help in the refolding of denatured proteins, thus protecting the cell from damage.

Post-translational chemical modifications	
Type	Amino acids (and terminals) modified
Addition of small chemical groups	
Acetylation	Lysine and N-terminal
Methylation	Lysine and arginine
Phosphorylation	Serine, threonine, tyrosine and histidine
Hydroxylation	Proline and lysine
Addition of sugar residues	
O-linked glycosylation	Serine and threonine
N-linked glycosylation	Asparagine
Addition of lipids	Cysteine, N-terminal and C-terminal

Table 3.5 Common chemical modifications to proteins

Protein structure and function

The sequence of amino acids in a polypeptide chain, i.e. its primary structure, determines how it folds into its final three-dimensional structure, which in turn governs its biological role.

Some proteins have several different isoforms (subtypes). Protein isoforms are expressed from different genes, or expressed from the same gene but the mRNA undergoes different splicing. They have a different primary sequence but their overall tertiary or quaternary structure is similar and they carry out the same biological function.

The three primary roles of proteins are:

- structural
- binding
- catalytic

The two major classes are fibrous and globular proteins.

> Prions are infectious protein molecules that are able to disrupt the three-dimensional structure of other proteins and induce them to fold abnormally. They usually affect proteins in the brain, producing protein aggregates that damage neuronal cells. Prions cause various progressive neurodegenerative disorders, such as Creutzfeldt–Jakob disease.

Peptide bonds

Amino acids are linked in polypeptide chains by peptide bonds (see page 35), so the amino group of one amino acid molecule interacts with the carboxyl group of the next. Therefore the two ends of a polypeptide chain differ.

- One end (the N terminal) has a free amino group
- The other end (the C terminal) has a free carboxyl group

All polypeptides have a backbone of peptide bonds, nitrogen and carbon. Structural and functional variability is provided by the amino acid side chains, which are free to interact either with each other or with other compounds to form the final three-dimensional structure of the protein.

Protein three-dimensional structure

The three-dimensional structures of proteins (see page 35) are described as:

- secondary (local folding)
- tertiary (overall folding)
- quaternary (for combinations of multiple polypeptide chains)

These structures are maintained by non-covalent interactions involving both the backbone of the polypeptide chain and the amino acid side chains. These include hydrogen bonds, van der Waals' forces, ionic bonds and hydrophobic interactions (see page 27).

Protein structure may be further stabilised, more often in extracellular proteins, by covalent bonds such as disulphide bonds (see page 27).

Secondary structure

The secondary structure of a protein is the localised folding which occurs within regions of the polypeptide chain. It is governed by the flexibility of the polypeptide backbone. Rotation of the peptide bond is possible around the α-carbon only, which limits folding of the polypeptide chain.

This creates regular or periodic secondary structures, in which the spatial relationship between amino acids is the same and is governed by the angles of rotation around the α-carbon. The two most common secondary structures are α helices and β sheets (see page 35).

Secondary structures are stabilised by hydrogen bonds between atoms in the polypeptide backbone. The amino acid side chains have no role in bonding, but they influence secondary structure by governing how closely the amino acids pack together. Proline is often found in β turns (180° changes in direction), because this amino acid is relatively inflexible.

Tertiary structure

Tertiary structure is the overall folding of the whole polypeptide chain, and is determined by amino acid sequence and the local environment. It is controlled primarily by interactions between amino acid side chains. However, hydrophilic or hydrophobic conditions also affect tertiary structure by determining which amino acid side chains are exposed on the protein's surface.

Once folded, many proteins contain multiple domains (parts of the protein with a discrete structure and function). For example, membrane-bound receptors contain membrane-binding domains, intracellular domains and ligand-binding domains.

Quaternary structure

Quaternary structure is how multiple polypeptide chains (subunits) bond together within a protein. Multi-subunit proteins often contain two to six polypeptide chains of the same or different types. The polypeptide chains are held together by non-covalent interactions between the amino acid side chains on adjacent chains.

Fibrous proteins

Fibrous proteins have an elongated, filamentous structure. They usually have a structural role in cells and tissues, and are commonly found in connective tissue, muscle tissue and hair. These proteins also make up the cytoskeleton. They confer tensile strength or elasticity to tissues, essentially holding cells and tissues together (**Table 3.6**).

Fibrous proteins typically:

- have an α-helical secondary structure
- have little or no tertiary structure
- are insoluble
- contain multiple subunits that align to form fibrous structures

Collagen is the most abundant of the fibrous proteins. It is the main structural component of the extracellular matrix, the scaffolding between cells.

The formation of collagen releases by-products that are useful markers of collagen production. For example, increased procollagen type 1 N-terminal peptide indicates increased bone formation.

Globular proteins

Globular proteins are more numerous than fibrous proteins, and are involved in all chemical cellular processes, including transport, synthesis and catabolism, most often as enzymes (see page 20). Every globular protein has a specific compact tertiary structure necessary for its biological role. The tertiary structure creates domains that permit specific binding of a wide range of molecules and elements.

Plasma proteins

Plasma contains hundreds of soluble globular proteins. These are broadly classified as follows.

- Immunoglobulins: produced by the immune system and involved in the immune response

Fibrous proteins	
Protein	Function
Extracellular matrix components	
Collagen	Structural: tissue architecture and strength
Elastin	Provides elasticity
Fibrillin	Gives stability to elastic fibres
Fibronectin	Cell adhesion, cell migration, cell structure and linkage of other components of the extracellular matrix
Laminins	Basement membrane component: anchors cells and other extracellular matrix molecules
Proteoglycans	Give structural support to tissues, protect against compressive forces, provide hydration and used in cell signalling
Cytoskeletal components	
Actin, keratin, myosin, desmin, neurofilaments, lamins and tubulin	Provide cell structure and shape, and used in intracellular transport, movement and cell division

Table 3.6 Common fibrous proteins

- Transport proteins: synthesised primarily by the liver and transport many different types of molecule
- Other globular proteins: these include fibrinogen and other coagulation factors, enzymes, enzyme inhibitors and peptide hormones

Albumin is the most abundant plasma protein. It has a number of important functions.

- It maintains blood oncotic pressure
- It binds and transports drugs, thus determining the amount of free active drug available
- It binds and transports steroid hormones, fatty acids, unconjugated bilirubin and cations such as calcium and hydrogen

The major plasma proteins are often classified as α-, β- and γ-globulins, according to their size and charge. The classification is based on the different regions of protein migration during electrophoresis, a method of separating proteins in an electric field.

Measurement of different plasma proteins is useful in the diagnosis and monitoring of a wide range of disorders (**Table 3.7**). Several disorders are associated with inherited defects in plasma-binding proteins. Other plasma proteins are useful tumour markers.

Acute phase proteins

The most common changes in plasma protein concentration occur as a result of the acute phase response. This response is a non-specific reaction in inflammation caused by infection or tissue injury.

Plasma proteins			
Classification	Protein	Function	Clinical significance
Albumin	Albumin	Maintains plasma oncotic pressure	Low albumin levels cause oedema
		As a general transport protein, for example for fatty acids, steroids, haem, bilirubin, biliverdin, divalent and trivalent cations (e.g. Ca^{2+}), drugs and hormones	
	Transthyretin	General transport protein	Low levels in protein malnutrition
α_1-Globulins	α_1-Antitrypsin	Serine protease inhibitor	Deficiency arising from inherited variants causes emphysema and liver disease
	α_1-Fetoprotein	Fetal albumin analogue	In pregnancy:
			decreased levels associated with fetal trisomy 18 or 21
			Increased levels associated with neural tube defects
			Non-pregnancy: tumour marker
α_2-Globulins	Caeruloplasmin	Copper transport	Inherited deficiency causes Wilson's disease
	Haptoglobin	Binds haemoglobin	Low levels in haemolysis
β-Globulins	Transferrin	Iron transport	High levels in iron deficiency
	C-reactive protein	Activates complement pathway	Sensitive positive acute phase protein
γ-Globulins	Immunoglobulins G, A and M	Immune response	Increased levels in monoclonal gammopathies

Table 3.7 Major plasma proteins and their clinical significance

During the acute phase response, there are characteristic changes in the concentration of several plasma proteins (**Table 3.8**).

- Some of these proteins increase in concentration (positive acute phase proteins)
- Others decrease in concentration (negative acute phase proteins)

Major acute phase proteins	
Positive	Negative
α1-Antitrypsin	Albumin
Caeruloplasmin	Cortisol-binding globulin
C-reactive protein	Retinol-binding protein
Fibrinogen	Transthyretin
Ferritin	Transferrin
Haptoglobin	
Serum amyloid A	

Table 3.8 Major positive (increased plasma concentration) and negative (decreased plasma concentration) acute phase proteins

Protein turnover

All proteins are subject to continuous degradation and synthesis. This protein turnover is required for the maintenance of normal tissue function and structure. It allows replacement of damaged proteins, regulates cellular processes and allows the cell to rapidly adapt to changes in its environment by removing proteins whose function is no longer required.

The rate of turnover varies greatly between proteins and is expressed as the half-life (the time for half of the protein molecules to be degraded).

- Plasma proteins tend to have short half-lives
- The structural proteins of connective tissue are more stable and therefore have longer half-lives

Proteolysis

Most proteins are too large to be filtered by the glomerular membrane in the kidney and excreted in the urine. Therefore the major mechanism for the removal of unwanted proteins is proteolysis, the degradation of proteins into their respective amino acids. Proteolysis is also vital for the utilisation of dietary proteins which cannot be absorbed and utilised by the body until they are broken down into their respective amino acids.

The amino acids released by proteolysis have one of two fates (**Figure 3.12**):

- they contribute to the pool of essential amino acids required for the synthesis of proteins and other nitrogenous compounds
- they are further degraded and used for energy metabolism

Free amino acids in the blood are small enough to be filtered by the kidney; however, most are reabsorbed by the tubular cells. Therefore urine usually contains only trace amounts of protein (20–150 mg/24 h) and amino acids.

Albumin is too large to be filtered by the kidney, so it is not normally excreted in the urine. Microalbuminuria, the detection of small amounts of albumin in the urine, is a sensitive and early indicator of damage to the glomerular membrane and kidney disease.

Proteases

Proteins are degraded by a large group of enzymes called proteases, which catalyse

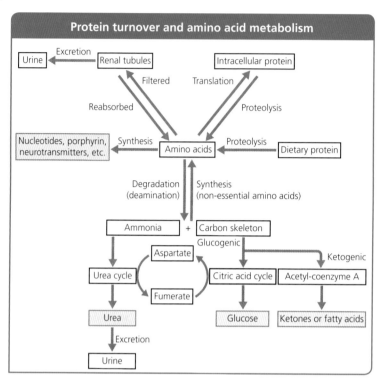

Figure 3.12 Protein turnover and amino acid metabolism.

hydrolysis of the peptide bond. Each protease varies in its substrate specificity.

- Some proteases (endopeptidases) cleave peptide bonds within the protein molecule, often next to specific amino acids only
- Others (exopeptidases) cleave peptide bonds at either the C-terminal (carboxypeptidases) or the N-terminal (aminopeptidases)

There are six groups of proteases, classified by the residue in their active which participates in the hydrolytic reaction (**Table 3.9**).

To regulate their activity, proteases are often activated or inhibited through cleavage by other proteases. An important example is trypsin, a digestive enzyme which is secreted as an inactive protein called trypsinogen. Trypsinogen is cleaved to trypsin by enteropeptidase, a serine protease. Additionally the activity of some proteases is inhibited by protease inhibitors.

Common proteases	
Classification	Example
Serine proteases	Trypsin: selectively cleaves after lysine or arginine
	Chymotrypsin: selectively cleaves after tyrosine, phenylalanine or tryptophan
	Elastase: selectively cleaves after alanine, glycine or valine
	Thrombin
	Plasmin
Threonine proteases	Proteasome subunits
Cysteine proteases	Papain
	Cathepsins
Aspartate proteases	Pepsin
	Renin
Metalloproteinases	Carboxypeptidases
	Matrix metalloproteases (e.g. collagenase)
Glutamic acid proteases	Scytalidoglutamic peptidase (only found in fungi)

Table 3.9 Common proteases grouped by the catalytic residue in their active site

The protease inhibitor α_1-antitrypsin inhibits the activity of elastase. Therefore inherited α_1-antitrypsin deficiency often causes emphysema because of increased elastase activity and the associated reduced amount of elastin in lung tissue.

Cellular proteolysis

Most protein degradation takes place within the cell through one of two mechanisms:

- Degradation in the lysosome of the cell
- Degradation by proteasomes (protease complexes) in the cytoplasm; proteins are targeted to the proteasome by the covalent addition of an ubiquitin peptide (ubiquitination is used by the cell to mark proteins for destruction)

Amino acid degradation

Organisms have no mechanism for storing amino acids, so excess amino acids must be degraded. Essentially, the degradation of amino acids is the reverse of amino acid synthesis. It involves removal of the amino group (deamination) to produce ammonia and a carbon skeleton. The ammonia is removed by the urea cycle, and the carbon skeleton is used to provide a source of energy for the cell.

Deamination

Only a few amino acids are directly deaminated:

- glutamate
- glutamine
- serine
- threonine

Therefore the first step in the degradation of the other amino acids is transfer of the amino group by aminotransferases to generate one of these amino acids. Generally, amino groups are transferred to α-ketoglutarate to generate glutamate. Ammonia is then released from glutamate by glutamate dehydrogenase.

Most of the ammonia generated is converted to urea in the liver through the urea cycle and excreted in the urine. Free ammonia is extremely toxic, because it can diffuse into brain

cells and react with α-ketoglutarate, which then inhibits the citric acid cycle and reduces ATP production. This is why most ammonia is transported to the liver as either glutamine or alanine through the alanine cycle (**Figure 3.13**).

The urea cycle

Urea is generated in liver cells by the urea cycle and results in the excretion of two amino groups for every molecule of urea. One amino group is provided by the ammonium ion, and the other is from aspartate (**Figure 3.14**).

The first step in the urea cycle is the generation of carbamoyl phosphate from ammonia and bicarbonate. This reaction is catalysed by carbamoyl-phosphate synthetase I, which requires N-acetyl glutamate as an activator (see **Figure 3.14**). The synthesis of N-acetyl glutamate by N-acetyl glutamate synthetase is upregulated by arginine, an intermediate in the urea cycle.

Carbamoyl phosphate then reacts with ornithine and aspartate to produce argininosuccinate, which is subsequently cleaved to arginine and fumarate. Fumarate is recycled back to aspartate by the citric acid cycle (see **Figure 3.14**) and arginine is hydrolysed to urea, resulting in the regeneration of ornithine.

A 78-year-old woman is admitted to the emergency department after being found collapsed in her home. On admission, her serum urea and electrolytes results were as follows.

- Sodium: 149 mmol/L (reference range, 133–146 mmol/L)
- Potassium: 5.3 mmol/L (reference range, 3.5–5.3 mmol/L)
- Urea: 22 mmol/L (reference range, 2.5–7.8 mmol/L)
- Creatinine: 173 µmol/L (reference range, 50–130 µmol/L)

The increased serum urea and creatine are consistent with an acute kidney injury caused by dehydration. Dehydration results in poor renal perfusion, leading to reduced glomerular filtration and excretion of waste products.

The increased serum sodium concentration is also consistent with dehydration. This patient needs rapid intravenous fluid replacement therapy with crystalloids.

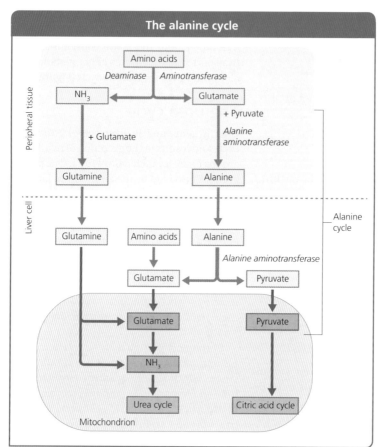

Figure 3.13 The alanine cycle: amino acid degradation and the transport of ammonia to liver cells.

Metabolism of the carbon skeleton

The carbon skeletons of amino acids are converted to one of seven metabolic intermediates:

- pyruvate
- oxaloacetate
- fumarate
- succinyl coenzyme A
- α-ketoglutarate
- acetyl coenzyme A
- acetoacetyl coenzyme A

The amino acids that are degraded to acetyl coenzyme A or acetoacetyl coenzyme A are called ketogenic amino acids, because they are ultimately metabolised to ketones or fatty acids. The amino acids degraded to the other intermediates are called glucogenic amino acids, because they are potentially metabolised

to glucose. Some of the amino acids are degraded to more than one of the seven intermediates, and are both glucogenic and ketogenic (**Table 3.10**).

Disorders of amino acid degradation

Inherited inborn errors of metabolism that disrupt amino acid degradation are broadly classified into two groups:

- those that affect the urea cycle and the removal of ammonia (see **Table 3.1**)
- those that affect the degradation pathways of the carbon skeletons (**Table 3.11**)

The disorders all result from an enzyme deficiency, which usually causes a build-up of upstream toxic intermediates. An important example is phenylketonuria, caused

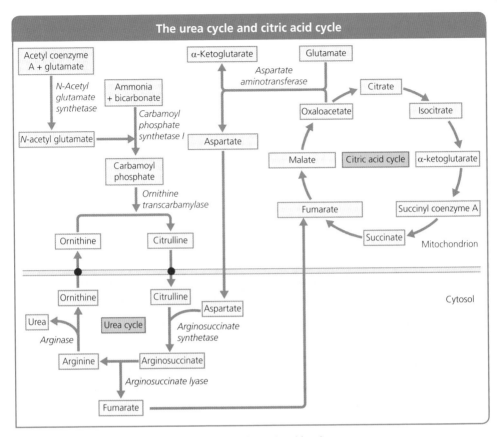

Figure 3.14 The urea cycle and its integration with the citric acid cycle.

Glucogenic, ketogenic and glucogenic-ketogenic amino acids

Glucogenic	Ketogenic	Glucogenic and ketogenic
Arginine	Leucine	Alanine
Asparagine	Lysine	Cysteine
Aspartate	Tryptophan	Glycine
Glutamate		Isoleucine
Glutamine		Phenylalanine
Histidine		Serine
Methionine		Threonine
Proline		Tyrosine
Valine		

Table 3.10 Amino acid degradation and the fate of the carbon skeleton

by deficiency of the enzyme phenylalanine hydroxylase, which converts phenylalanine to tyrosine. Deficiency of phenylalanine hydroxylase causes excess phenylalanine to accumulate which is toxic to neuronal cells.

Disorders in the synthetic pathways and the transport of amino acids also exist. An important example is the disorder cystinuria, caused by a deficiency of the renal transporter for the dibasic amino acids cysteine, orinthine, arginine and lysine (COAL). Deficiency of the transporter prevents reabsorption of these amino acids in the kidney and they are excreted in the urine. Cysteine then precipitates in the urine to form renal stones.

Primary disorders of amino acid degradation		
Disorder	Amino acid pathway affected	Amino acid increased
Phenylketonuria	Phenylalanine	Phenylalanine
Tyrosinaemia	Tyrosine	Tyrosine
Alkaptonuria	Tyrosine	Homogenistic acid
Homocystinuria	Methionine	Homocysteine and methionine
Histidinaemia	Histidine	Histidine
Maple syrup urine disease	Leucine, isoleucine and valine (branched chain amino acids)	Leucine, isoleucine, valine and corresponding ketoacids
Non-ketotic hyperglycinaemia	Glycine	Glycine
Hyperprolinaemia	Proline	Proline

Table 3.11 Inborn errors of amino acid degradation

Answers to starter questions

1. A change in the DNA sequence of a gene will only affect the function of a protein if it: changes the three dimensional shape of the protein or affects the ability of the protein to interact with other compounds. Therefore, the change must occur in a coding region of the gene, alter the genetic code and result in a change in protein structure.

2. The three dimensional shape of a protein is governed by its sequence of amino acids and post-translational modifications. Interactions between the different amino acid side chains, which have different electrochemical and bond-forming properties, determine how the protein chain folds upon itself. Proteins called chaperones also facilitate folding.

3. A change in protein structure can lead to disease by either: preventing proper function of the protein, for example by causing a reduction in binding affinity, a reduction in enzyme activity or an inability to form quaternary structure, or by causing damage to tissues and organs by the accumulation of misfolded protein aggregates within cells and tissues.

4. The plasma protein albumin plays a major role in maintaining the oncotic pressure within blood vessels – the main force that retains water within the vascular compartment. A decrease in blood albumin levels causes a drop in the intravascular oncotic pressure and water moves from the vascular space to the interstitial space causing oedema and the abdominal cavity causing ascites.

5. Monosodium glutamate is the sodium salt of the non-essential amino acid glutamic acid. It improves the overall palatability of a wide range of foods by acting on the taste receptors as glutamate. These receptors confer the taste umami, which, along with sweet, salt, sour, and bitter, is one of the five basic tastes. Umami acts to blend and balance out the other tastes, producing a more rounded pleasant taste.

Chapter 4
Carbohydrates

Starter questions

Answers to the following questions are on page 122.

1. Why is fructose a 'quicker' source of energy than glucose?
2. What is the difference between the D- and L-forms of glucose?
3. Why is the brain solely dependent on glucose for energy?
4. Is muscle burn caused by a build-up of lactic acid?
5. Why are mitochondria considered the powerhouses of cells?
6. Why does cyanide poisoning work so quickly?

Introduction

Carbohydrates are molecules containing carbon, hydrogen and oxygen. As the name implies, they are generally hydrates of carbon, and as in water, they contain hydrogen and oxygen in a ratio of 2:1. They are structurally termed saccharides (Latin: saccharum, 'sugar') and are divided into four chemical groups: mono-, di-, oligo- and polysaccharides.

Although a common source of energy, carbohydrates are not an essential nutrient, because humans are able to obtain 100% of their daily energy requirement from protein and fat. Neither are carbohydrates essential for the synthesis of other molecules. However, they are more readily converted than protein or fat into the key energy monosaccharide: glucose.

When digested, all carbohydrates are broken down to glucose, which is then transported in the blood to cells for energy production. Carbohydrate is one of the main products of photosynthesis in plants, predominantly glucose and is the main fuel for cellular respiration to produce energy, carbon dioxide and water.

Case 3 Collapsed and unresponsive

Presentation

Charles Lee, aged 32 years, presents to Dr Sloane in the emergency department. Mr Lee has collapsed and is unresponsive. He has a long history of self-neglect and alcohol misuse.

Clinical examination identified a pale, underweight man who felt clammy to the touch. Dr Sloane smelt alcohol. As Mr Lee was unresponsive he was unable to question him to his lifestyle and any current medications. There was no sign of trauma and blood pressure and heart rate were stable (110/70 mmHg and 65 bpm respectively).

Dr Sloane orders blood tests to assess Mr Lee's nutritional status and liver function. Based upon his history the collapse is most likely to be the result of alcohol-dependent nutritional deficiencies and liver dysfunction.

Analysis

The blood test results (**Table 4.1**) show:

- low serum glucose (hypoglycaemia)
- markedly increased γ-glutamyl transferase

Blood test results		
Test	Result	Reference range
Glucose (mmol/L)	1.9	3.5–5.0
γ-Glutamyl transferase (U/L)	352	<35
Potassium (mmol/L)	2.6	3.5–5.3
Magnesium (mmol/L)	0.40	0.70–1.0
Phosphate (mmol/L)	0.34	0.7–1.40

Table 4.1 Blood test results for a man who has collapsed and is unresponsive

Hypoglycaemia: causes, investigation and treatment

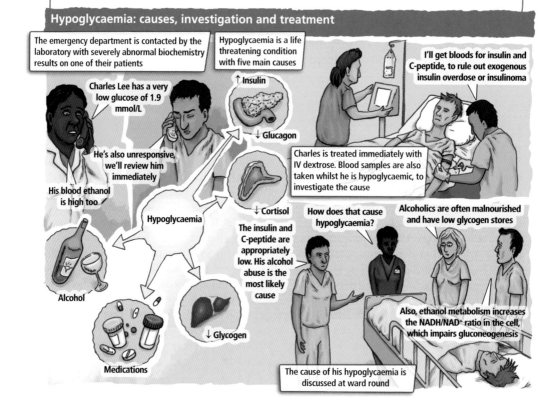

The emergency department is contacted by the laboratory with severely abnormal biochemistry results on one of their patients

Charles Lee has a very low glucose of 1.9 mmol/L

He's also unresponsive, we'll review him immediately

His blood ethanol is high too

Hypoglycaemia is a life threatening condition with five main causes

↑ Insulin

↓ Glucagon

↓ Cortisol

Hypoglycaemia

Alcohol

↓ Glycogen

Medications

I'll get bloods for insulin and C-peptide, to rule out exogenous insulin overdose or insulinoma

Charles is treated immediately with IV dextrose. Blood samples are also taken whilst he is hypoglycaemic, to investigate the cause

The insulin and C-peptide are appropriately low. His alcohol abuse is the most likely cause

How does that cause hypoglycaemia?

Alcoholics are often malnourished and have low glycogen stores

Also, ethanol metabolism increases the NADH/NAD⁺ ratio in the cell, which impairs gluconeogenesis

The cause of his hypoglycaemia is discussed at ward round

Case 3 continued

- decreased potassium (hypokalaemia), magnesium (hypomagnesaemia) and phosphate (hypophosphataemia)

In this clinical context, the probable explanations are hypoglycaemia reflecting the inability to mount a glyconeogenetic response due to a malnourished state, high γ-glutamyl transferase as a result of alcoholic liver damage, and lowered electrolytes secondary to nutritional deficiencies.

Further case

To aid Dr Sloane's differential diagnosis further laboratory tests were requested on Mr Lee to measure insulin and C-peptide. Both were undetectable indicating a non-insulin mediated hypoglycaemia.

Mr Lee is admitted to hospital for intravenous replacement of potassium, magnesium and phosphate. Glucose is also given intravenously. After several hours he is sitting up in bed, alert and chatting to the doctor.

Further analysis

The insulin and C-peptide measurements were indicated by Mr Lee's hypoglycaemia to confirm that excess insulin is not responsible for his condition. C- (connecting-) peptide is a by-product of the breakdown of proinsulin to active insulin, therefore its concentration is used to assess insulin production.

Hypoglycaemia is common in patients who consume excessive amounts of alcohol without adequate nutrition. In this group of patients, the condition is a consequence of:

- low glycogen stores
- impaired citric acid cycle and gluconeogenesis; ethanol metabolism by alcohol dehydrogenase reduces NAD^+ to NADH; the next step in the metabolism of alcohol by aldehyde dehydrogenase also reduces NAD^+ to NADH thereby increasing the NADH/NAD^+ ratio. This change affects gluconeogenesis

This change in NADH negatively affects enzymes in the gluconeogenesis pathway. Conversion of lactate to pyruvate is inhibited and lactate production is favoured; production of oxaloacetate from malate is inhibited. However other mechanisms for glucose production such as glycogenolysis can still occur. Mr Lee has a poor nutritional intake so glycogen stores are minimal. Alcohol misuse is associated with nutritional deficiencies resulting from a poor diet and inhibition of digestive enzymes by alcohol will impair nutrient absoprtion. These lead to electrolyte deficiencies requiring oral or intravenous supplementation.

Mr Lee's collapse was caused by hypoglycaemia secondary to alcohol inhibiting gluconeogenesis. He is referred to an alcohol withdrawal programme, advised on eating and lifestyle changes and prescribed multi-vitamins to help correct nutritional deficiencies.

> γ-**Glutamyl transferase concentration is increased in 75% of patients with long-term alcohol misuse.** This result indicates oxidative damage to the liver.

Chemical energy

Chemical energy is energy stored in the bonds of chemical compounds. This energy is released in chemical reactions.

Food is an example of stored chemical energy. Digestion breaks down the molecules in food into smaller components. Energy is released by the breaking of bonds during the chemical reactions in this process.

Carbohydrates are the central molecules of metabolic energy in all forms of organism; they are used to both store and generate energy. Their widespread use is probably partly the consequence of the development of photosynthesis by cyanobacteria about 3.6 billion years ago. Photosynthesis harnesses the energy of sunlight to form chemical bonds, and glucose is one of its products.

Food energy

Energy in food is released by the metabolic pathways described in this chapter, and is measured in kilocalories or kilojoules (**Table 4.2**). Carbohydrate, protein and fat differ in structure, so they are broken down in different pathways. However, their metabolites enter shared pathways, the final common pathways that release energy.

The production, storage and use of energy are fundamental to cells; they also require energy to do all their work. Therefore an understanding of biochemical energetics provides the basis for an understanding of metabolism (see page 31).

Monosaccharides

Monosaccharides are the simplest carbohydrates, because they cannot be hydrolysed to smaller carbohydrates. They all have the general formula $(C.H_2O)_n$ and include glucose, fructose and galactose.

The following characteristics are used to classify monosaccharides (**Figure 4.1**).

■ Carbonyl group: if this is an aldehyde, the monosaccharide is an aldose
■ Number of carbon atoms: three for trioses, four for tetroses, five for pentoses and six for hexoses
■ Chiral nature: the classification of D or L is based on the orientation of the asymmetrical carbon furthest from the carbonyl group

  ■ D-sugars have a hydroxyl group on the right
  ■ L-sugars have a hydroxyl group on the left (easily remembered as 'l' for left)

As an example, under this classification D-glucose is an aldohexose.

Monosaccharides, predominately glucose, are the major source of fuel for metabolism. They are broken down in the cytoplasm by the citric acid cycle, then further utilised by mitochondria to produce adenosine triphosphate (ATP). When not required,

Energy content of foods		
Component	Energy (kcal/g)	Energy (kJ/g)
Carbohydrate	4	17
Fat	9	37
Protein	4	17
Fibre	2	8
Alcohol	7	29

The joule is the most widely SI unit used to measure energy

Table 4.2 Energy content of major food groups

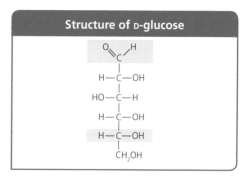

Structure of D-glucose

Figure 4.1 Structure of D-glucose. Monosaccharides are classified by carbonyl group (orange), number of carbon atoms and chiral nature. The classification of D or L is based on the orientation of the asymmetrical carbon furthest from the carbonyl group (blue).

monosaccharides are converted to space-efficient, insoluble storage polysaccharides such as glycogen.

Disaccharides

Disaccharides are two monosaccharaides joined by a covalent bond formed by a dehydration reaction. The reaction results in the loss of hydrogen from one monosaccharide and a hydroxyl group from the other.

- Sucrose (table sugar) is a disaccharide formed from D-glucose and D-fructose
- Lactose is formed from D-galactose and D-glucose

Oligosaccharides

Oligosaccharides are polymers of monosaccharides. They are generally O-linked to amino acid side chains in proteins or lipids. O-linked glycosylation is when glycans (sugars) are attached to the hydroxyl oxygen of the amino acids serine, threonine, tyrosine or hydroxylysine and hydroxyproline. The glycans can also be O-linked to oxygens on lipids.

Oligosaccharides differ from polysaccharides in the number of linked monosaccharide units. Oligosaccharides contain two to ten, whereas polysaccharides contain hundreds.

> **Sweetness is caused by the activation of taste receptors on the tongue by hydroxyl groups with certain orientations.** Through evolution, humans developed their sensitivity and attraction to sweetness because of its value as a readily metabolised source of abundant energy.

> **A kilocalorie is commonly referred to as a calorie,** and is the energy required to increase the temperature of 1 g of water by 1°C. A kilojoule is equivalent to 4.2 kilocalories.

Energy transfer

The body transfers energy by breaking and making bonds. Glucose is the main molecule of energy exchange. However, it is ATP, and the phosphate–phosphate bonds it contains, that directly supplies chemical reactions with the energy they need.

Adenosine triphosphate

Adenosine triphosphate (ATP) is the body's main currency of energy; it is an adenosine molecule (adenine ring and a ribose sugar) attached to three phosphate groups (**Figure 4.2**). Energy is released by hydrolysis of the 3rd phosphate group, whose removal produces adenosine diphosphate (ADP). ADP absorbs energy during cellular processes and thus regains a phosphate group, regenerating ATP.

> **The total amount of ATP in the human body is about 0.1 mol.** The energy used daily by an average-sized adult requires hydrolysis of 200–300 mol of ATP. To achieve this, each molecule of ATP is recycled 2000–3000 times during the day.

Phosphates are high-energy molecules. They release high levels of energy when individual phosphate groups are removed.

Figure 4.2 Structure of adenosine triphosphate.

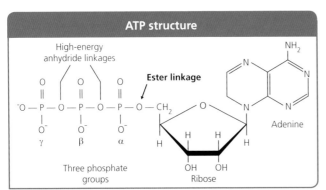

Energy for reactions

The dephosphorylation reaction of ATP to ADP is frequently coupled to another reaction to exploit the release of energy. Release of phosphate is exothermic (gives off heat) and can be joined to an endothermic reaction (one that requires energy or heat). The phosphate group is transferred to another compound (phosphorylation) to produce ADP, phosphate and energy.

The phosphate bond in ATP contains sufficient energy to supply most reactions. When more energy is needed, ATP is able to release two phosphate groups. This produces adenosine monophosphate (AMP) and pyrophosphate, which has two phosphate groups.

Other energy currencies

Although ATP is the main energy carrier, other nucleotide phosphates are also used as energy currencies. The citric acid cycle rephosphorylates only ADP. However, it can transfer phosphate from ATP to a nucleotide diphosphate, commonly guanosine diphosphate (GDP) (to form guanosine triphosphate, GTP). GTP can be used to supply energy for protein synthesis and gluconeogenesis. It is also essential in G-protein–linked signal transduction (see page 19).

Electron transport and oxidative phosphorylation

In mitochondria, the main site of ATP production, coenzymes transfer the energy from products of metabolism to ATP. They are known as redox coenzymes, because they couple reduction and oxidation reactions. In simple terms, they are vital to the transfer of electrons and protons, and during this process produce a large amount of free energy used to form ATP from ADP.

> Remember that an oxidation reaction involves loss of hydrogen or electrons, and reduction is gain of hydrogen or electrons. A simple mnemonic is OIL RIG (oxidation is loss, reduction is gain).

Redox coenzymes

In metabolism, specific enzymes catalyse oxidation. Cofactors of these enzymes, (coenzymes), usually act as carriers for the products of reactions.

In metabolism, three key coenzymes are responsible for the transduction of energy:

- nicotinamide adenine dinucleotide (NAD^+)
- flavin adenine dinucleotide (FAD)
- flavin mononucleotide (FMN)

During energy metabolism, i.e. the series of reactions that produce or use ATP, electrons are transferred from carbohydrates and fats to these coenzymes, thereby reducing them. The reduced products are NADH, $FADH_2$ and $FMNH_2$, respectively.

The hydrogen gained by NAD^+ from NADH can be transferred to FAD. The reduced $FADH_2$ enables NADH to return to its oxidised form (NAD^+). Electrons are moved through a sequence of reactions using the coenzymes to enable the transfer of hydrogen to oxygen, forming water.

Electron transport system and oxidative phosphorylation

This chain of events is the electron transport system. The system also drives the transport of protons from the mitochondrial matrix to the intermembrane space of mitochondria. This proton transport generates potential energy in the form of a pH gradient and an electrical potential across the membrane. Protons are able to flow back across the membrane through ATP synthase.

The ATP synthase uses the energy to generate ATP from ADP in a phosphorylation reaction; this process is known as oxidative phosphorylation. Oxidative phosphorylation is the metabolic pathway by which the mitochondria, the enzymes and the energy released during the electron transport system reform ATP (see page 113).

Pathways of energy metabolism

Carbohydrate metabolic pathways are the central pathways of energy metabolism. They are based on the synthesis, storage and production of glucose (**Figure 4.3**). The energy generated is used to drive other biochemical reactions.

Glucose circulates in the bloodstream, and its availability determines which of the carbohydrate pathways are active. Glucose availability is determined by the following processes.

- Glycolysis: the breakdown of glucose
- The pentose phosphate pathway: the conversion of glucose to the sugars used to synthesise nucleotides and nucleic acids; this generates no ATP but a large amount of the reduced form of nicotinamide adenine dinucleotide phosphate (NADPH)
- Gluconeogenesis: the synthesis of glucose from non-carbohydrates when levels are low
- The electron transport system and oxidative phosphorylation: the use of glucose to produce ATP
- Glycogen production: glycogenesis (when glucose levels are high)
- Glycogen breakdown: glycogenolysis (when glucose levels are low)

The coordination of these pathways is called glucose homeostasis.

> **Tubes used to collect blood samples for the measurement of glucose concentration (a very common test) contain an inhibitor of glycolysis.** This inhibitor, usually fluoride, prevents still-active red blood cells from breaking down the glucose present in the blood.

Glucose homeostasis

Cells in the Islets of Langerhans monitor glucose levels. Blood glucose concentration is kept within a normal range of 3.5–6.0 mmol/L mainly by the action of two pancreatic hormones: glucagon and insulin.

- Glucagon is released by pancreatic alpha cells when glucose levels are low. It stimulates glycogenolysis in liver cells, and gluconeogenesis in liver and kidney cells, when glycogen is depleted
- Insulin is released from pancreatic beta cells when glucose levels are high, and

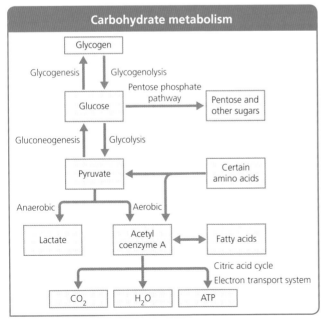

Figure 4.3 Overview of carbohydrate metabolism.

Carbohydrate metabolism diagram:
- Glycogen
  - Glycogenesis / Glycogenolysis
- Glucose
  - Pentose phosphate pathway → Pentose and other sugars
  - Gluconeogenesis / Glycolysis
- Pyruvate ← Certain amino acids
  - Anaerobic → Lactate
  - Aerobic → Acetyl coenzyme A ↔ Fatty acids
    - Citric acid cycle
    - Electron transport system
    - CO_2 / H_2O / ATP

acts on all cells to increase glucose uptake by facilitated diffusion through glucose transporter type 4 (GLUT4) membrane transporters; insulin also acts on liver cells to increase glycogenogenesis

Other hormones also influence blood glucose levels (**Table 4.3**).

Disorders of glucose homeostasis will result in either hypoglycaemia (low blood glucose) or hyperglycaemia (high blood glucose). Signs and symptoms of both are shown in **Figure 4.4**.

Diabetes

Diabetes is a group of metabolic diseases predominantly in which either the production of insulin is deficient (type 1 diabetes) or cells have increased resistance to it (type 2 diabetes) (**Table 4.4**). Both these types of diabetes increase blood glucose, which will result in the following:

- Glycosuria: glucose in urine, as the renal threshold for glucose reabsorption is exceeded

Hormones that affect blood glucose			
Hormone	Tissue of origin	Metabolic effect(s)	Effect on blood glucose
Insulin*	Pancreas (beta cells)	Stimulates glycogenesis	Decrease
		Enhances glucose uptake by cells	
		Antagonistic to gluconeogenesis	
		Enhances synthesis of fatty acids and proteins	
Glucagon*	Pancreas (alpha cells)	Stimulates glycogenolysis	Increase
		Enhances synthesis of glucose from non-carbohydrate precursors (amino acids and fatty acids)	
Cortisol	Adrenal cortex	Stimulates gluconeogenesis	Increase
		Facilitates activation of glycogen phosphorylase (essential for the effects of adrenaline on glycogenolysis)	
		Antagonises insulin	
Adrenaline (epinephrine)	Adrenal medulla	'Fight or flight' response	Increase
		Enhances glycogenolysis	
		Increases release of fatty acids from adipose tissue	
Growth hormone	Anterior pituitary	Antagonises insulin	Increase
		Decreases rate at which cells use carbohydrate for energy	
Somatostatin (growth hormone–inhibiting hormone)	Pancreas (delta cells)	Inhibits secretion of insulin and glucagon	Decrease
Thyroxine	Thyroid gland	Enhances glycogenolysis	Increase
		Stimulates the use of carbohydrates as an energy source	

*Main hormones in glucose homeostasis.

Table 4.3 Hormones that affect blood glucose concentration

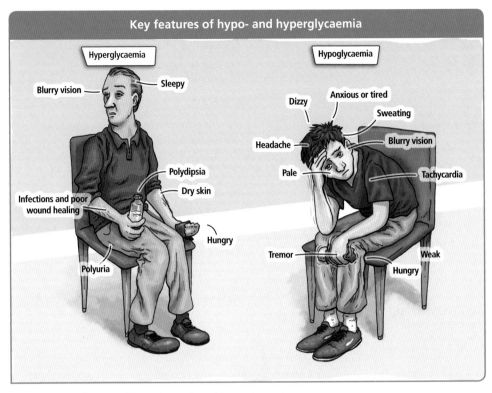

Figure 4.4 Key features of hypoglycaemia and hyperglycaemia.

- Polyuria: excess water excretion as it 'follows' the hypertonic urine with excess glucose
- Dehydration: decreased blood volume as water is lost from the blood, followed by water leaving the cells to maintain fluid balance
- Polydipsia: increased thirst

Diabetes causes long-term complications from glucose-induced vascular disease. This condition results from high levels of glucose damaging structural proteins, disrupting fluid balance and generating increased cell damage from free radicals (reactive atoms or molecules with an unpaired electron that are a by-product of an overwhelmed electron transport system).

Complications of chronic glucose damage include poor wound healing, retinopathy, nephropathy and neuropathy, as well as cardiovascular and cerebrovascular disease.

Classification of diabetes			
Type	Description	Information on groups affected	Treatment
Type 1 diabetes	Autoimmune disease that destroys pancreatic beta cells Absence or deficiency of insulin production	Onset usually in childhood (juvenile diabetes)	Insulin
Type 2 diabetes	Insulin resistance: insulin is produced but not used as effectively	Previously called adult onset diabetes, but with the increasing prevalence of obesity, an increasing number of young adults and children are being diagnosed	Dietary modification and exercise Oral medications to improve insulin sensitivity Insulin
Gestational diabetes	Increased insulin resistance as a result of placental hormone production Insulin requirement doubled to tripled by growth of fetus	Affects 3–5% of all pregnancies and develops in 2nd and 3rd trimester	Diet and exercise Rarely insulin
Latent autoimmune diabetes of adulthood (occasionally referred to as type 1.5 diabetes)	Classified as type 2 but lacks the classic symptoms More typical physique of type 1 but does not require insulin in early stages	Adulthood	Insulin requirement may rapidly develop
Maturity onset diabetes of the young	Similar to type 2 diabetes, with strong genetic risk Not linked to obesity More than 10 different genetic mutations for this condition have been identified	Adults aged < 25 years	Depends on type, but most common type (caused by *HNF1A* gene; about 70% of cases) treated with sulfonylurea pills to increase insulin production
Type 3 diabetes	A form of Alzheimer's disease that results from insulin resistance in the brain Patients with type 2 diabetes have increased risk of developing Alzheimer's disease	Late adulthood	As for types 1 and 2
Steroid-induced diabetes	Treatment with corticosteroids potentially will increase insulin resistance, particularly in people at high risk of developing type 2 diabetes	Long-term steroid treatment	As for type 2

Table 4.4 Classification of diabetes

Glucose breakdown

The breakdown of glucose (glycolysis) is essential, because glucose is the main source of energy for cells. Glycolysis is the first step of cellular respiration (the reactions in a cell that produce energy from nutrients) and is also a central metabolic pathway, with intermediate metabolites that link to other pathways including those of fat and protein metabolism.

Glycolysis occurs in the cytosol of the cells of all organisms (with rare exceptions) to convert one molecule of glucose to two pyruvate molecules, two ATP molecules, hydrogen ions, water and heat:

$$\text{D-Glucose} + 2\,\text{NAD}^+ + 2\,\text{Pi} + 2\,\text{ADP}$$
$$\downarrow$$
$$2\text{Pyruvate} + 2\,\text{NADH} + 2\,\text{ATP} + 2\,\text{H}^+ + 2\,\text{H}_2\text{O}$$
$$+ \text{heat}$$

The fate of pyruvate depends on whether oxygen is present.

- In the presence of oxygen, pyruvate enters aerobic respiration and is converted to acetyl coenzyme A, which then enters the citric acid cycle in mitochondria
- In the absence of oxygen, anaerobic respiration converts pyruvate to lactic acid to be excreted from the cell and to regenerate the NAD$^+$ needed for glycolysis

Glycolysis has many steps but yields only two moles of ATP per mole of glucose. Most ATP is generated in the mitochondria from the electron transport system.

> The glycolytic pathway occurs in every cell of the body, because all cells catabolise glucose for energy. Other monosaccharides can also be metabolised by the pathway, including fructose, galactose and mannose.

Glycolytic pathway

Nine reactions convert 6-carbon glucose to two 3-carbon pyruvate molecules (**Table 4.5**). The energy released by breaking the carbon–carbon bond is used to produce two molecules of ATP (from ADP) and two molecules of NADH (from NAD$^+$).

Glycolysis in nine steps

Step	Reaction	Product(s)	Enzyme	Generates (+) or uses (−) ATP[†]
1	Phosphorylation	Glucose 6-phosphate	Hexokinase	−
2	Conversion	Fructose 6-phosphate	Phosphoglucose isomerase	
3	Phosphorylation	Fructose 1,6-bisphosphate	Phosphofructokinase	−
4	Cleavage	Dihydroxyacetone phosphate + Glyceraldehyde 3-phosphate (1st product)		
	Conversion	Glyceraldehyde 3-phosphate (2nd product)	Triose phosphate isomerase	
5*	Oxidation coupled to phosphorylation	1,3-Bisphosphoglycerate	Glyceraldehyde 3-phosphate dehydrogenase	
6*	Dephosphorylation	3-Phosphoglycerate	Phosphoglycerate kinase	++
7*	Rearrangement	2-Phosphoglycerate	Phosphoglycerate mutase	
8*	Dehydration	Phosphoenolpyruvate	Enolase	
9*	Dephosphorylation	Pyruvate	Pyruvate kinase	++

ATP, adenosine triphosphate.

*One molecule of glucose produces two molecules of glyceraldehyde phosphate. Steps 5–9 are for two molecules of glyceraldehyde 3–phosphate.

†For one molecule of glucose, two ATP are used and four are produced, giving a net gain of two ATP.

Table 4.5 Summary of glycolysis

Investment stage

The first three steps of glycolysis are the 'investment' stage: energy is invested in the processes for the outcome at the end of the pathway.

Step 1: phosphorylation

The first step of glycolysis (**Figure 4.5**) is phosphorylation of the glucose ring, a reaction catalysed by hexokinase. A phosphate group from ATP is added to carbon 6 of the glucose molecule to produce glucose 6-phosphate. This step 'traps' glucose in the cell, because the negatively charged phosphate prevents it from crossing the cell's plasma membrane through glucose transporters. A magnesium ion is required to form a complex with ATP.

Step 2: rearrangement of the carbon ring

Glucose 6-phosphate is converted into fructose-6-phosphate in a reaction catalysed by phosphoglucose isomerase. This rearranges the six-membered carbon ring into a five-membered ring, so that carbon 1 becomes external to the ring structure.

Step 3: phosphorylation

Carbon 1 is phosphorylated by phosphofructokinase-1 to produce fructose 1,6-bisphosphate. This reaction requires ATP and is irreversible. As in step 1, magnesium is required as an enzyme cofactor.

Step 4: splitting

Fructose 1,6-bisphosphate is cleaved in the middle to produce two 3-carbon molecules. This is a freely reversible reaction producing dihydroxyacetone phosphate and glyceraldehyde 3-phosphate. Only glyceraldehyde 3-phosphate, two per molecule of glucose, continues in the glycolytic pathway, with dihydroxyacetone phosphate converted to glyceraldehyde 3-phosphate by triose phosphate isomerase.

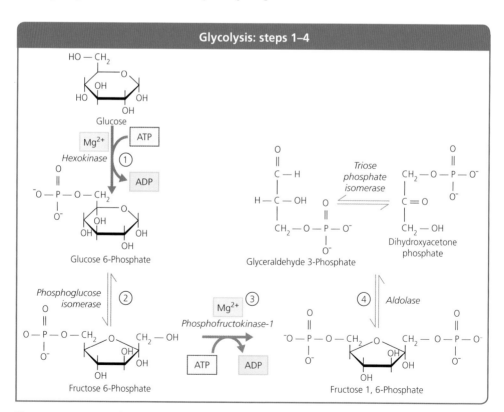

Figure 4.5 Steps 1–4 of glycolysis: the investment stage. One mole of glucose is converted to two moles of glyceraldehyde 3-phosphate. ADP, adenosine diphosphate; ATP, adenosine triphosphate.

Yield stages

The next steps of the pathway (**Figure 4.6**) are considered the 'yield' stages: 4 moles of ATP are produced for an overall gain of 2 moles of ATP, because 2 were used in steps 1 and 3.

Step 5: oxidation and phosphorylation

Glyceraldehyde 3-phosphate is converted to 1,3-bisphosphoglycerate by glyceraldehyde 3-phosphate dehydrogenase in two reactions (**Figure 4.7**).

1. Oxidation of glyceraldehyde 3-phosphate at the carbon 1 position and simultaneous reduction of NAD+ to NADH
2. Phosphorylation: transfer of phosphate from 1,3-bisphosphoglycerate to the oxidised form of glyceraldehyde 3-phosphate

The steps are linked, because energy released from the first exergonic oxidation reaction drives the second endergonic phosphorylation reaction.

Step 6: dephosphorylation

Next, 1,3-bisphosphoglycerate is converted to 3-phosphoglycerate by phosphoglycerate kinase, which removes a phosphate and transfers it to ADP to produce ATP. This is the first step in the production of ATP, with two moles of ATP produced for each mole of glucose. Two moles were used in steps 1 and 3, so at this point in the pathway there is a net balance of zero ATP.

Step 7: phosphate rearrangement

Phosphoglycerate mutase moves the position of a phosphate so that 3-phosphoglycerate becomes 2-phosphoglycerate. Initially a

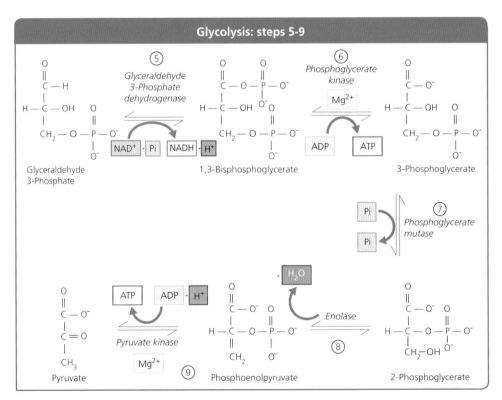

Figure 4.6 Continuation of the glycolytic pathway (steps 5–9): the yield stages. Only the processing of one glyceraldehyde 3-phosphate is shown, but for every glucose molecule entering the pathway, two glyceraldehyde 3-phosphates are produced. ADP, adenosine diphosphate; ATP, adenosine triphosphate; NAD+, nicotinamide adenine dinucleotide (oxidised form); NADH, nicotinamide adenine dinucleotide (reduced form), Pi, inorganic phosphate.

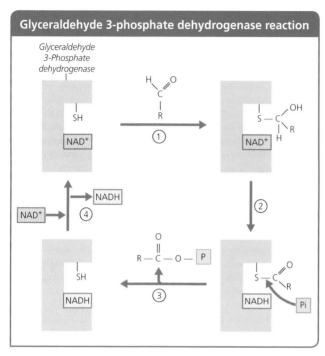

Glyceraldehyde 3-phosphate dehydrogenase reaction

Figure 4.7 The glyceraldehyde 3-phosphate dehydrogenase reaction. ① The active site of the sulfhydryl group of the enzyme forms a thiohemiacetal adduct with glyceraldehyde 3-phosphate. ② The thiohemiacetal is oxidised to a thioester by nicotinamide adenine dinucleotide (NAD+), also bound in the active site. ③ Phosphate enters the active site and displaces the thiol group through a phosphorylase reaction; this yields 1,3-bisphosphoglycerate and regenerates the sulfhydryl group. ④ The enzyme exchanges NADH for NAD+, thus completing the cycle. Pi, inorganic phosphate.

phosphate is added to carbon 2, and then the group on carbon 3 is removed.

Step 8: dehydration

The 2-phosphoglycerate is dehydrated (i.e. loses a water molecule) to become phosphoenolpyruvate in a reaction catalysed by enolase.

Step 9: dephosphorylation

The final step of glycolysis converts phosphoenolpyruvate into pyruvate with the help of pyruvate kinase. This enzyme transfers the phosphate group from carbon 2 to ADP, yielding ATP. Because there are two molecules of phosphoenolpyruvate, two molecules of ATP are generated.

End of glycolysis

By the end of glycolysis, for every molecule of glucose that entered the pathway there is a net gain of two moles of ATP, because 4 were generated but 2 were used. The nine steps of glycolysis are anaerobic, i.e. oxygen is not required to produce pyruvate.

The fate of pyruvate depends on the cell type, whether mitochondria are present, and the amount of oxygen available.

The NAD+ used to oxidise glyceraldehyde 3-phosphate in step 5 is essential in glycolysis, therefore the resulting NADH must be reoxidised to NAD+. This occurs in both the aerobic and the anaerobic pathways of pyruvate metabolism.

> **Mature red blood cells contain no mitochondria.** Therefore they rely entirely on glycolysis and the subsequent anaerobic metabolism of pyruvate for their energy.

Anaerobic metabolism of pyruvate

In anaerobic conditions, such as poor perfusion or in muscle during oxygen depletion, lactate dehydrogenase transfers the hydrogen molecule from NADH to pyruvate (**Figure 4.8**) to produce lactate and NAD+. The

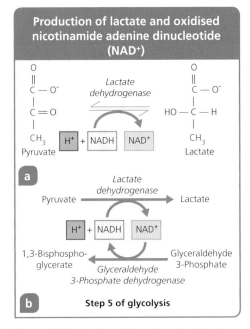

Production of lactate and oxidised nicotinamide adenine dinucleotide (NAD+)

a

b **Step 5 of glycolysis**

Figure 4.8 Production of lactate and oxidised nicotinamide adenine dinucleotide (NAD+). (a) Anaerobic metabolism of pyruvate to produce lactate. (b) Recycling of reduced nicotinamide adenine dinucleotide (NADH) during anaerobic glycolysis, which enables regeneration of NAD+ for use in step 5 of the glycolysis pathway.

carbon double bond in pyruvate is reduced to a hydroxyl group (C–O–H) in lactate.

All cells have lactate dehydrogenase, because it is an essential reaction to restore cellular NAD+ in the absence of oxygen.

> **Lactate is cleared by the lactic acid (or Cori) cycle.** It leaves the muscle cells via shuttling into the bloodstream and is converted in the liver to glucose by gluconeogenesis.

Aerobic metabolism of pyruvate

In cells with mitochondria and in the presence of enough oxygen, pyruvate is converted by the citric acid cycle (see page 110) into carbon dioxide and water. It is initially converted to acetyl coenzyme A, which enters the cycle to produce carbon dioxide.

The NADH and $FADH_2$ produced in the cycle then enter the electron transport system to form water and energy as ATP (see page 113). The NADH is reoxidised in the mitochondria to NAD+, ready for glycolysis. Aerobic metabolism is up to 15 times more efficient than anaerobic metabolism.

The pentose phosphate pathway

The pentose phosphate pathway, also known as the hexose monophosphate shunt, occurs in the cytosol of all cells. It is an alternative pathway for glucose oxidation, and although it generates no ATP, it produces over half the body's NADPH.

The main role of the pentose phosphate pathway is to produce five carbon sugars (pentoses) used in nucleotide and amino acid synthesis, as well as the NADPH necessary for reductive biosynthetic reactions, including the production of fatty acids. The pentose phosphate pathway is most active in the liver, adrenal cortex and mammary glands .

NADPH

The reduced form of nicotinamide adenine dinucleotide phosphate is an important coenzyme that prevents oxidative stress in cells. NADPH achieves this by donating electrons used to reduce glutathione, in a reaction catalysed by glutathione reductase.

Reduced glutathione is subsequently used to reduce damaging hydrogen peroxide (H_2O_2) to water, in a reaction catalysed by glutathione peroxidase. Without NADPH, reactive H_2O_2 is converted to free radicals that damage many components of the cell.

The pentose phosphate pathway and glycolysis

The pathway branches from the glycolytic pathway (see **Figure 4.5**) after step 1 after production of glucose 6-phosphate. It is a 'shunt' through its link to glycolysis, because when pentoses are not needed for biosynthetic reactions, the pentose phosphate intermediates are shunted back into the main glycolysis pathway by conversion into fructose 6-phosphate and glyceraldehyde 3-phosphate.

> **Synthesis of deoxyribonucleic acid (DNA) and ribonucleic acid (RNA) depends on the pentose phosphate pathway.** This is because the nucleotides that form their backbone are based on the 5-carbon sugars ribose (in RNA) and deoxyribose (in DNA).

Stages of the pentose phosphate pathway

The pentose phosphate pathway has two stages.

1. An irreversible redox (reduction–oxidation reaction) stage produces NADPH and pentose phosphates (**Figure 4.9**)
2. A reversible interconversion stage converts excess pentose phosphates into glycolytic pathway intermediates (**Figure 4.10**)

Stage 1: redox

Overall, the redox stage produces two moles of NADPH per mole of glucose 6-phosphate.

Step 1: oxidation

Glucose 6-phosphate is converted to 6-phosphogluconic acid lactone, and NADP⁺ is reduced to NADPH. Glucose 6-phosphate dehydrogenase oxidises the aldehyde group of glucose 6-phosphate to the acid.

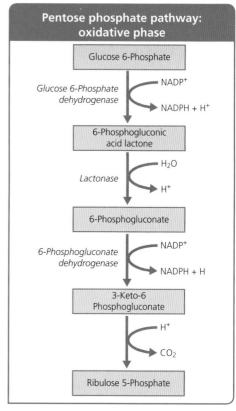

Pentose phosphate pathway: oxidative phase

Figure 4.9 The oxidative phase of the pentose phosphate pathway. These initial reactions are irreversible and produce two nicotinamide adenine dinucleotide phosphate (reduced form; NADPH). NADP⁺, nicotinamide adenine dinucleotide phosphate (oxidised form).

Step 2: hydrolysis

Next, 6-phosphogluconic acid lactone is hydrolysed to 6-phosphogluconate by lactonase.

Step 3: decarboxylation

Oxidative decarboxylation of 6-phosphogluconate, catalysed by 6-phosphogluconate dehydrogenase, produces ribulose 5-phosphate through an intermediate of 3-keto-6-phosphogluconate.

One mole of carbon dioxide and one mole of NADPH are produced in this reaction.

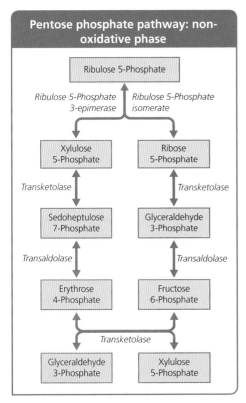

Pentose phosphate pathway: non-oxidative phase

Ribulose 5-Phosphate

Ribulose 5-Phosphate 3-epimerase | Ribulose 5-Phosphate isomerate

Xylulose 5-Phosphate | Ribose 5-Phosphate

Transketolase | *Transketolase*

Sedoheptulose 7-Phosphate | Glyceraldehyde 3-Phosphate

Transaldolase | *Transaldolase*

Erythrose 4-Phosphate | Fructose 6-Phosphate

Transketolase

Glyceraldehyde 3-Phosphate | Xylulose 5-Phosphate

Figure 4.10 The non-oxidative phase of the pentose phosphate pathway.

Glucose 6-phosphate dehydrogenase deficiency is an X-linked recessive disease. The disease causes cells to have reduced levels of NADPH and glutathione that protect against reactive oxygen species, rendering them prone to oxidative damage. Red blood cells are particularly susceptible, and patients present with haemolytic anaemia in response to infections or the use of certain medications, such as aspirin.

Glucose 6-phosphate dehydrogenase, confers protection against malaria infection, potentially because the malarial parasite is cleared more rapidly by the spleen due to the haemolysis.

The redox stage maintains high levels of NADPH, giving a cytoplasmic NADPH:NADP+ ratio of 100. Interestingly, the ratio of NADH:NAD+ in the cytoplasm is the reverse, about 0.01 – due to the requirement of NAD+ in glycolysis. These two redox systems have different set points and are metabolised by different dehydrogenases; the pentose phosphate pathway enzymes will only use NADPH – generally using it as a reducing agent, whilst the glycolytic pathway dehydrogenases are specific for NADH, where it is used as an oxidising agent.

Stage 2: interconversion

Ribulose 5-phosphate is isomerised (i.e. interconverted) to ribose 5-phosphate in cells with active nucleic acid synthesis (see **Figure 4.10**), in which it is used to synthesise ATP and other ribonucleotides. In non-dividing cells, three molecules of ribulose 5-phosphate are converted into two fructose 6-phosphate molecules and one glyceraldehyde 3-phosphate (**Table 4.6**).

Shunt into cellular respiration

Fructose 6-phosphate and glyceraldehyde 3-phosphate are converted to pyruvate by glycolysis. Pyruvate, as when produced in glycolysis, is then metabolised aerobically or anaerobically, depending on cellular conditions (see page 106).

Pyruvate dehydrogenase converts the pyruvate from glycolysis into acetyl coenzyme A, which can then enter the citric acid cycle. Pyruvate dehydrogenase deficiency is a congenital deficiency that results in a lack of energy generated by the citric acid cycle and an accumulation of lactate. Primary biliary cirrhosis is an autoimmune condition in which antimitochondrial antibodies against pyruvate dehydrogenase complex are detected. It manifests with jaundice, cirrhosis and xanthoma.

Pentose phosphate pathway: non-oxidative phase		
Reaction	Product(s)	Enzyme
Ribulose 5-phosphate	Ribose 5-phosphate	Ribulose 5-phosphate isomerase
Ribose 5-phosphate	Xylulose 5-phosphate	Ribulose 5-phosphate 3-epimerase
Xylulose 5-phosphate + ribose 5-phosphate	Glyceraldehyde 3-phosphate + sedoheptulose 7-phosphate	Transketolase
Glyceraldehyde 3-phosphate + sedoheptulose 7-phosphate	Erythrose 4-phosphate + fructose 6-phosphate	Transaldolase
Xylulose 5-phosphate + erythrose 4-phosphate	Glyceraldehyde 3-phosphate + fructose 6-phosphate	Transketolase

Table 4.6 Summary of reactions in the non-oxidative phase of the pentose phosphate pathway

The citric acid cycle

The citric acid cycle (also known as the tricarboxylic acid cycle or Krebs cycle) is the central pathway that interconnects the metabolic pathways of carbohydrates, protein and fat. It enables carbon atoms from amino acids to be converted into glucose, but those from lipolysis are unable to be diverted into gluconeogenesis. This means that animals cannot use fat stores to make glucose; instead, in the starvation state, fats are broken down to ketone bodies as an alternative metabolic fuel.

The citric acid cycle occurs in mitochondria and consists of a repeating cycle of eight reactions that generate energy from acetyl coenzyme A.

Acetyl coenzyme A

Acetyl coenzyme A is an acetyl group attached to a coenzyme A molecule. The coenzyme A molecule is a large molecule containing ADP, with two side chain groups to which the acetyl groups attach. It is considered a carrier of acetyl groups, more importantly the carbon atoms within the acetyl group to the citric acid cycle. Here they are oxidised for energy production.

Acetyl coenzyme A is derived from three metabolic precursors.

■ Carbohydrates undergo glycolysis to produce pyruvate, which is decarboxylated to acetyl coenzyme A by pyruvate dehydrogenase

■ Fats are converted to free fatty acids, which are oxidised in the mitochondria to acetyl coenzyme A
■ Proteolysis of proteins produces amino acids, which are metabolised to acetyl coenzyme A

Stages of the citric acid cycle

The citric acid cycle begins with the reaction between acetyl coenzyme A and oxaloacetate, a 4-carbon molecule (**Figure 4.11**). This forms the 6-carbon citric acid after which the cycle is named.

In summary, through the cycle, two of the six carbons are removed as carbon dioxide to yield the 4-carbon oxaloacetate, which starts the cycle again.

Each cycle produces three NADH, one $FADH_2$ and one GTP for every molecule of acetyl coenzyme A.

Step 1: aldol condensation

Acetyl coenzyme A is joined to oxaloacetate to form citric acid in a reaction catalysed by citrate synthase. Once citric acid is formed, the coenzyme A is released from the complex.

Step 2: dehydration

The second step is removal of a water molecule from the oxaloacetate end of the molecule; the water molecule is moved to

The citric acid cycle

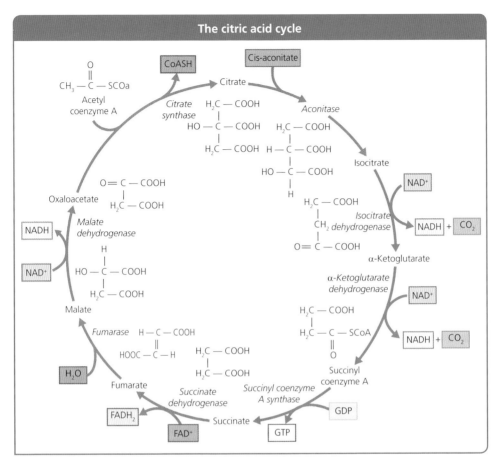

Figure 4.11 The citric acid cycle (also known as the tricarboxylic acid cycle or Krebs cycle), a sequence of eight enzymatic reactions. CoASH, coenzyme A FAD+, flavin adenine dinucleotide (oxidised form); FADH₂, flavin adenine dinucleotide (reduced form); NAD+, nicotinamide adenine dinucleotide (oxidised form); NADH, nicotinamide adenine dinucleotide (reduced form); SCoA, succinyl coenzyme A.

carbon 4 on the molecule to form isocitrate. This reaction is catalysed by aconitnase, an iron-sulphur protein, which is specific for the movement of water from carbon 3 to carbon 4.

Step 3: oxidation and decarboxylation

The enzyme isocitrate dehydrogenase then catalyses oxidation of the OH group at carbon 4 to yield an intermediate from which a carbon dioxide molecule is removed to form α-ketoglutarate. This third reaction generates NADH from NAD+.

Step 4: decarboxylation

The α-ketoglutarate loses a carbon dioxide molecule and is replaced by coenzyme A to form succinyl coenzyme A. This decarboxylation occurs with the help of NAD+, which is converted to NADH, and α-ketoglutarate dehydrogenase.

Step 5: substrate level phosphorylation

In step 5, succinyl coenzyme A is attacked by a free phosphate group, which releases the coenzyme A and succinate. The phosphate group is transferred to GDP to produce a molecule of GTP. GTP is similar in structure and energy to ATP, and its synthesis occurs similarly to that of ATP. This reaction is catalysed by succinyl coenzyme A synthetase.

Cofactors are non-protein compounds or elements which are required for biological activity. Cofactors are ionorganic ions such as magnesium or organic cofactors including heme or flavin. Organic cofactors can be coenzymes or prosthetic groups. They include the following:

- NADH: involved in redox reaction transporting electrons between two reactions. Key in beta oxidation, glycolysis and citric acid cycle

- NADPH: reducing agent in lipid and nucleic acid synthesis and protects against reactive oxygen species allowing regeneration of glutathione

- FADH: primary role is transport of electrons (energy) through electron transport chain.

Step 6: oxidation

Succinate then undergoes removal of two hydrogens by succinate dehydrogenase. A molecule of FAD^+, a coenzyme similar to NAD^+, is reduced to $FADH_2$ by accepting the two hydrogens. FAD^+ and NAD^+ carry out the same oxidation and reduction reactions but work on different classes of molecule.

- FAD^+ oxidises carbon–carbon double and triple bonds
- NAD^+ oxidises carbon–oxygen bonds

The product from the step 6 reaction is fumarate.

Step 7: hydration

Fumarate undergoes addition of a water molecule to form L-malate, a reaction catalysed by fumarase.

Step 8: oxidation

In the final step of the citric acid cycle, L-malate is then oxidised to regenerate oxaloacetate, using NAD^+ to produce NADH.

Overall, one citric acid cycle:

- reduces three molecules of NAD^+ to NADH
- reduces one molecule of FAD^+ to $FADH_2$
- produces one molecule of GTP

These reduced coenzymes are then subjected to the next stage of metabolism: oxidative phosphorylation. Ultimately, each NADH produces three ATP, and each $FADH_2$ produces two ATP. Overall 12 ATP equivalents are produced per mole of acetyl coenzyme A.

Oxidative phosphorylation

Mitochondria are the powerhouses of cells, because they are the site of both the citric acid cycle (in the matrix) and oxidative phosphorylation, the process by which the vast majority of ATP is formed. Oxidative phosphorylation is a series of redox reactions along proteins in the inner mitochondrial membrane: the electron transport system (or 'chain'). Electrons are conducted through these proteins, from electron donors to acceptors, and finally passed to oxygen.

These redox reactions release energy, which is ultimately collected to reform ATP, the base unit of chemical energy used in all aerobic organisms.

Transmembrane potential

The energy derived from the conduction of electrons along the electron transport system is used to drive the transport of protons (H^+) from the mitochondrial matrix to the intermembrane space. This movement of protons generates a transmembrane pH gradient and electric potential (a store of energy), which is then harvested by letting them back down their electrochemical gradient to the other side.

Harvesting the potential energy

The 'harvest' of energy occurs as the protons pass down their gradient through the large transmembrane ATP synthase enzyme. This enzyme has a rotary subunit that is moved by the protons, so that energy is collected as in a turbine. This kinetic energy is used to form a phosphate–phosphate bond by hydrolysing ADP to a third phosphate group and forming ATP.

The electron transport system pathway

The electron transport system consists of four large protein complexes and two small independent components called ubiquinone (coenzyme Q_{10}) and cytochrome c.

Electrons enter the electron transport system at:

- complex I (for electrons from NADH)
- complex II (for electrons from $FADH_2$)

These pathways meet at ubiquinone, which is the start of the common electron transport system. The common pathway consists of complex III, cytochrome c and complex IV. The final electron acceptor is molecular oxygen, which is reduced to water. Protons are pumped from the matrix and into the intermembrane space by complexes I, III and IV (**Figure 4.12**).

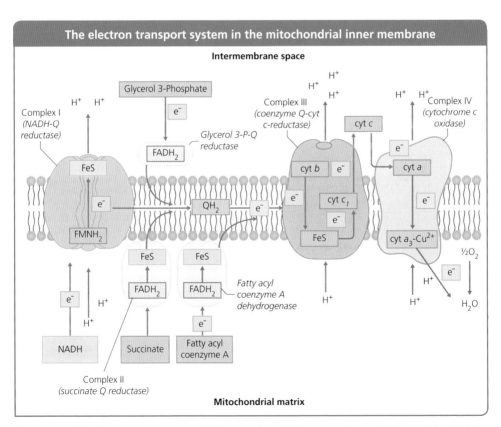

Figure 4.12 The electron transport system in the mitochondrial inner membrane. FeS, iron sulphur; $FADH_2$, flavin adenine dinucleotide (reduced form); FMN, flavin mononucleotide; $FMNH_2$, flavin mononucleotide (reduced form); NADH, nicotinamide adenine dinucleotide (reduced form).

> The amount of chemical energy (ATP) synthesised during the electron transport system per electron pair depends on when they join the chain:
>
> - an electron pair from NADH passes through complexes I, III and IV to produce three moles of ATP
> - from $FADH_2$, only two moles of ATP are synthesised, because they join at complex II and bypass complex I

Step 1a: complex I

Complex I is also known as NADH-Q reductase or NADH dehydrogenase. It is a flavoprotein; it contains a nucleic acid derivative of riboflavin called flavin mononucleotide (FMN). FMN acts as a dehydrogenase and can transfer one or two electrons, making it a strong oxidising agent.

NADH is oxidised, and the electrons taken from it are transferred through FMN and iron-sulphur complexes to ubiquinone. Complex I contributes enough energy to the proton gradient to produce one mole of ATP.

Step 1b: complex II

Complex II contains three different flavoproteins, each of which can be a point of entry for electrons into the electron transport pathway (**Table 4.7**). Complex II does not transport protons across the membrane (**Figure 4.12**) and therefore does not contribute to the proton gradient.

Step 2: ubiquinone

Ubiquinone is the start of the common pathway; it accepts one or two electrons from complex I or II and transfers them to complex III. Ubiquinone is a small lipid-soluble compound that contains a side chain of 10 isoprene units (hence its other name, coenzyme Q_{10}).

Step 3: complex III

Complex III is an oligomer of eight peptides containing cytochrome b, an iron-sulphur centre and cytochrome c_1; it is also known as ubiquinone–cytochrome c reductase. It oxidises ubiquinone and reduces cytochrome c. Its transport of two electrons to cytochrome c yields sufficient energy and proton movement to produce one mole of ATP.

Step 4: cytochrome c

Cytochrome c is a small mobile haem protein, but unlike haemoglobin, it is not involved in oxygen transport. Instead, it shuttles electrons from complex III to complex IV. The reduction of the iron in cytochrome c from Fe^{3+} to Fe^{2+} changes its conformation so that electrons are transferred to cytochrome a in complex IV.

Step 5: complex IV

Complex IV (cytochrome c oxidase) oxidises cytochrome c, and conducts the electrons through cytochromes a and $a3$ of complex IV, before being used to reduce oxygen to water.

Complex II flavoproteins		
Flavoprotein complex	Oxidation step	Reduction step
Succinate Q reductase	Oxidises succinate to fumarate	Reduces FAD^+ to $FADH_2$
Glycerol-3-phosphate Q reductase	Oxidises cytoplasmic glycerol 3-phosphate to dihydroxyacetone phosphate	Reduces FAD^+ to $FADH_2$
Fatty acyl coenzyme A	Catalyses first step in mitochondrial oxidation of fatty acids	Reduces FAD^+ to $FADH_2$

FAD^+, flavin adenine dinucleotide (oxidised form); $FADH_2$, flavin adenine dinucleotide (reduced form).

Table 4.7 Three flavoproteins in complex II of the electron transport pathway

Copper is a key component of such oxidising enzymes, because three atoms are required for the redox-active cofactor for complex IV. Complex IV pumps protons out of the mitochondrial matrix and into the intermembrane space, enabling synthesis of another mole of ATP.

> **Sugar consumption has increased from 5 kg per person per year in the 1800s to about 70 kg in the last decade.** Excessive sugar consumption underlies the modern epidemics of obesity, diabetes and vascular disease. Different theories of sugar toxicity include:
>
> ■ an increase in reactive oxygen species, which damage cells and tissues
>
> ■ the formation of spontaneous disruptive and permanent bonds with proteins and lipids, including the advanced glycated end products implicated in vascular disease

ATP–proton gradient

Complexes I, III and IV all produce protons as they pass electrons along to the next complex in the electron transport system. They are pumped out of the matrix into the intermembrane space. This movement of protons creates an electrochemical potential across the inner membrane.

The outside of the mitochondrion becomes more acidic and more positively charged than the matrix. This creates a flux of protons back into the matrix along the electrochemical gradient, through the ATP synthase complex. The membrane is impermeable to protons except through this complex.

ATP synthase

The ATP synthase complex is an example of rotary catalysis. It is composed of two major complexes (**Figure 4.13**).

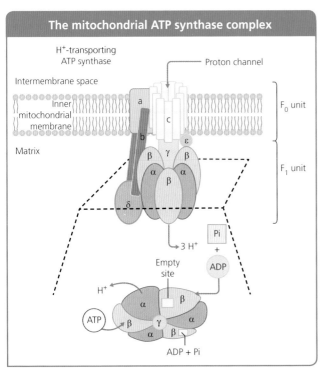

The mitochondrial ATP synthase complex

Figure 4.13 Structure of the mitochondrial adenosine triphosphate (ATP) synthase complex. The inner membrane component of the complex is F_0. It contains the proton channel and a stalk piece (δ) through which protons flow. The F_1-ATP synthase complex consists of a central γ subunit surrounded by alternating α and β subunits. The central γ unit rotates in response to the proton flux, which induces conformational changes. ADP, adenosine diphosphate; Pi, inorganic phosphate.

- An inner membrane component, which contains the proton channel (F_0)
- An ATP synthase complex (F_1), bound to F_0, with alternating α and β subunits; a central γ subunit physically rotates in response to the proton flux, like a waterwheel or turbine, and this rotation changes the shape of the α and β subunits so that they cyclically bind ADP and release ATP

> **Some chemicals are toxic because they disrupt the inner mitochondrial membrane and the electron transport system.** Examples are rotenone (an insecticide), cyanide and carbon monoxide.

Glycogen

Glycogen is a branched polysaccharide of glucose that is an energy storage molecule, predominantly in the liver and muscle cells. Small amounts are in the kidneys and intestine.

Glycogen is a quickly accessible source of glucose. It contains two glycosidic linkages: chains of α1-4-linked glucose residues with α1-6 branches about every four to six residues (**Figure 4.14**). This structure, with many branches and glucose residues, enables ready access for the enzymes that release glucose from glycogen.

Glycogenesis

Glycogen production (glycogenesis) occurs in the liver during and immediately after a meal, as well as in skeletal muscle during rest periods.

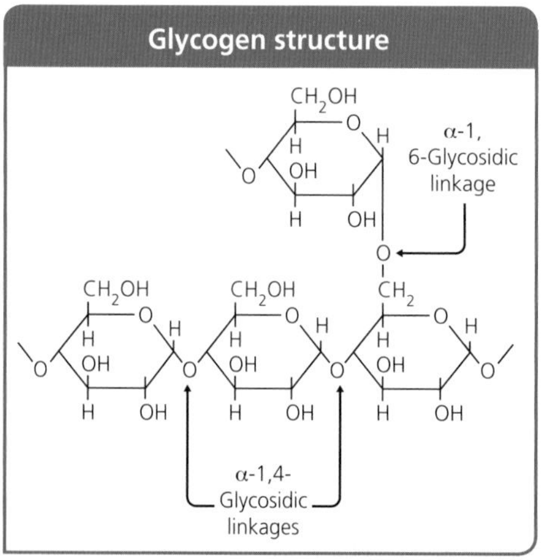

> **Muscle has twice the amount of glycogen as that in the liver.** However, unlike liver glycogen, muscle glycogen is not readily available for other tissues, because myocytes are unable to synthesise glucose 6-phosphate. Glucose 6-phosphate is necessary to generate glucose (for export via glucose transporter proteins) and organic phosphate. Without the enzymes, muscle glycogen remains for use in muscle tissue only.

Glycogenesis pathway

The pathway has four steps with four enzymes, and occurs in the cytosol of cells (**Figure 4.15**). Like the pentose phosphate pathway, glycogenesis starts after step 1 of glycolysis: the phosphorylation of glucose to glucose 6-phosphate by hexokinase in muscle and glucokinase in the liver.

Step 1: isomerisation

Glucose 6-phosphate is isomerised to glucose 1-phosphate by phosphoglucomutase.

Step 2: conversion

Glucose 1-phosphate reacts with uridine triphosphate to form uridine diphosphate (UDP)-glucose and pyrophosphate. This reaction is catalysed by UDP-glucose pyrophosphatase.

Glycogen structure

Figure 4.14 Glycogen structure, showing α-1,4 and α-1,6-glycosidic linkages.

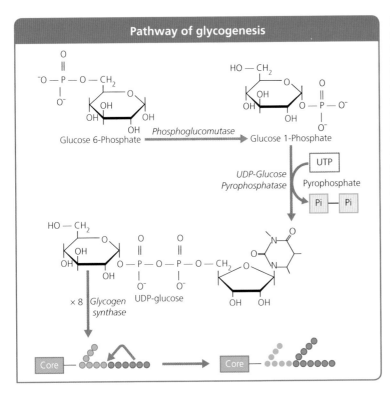

Figure 4.15 Pathway of glycogenesis. Glucose is transferred to glycogen in α1–4 linkages by glycogen synthase. When the chain exceeds eight residues, a glycogen-branching enzyme transfers some of the α1–4-linked sugars to an α1–6 branch. This enables further elongation of both of the α1–4 chains in turn until they become long enough for transfer by debranching enzymes. Pi, inorganic phosphate; UDP, uridine diphosphate; UTP, uridine triphosphate.

Step 3: hydrolysis

Pyrophosphate is rapidly hydrolysed to inorganic phosphate by pyrophosphatase.

Step 4: polymerisation

The final step is the action of glycogen synthase, which catalyses the formation of a glycoside bond between carbon 1 of the glucose on UDP-glucose and carbon 4 of a terminal glucose residue of glycogen, releasing the UDP. This process simply adds glucose on to a pre-existing glycogen fragment.

When there is no glycogen polymer to start this cascade, glycogenin (a protein primer) will initiate the reaction.

Control of glycogenesis

Glycogenesis is controlled by both allosteric and hormonal regulation.

Allosteric regulation

Allosteric regulation is when an effector molecule binds to a protein at a site, other than the active site - the allosteric site. This results in conformational change and can enhance activity (allosteric activator) or inhibit activity (allosteric inhibitor).

In the fed state, glycogen synthase in the liver is allosterically activated by glucose 6-phosphate and ATP.

Hormonal regulation

Insulin stimulates the activity of glycogen synthase, and therefore glycogenesis. Insulin is released by pancreatic beta cells when blood glucose is high.

Glycogen synthase is the target enzyme of glycogenesis regulation, because UDP-glucose pyrophosphorylase is also involved in the synthesis of glycoproteins and other sugars.

Glycogenolysis

Glycogen is gradually degraded between meals by glycogenolysis, releasing glucose to maintain blood glucose concentration. However, total hepatic stores of glycogen are barely sufficient for the maintenance of blood glucose during a 12-h fast. There is then a shift from glycogenolysis to de novo synthesis of glucose (gluconeogenesis).

Glycogenolysis pathway

The pathway has four steps with four enzymes, two of which cleave different types of glucose–glucose bonds:

- glycogen phosphorylase, which cleaves the core chain α1–4 linkages
- glycogen-debranching enzyme, which transfers 3–glucose sections of 4-residue branches, and then cleaves the remaining α1–6 branch to release free glucose

Step 1: debranching

The branching links are α1–6 linkages, cleaved by glycogen-debranching enzyme, which has both transglycosylase and glucosidase activity. Transglycosylase removes the last three of four glucose residues of a branch, and transfers them to another branch, thus exposing the final single α1–6 glucose molecule, which is then cleaved free by glucosidase.

Step 2: phosphorylation

This step is phosphorylation of the terminal α1–4 linked glucose residue by glycogen phosphorylase (**Figure 4.16**). This enzyme can cleave only the terminal glucose residues, uses phosphate and releases glucose 1-phosphate. Most glycogen breakdown is through this activity.

Step 3: isomerisation

Glucose 1-phosphate is converted to glucose 6-phosphate by phosphoglucomutase, a reverse of the initial steps in glycogenesis.

Release into the bloodstream

In the liver, the glucose is released from glucose 6-phosphate by glucose-6-phosphatase. It then exits through glucose transporter type 2 (GLUT2) into the blood.

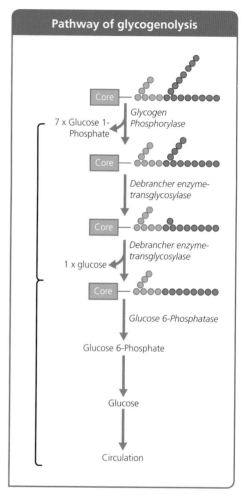

Pathway of glycogenolysis

7 x Glucose 1-Phosphate — Glycogen Phosphorylase

Core — Debrancher enzyme-transglycosylase

Core — Debrancher enzyme-transglycosylase

1 x glucose

Core — Glucose 6-Phosphatase

Glucose 6-Phosphate

Glucose

Circulation

Figure 4.16 Pathway of glycogenolysis. About 90% of glucose is released as glucose 1-phosphate, and the remainder as 'free' glucose from the α1–6 branching residues.

Control of glycogenolysis

Glycogenolysis in the liver is activated when glucose is in demand, either during the post-absorption state or in preparation for increased utilisation, i.e. during stress states. There are three hormonal activators of glycogenolysis (**Table 4.8**):

Hormonal control of glycogenolysis			
Hormone	Source	Initiator	Effect on glycogenolysis
Glucagon	Pancreatic alpha cells	Hypoglycaemia	Rapid activation
Adrenaline (ephinephrine)	Adrenal medulla	Stress or hypoglycaemia	Rapid activation
Insulin	Pancreatic beta cells	Hyperglycaemia	Inactivation
Cortisol	Adrenal cortex	Stress	Chronic activation

Table 4.8 Hormonal control of glycogenolysis

1. glucagon
2. adrenaline (ephinephrine)
3. cortisol

Glycogenolysis and glycogenesis are opposing pathways. Therefore activation of glycogenolysis is coordinated with inactivation of glycogenesis.

Glycogen storage diseases result from defects in glycogen synthesis or breakdown. These diseases arise as a result of a dysfunctioning enzyme in the pathway. The most common of the 12 is glucogen storage disease type I (von Gierke's disease), a lack of glucose 6-phosphatase. This condition affects 1 in 50,000 to 100,000 neonates and causes:

■ impaired liver glycogenolysis and gluconeogenesis

■ hypoglycaemia, liver and kidney problems, lactic acidosis and hyperlipidaemia

Gluconeogenesis

Gluconeogenesis is the generation of glucose from non-carbohydrate carbon substrates. It occurs primarily in the liver. The substrates are pyruvate, lactate, glycerol and a-keto acids (derived from amino acids).

In humans, the predominant precursors are lactate, glycerol, alanine and glutamine, which account for >90% of gluconeogenesis. These sources become important when liver glycogen is depleted, for example from strenuous exercise or prolonged fasting. The end product is adequate glucose for the brain and red blood cells, which rely on glucose as their energy source.

Drugs used to treat type 2 (insulin-resistant) diabetes target the gluconeogesis pathway. For example, metformin suppresses glucose production by the liver, increases insulin sensitivity and enhances peripheral uptake of glucose.

Gluconeogenesis pathway

The reactions are considered the reverse of glycolysis (**Table 4.9**). However, three steps of glycolysis are irreversible and must be overcome by distinct reactions:

■ step 1 (hexokinase)
■ step 3 (phosphofructokinse)
■ step 9 (pyruvate kinase)

Gluconeogenesis uses alternative reactions to make these steps. If the reactions were all reversible, gluconeogenesis would be considered highly endergonic. An endergonic reaction is an unfavourable reaction in terms of energy, because the reaction would require more energy to proceed than it would produce, resulting in an overall net loss of energy. In reverse, the steps of gluconeogesis are as follows.

Gluconeogenesis in nine steps				
Step	Reaction	Product(s)	Enzyme	Generates (+) or uses (-) ATP*
1	Carboxylation	Oxaloacetate	Pyruvate carboxylase	– ATP
2	Phosphorylation	Phosphoenolpyruvate	Phosphoenolpyruvate carboxykinase	– GTP
3	Hydration	2-Phosphoglycerate	Enolase	
4	Rearrangement	3-Phosphoglycerate	Phosphoglycerate mutase	
5	Phosphorylation	1,3-Bisphosphoglycerate	Phosphoglycerate kinase	
6	Conversion	Dihydroxyacetone phosphate + glyceraldehyde 3-phosphate	Glyceraldehyde 3-phosphate dehydrogenase	
		Fructose 1,6-bisphosphate	Triose phosphate isomerase	
7	Conversion	Fructose 6-phosphate	Fructose 1,6-bisphosphatase	- ATP
8	Conversion	Glucose 6-phosphate	Phosphoglucoisomerase	
9	Dephosphorylation	Glucose		

ATP, adenosine triphosphate; GTP, guanosine triphosphate.
*Per molecule of pyruvate (four ATP and two GTP molecules overall).

Table 4.9 Summary of gluconeogenesis

Step 1: conversion of pyruvate to phosphoenolpyruvic acid

This is a two-step process in which pyruvate carboxylase catalyses the carboxylation of pyruvate to form oxaloacetate. This reaction requires ATP to proceed.

Pyruvate carboxylase is present in mitochondria. Oxaloacetate is subsequently decarboxylated and phosphorylated to produce phosphoenolpyruvate, using GTP and the enzyme phosphoenolpyruvate carboxykinase.

There is an intermediate step in these two reactions, because oxaloacetate cannot cross the mitochondrial membrane. Oxaloacetate is converted into malate (in a reduction reaction using NADH) by malate dehydrogenase, which can pass through the membrane into the cytoplasm, where it is converted back to oxaloacetate (through oxidation, using NAD^+), again by malate dehydrogenase.

Steps 2–7: glycolysis reversal

The next six steps are the exact reversal of glycolysis, catalysed by enolase, phosphoglycerate mutase, phosphoglycerate kinase, glyceraldehyde 3-phosphate dehydrogenase, triosephosphate isomerase and aldolase (see **Table 4.9**).

Step 7: fructose 6-phosphate

Fructose 1,6-bisphosphatase converts fructose 1,6-bisphosphate to fructose 6-phosphate. The reaction uses one molecule of water and produces phosphate. This step is the rate-limiting step of gluconeogenesis. This is in contrast to glycoslysis, in which fructose 6-phosphate is converted to fructose 1,6-bisphosphate by phosphofructokinase-1.

Step 8: glucose 6-phosphate

Phosphoglucoisomerase converts fructose 6-phosphate into glucose 6-phosphate, which is then used in other metabolic pathways or continue through gluconeogenesis.

Step 9: glucose

The final stage of the pathway is dephosphorylation of glucose 6-phosphate into free glucose and an inorganic phosphate. Glucose 6-phosphate cannot be transported out of the cell until this dephosphorylation occurs.

This step is not a reversal of the start of glycolysis, in which glucose and ATP are converted into glucose 6-phosphate by hexokinase.

Control of gluconeogenesis

The three steps in the gluconeogenesis pathway (see page 119) are the regulatory stages in the control of gluconeogenesis. In glycolysis, the enzyme pyruvate kinase is replaced by phosphoenolpyruvate carboxykinase, phosphofructokinase by fructose 1,6-bisphosphatase, and hexokinase by glucose 6-phosphatase. These three key steps are vital in energy conservation, because:

- when excess energy is available, gluconeogenesis is inhibited
- when energy is required, the pathway will be activated

By having these three regulatory steps, the process of gluconeogenesis goes from an energonic pathway to an exergonic pathway that can occur spontaneously:

$$2\,\text{pyruvates} + 4\,\text{ATP} + 2\,\text{GTP} + 2\,\text{NADH} + 4\,H_2O$$
$$\downarrow$$
$$\text{glucose} + 4\,\text{ADP} + 2\,\text{GDP} + 6\,\text{Pi} + 2\,\text{NAD}^+ + 2\,H^+$$

These key regulation steps ensure that glycolysis and gluconeogenesis are coordinated so that only one pathway is active when required. If both directions were active, then the overall net result would be hydrolysis of two ATP molecules and two GTP molecules per cycle.

Other fuels: fructose and galactose

Fructose and galactose are sugars that provide a source of glucose, independently of glycogenolysis and gluconeogenesis.

Fructose

Fructose (**Figure 4.17**) is in honey, fruit and root vegetables, and is absorbed directly into the bloodstream after digestion. It is one of the three main dietary monosaccharides, along with glucose and galactose. Combined with glucose, it forms sucrose, the disaccharide of common table sugar.

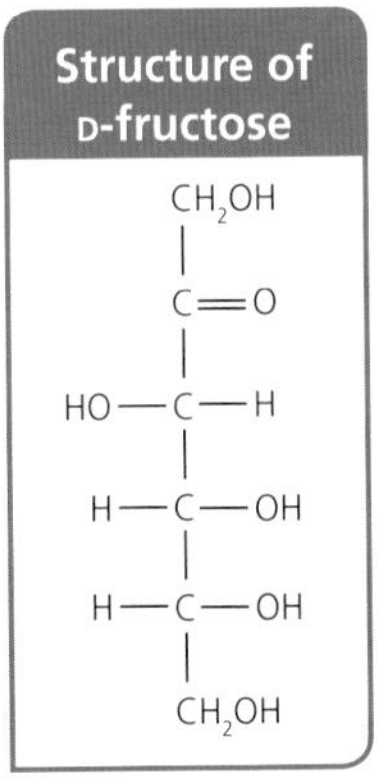

Unlike glucose, insulin is not needed for fructose to enter cells. Instead, it enters cells by facilitated diffusion (glucose transporter 5 GLUT5).

Glycolytic pathway

Fructose enters the glycolytic pathway (see page 104) through two routes.

- Fructose is converted to fructose 1-phosphate by fructokinase in the liver; fructose 1-phosphate is then split into dihydroxyacetone phosphate and glyceraldehyde by fructose 1-phosphate aldolase, and both molecules are converted into glyceraldehyde 3-phosphate
- Fructose in converted to fructose 6-phosphate by hexokinase in muscle and adipose tissue

Fructose is metabolised, predominantly in the liver, by the first of these pathways. The glyceraldehyde 3-phosphate is then used to replenish liver glycogen stores or for triglyceride synthesis.

Structure of D-fructose

CH₂OH
|
C=O
|
HO—C—H
|
H—C—OH
|
H—C—OH
|
CH₂OH

Figure 4.17 The structure of D-fructose.

Fructose is converted to glycogen only in an energy-depleted state, as a ready store of glucose in the liver. It is usually converted into liver fat. This might explain why studies in the 1980s of fructose-based sweeteners showed that a high-fructose diet in patients with type 2 diabetes induces high levels of blood triglycerides. Increased triglyceride levels are associated with an increased risk of atheroma formation, heart disease and stroke.

Structure of D-galactose

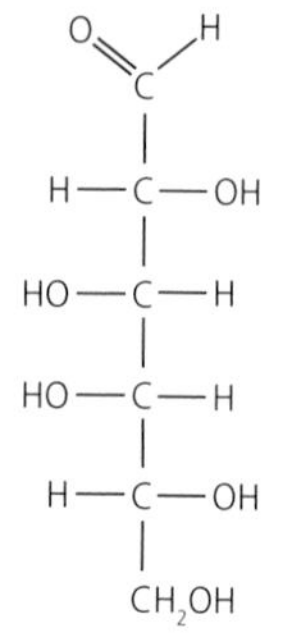

Figure 4.18 The structure of D-galactose.

Galactose

Galactose (**Figure 4.18**) is a monosaccharide. However, it is predominantly present as a disaccharide in milk (lactose) and a part of polysaccharide gums in plants.

When digested, galactose enters the circulation by cotransport with sodium, using the same transporter as glucose, i.e. glucose transporter-1.

The metabolic pathway of galactose has four steps.

1. Phosphorylation by galactokinase to form galactose-1-phosphate
2. Conversion of galactose 1-phosphate to glucose 1-phosphate through UDP-glucose
3. Conversion of glucose 1-phosphate to glucose 6-phosphate by phosphoglucomutase
4. Glucose 6-phosphate enters the glycolytic pathway (see page 104)

Answers to starter questions

1. Fructose enters glycolysis at the level of the triose phosphate intermediates. This is after the steps controlled by the regulatory enzymes hexokinase and phosphofructokinase-1. As these are the two rate limiting steps, fructose will provide a rapid source of energy in both aerobic and anaerobic cells.

2. The D and L forms of glucose are optical isomers – molecules with the same molecular formula but different chemical structures. D-glucose is the dietary form of glucose and is used as the ubiquitous fuel in metabolism. L-glucose does not occur naturally but can be synthesised. It is not used as a source of energy as hexokinase cannot phosphorylate glucose in the L form.

3. The brain almost exclusively uses glucose as its energy substrate, for example, consuming almost 75% of the liver's production. Other energy substrates such as free fatty acids are unable to cross the blood-brain barrier. The brain has large ATP energy requirements, which it needs to power the ion pumps that maintain membrane potentials so that neurons remain in their excitable state. ATP is also needed for neurotransmitter synthesis, release and uptake and intracellular transport.

4. Anaerobic respiration producing lactic acid is likely one mechanism causing muscle burn during intense exercise. As oxygen levels become inadequate and cells are unable use mitochondria to produce enough ATP, pyruvate is instead converted to lactate in order to generate NAD+ needed for glycolysis. Lactate is a weak

Answers *continued*

acid. However, increased metabolism of ATP also results in increased proton (i.e. acid) production and the increased carbon dioxide produced in cellular respiration contributes to a marginally lower pH. The nerves near the muscles sense the resulting acidic environment as a burning sensation.

5. Mitochondria are unique and essential organelles that produce most of the cell's energy. They do this by breaking down glucose and utilizing a high-energy electron passing along a system of 5 protein complexes in the inner membrane to generate an electrochemical gradient of protons across the membrane. As the protons finally pass down their gradient, through the ATP synthase enzyme, the electrochemical energy is converted to kinetic energy and then to chemical energy as ADP is phosphorylated to ATP. This means one molecule of glucose produces up to 38 molecules of ATP.

6. Cyanide compounds are poisonous because they bind to the iron atom in the enzyme cytochrome c oxidase, a component of the fourth complex of the electron transport system in the mitochondria. Binding of cyanide blocks the electron transport and prevents sufficient ATP production. Highly metabolic tissues like neurons and heart muscle are particularly sensitive to this lack of aerobic respiration. Death will occur within seconds.

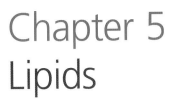

Chapter 5
Lipids

Starter questions

Answers to the following questions are on page 151.

1. Why is low-density lipoprotein (LDL) cholesterol 'bad' for you?
2. What does fat 'saturation' mean and why is it important?
3. How are lipids used as an energy source?
4. Why is it so biologically important that lipids are hydrophobic?
5. Why do steroids make good hormones?

Introduction

Lipids are molecules consisting of carbon, hydrogen and oxygen, principally linked by non-polar carbon–hydrogen (C–H) bonds. Their general lack of polarity is what makes lipids generally insoluble in water, whereas their polar hydrophilic head group makes them soluble in organic solvents.

However, some lipids also contain polar groups, such as sialic, phosphoryl, amino, sulfuryl and hydroxyl groups. These groups make these lipid molecules amphipathic by conferring both polar, soluble, water-loving (hydrophilic) and non-polar, fat-loving (lipophilic) properties. This combination of properties gives these lipids important functions in biology, for example the structure and function of membranes are attributable to the amphipathic nature of phospholipids.

Lipids are diverse in structure and function but have four main roles in the body. They:

- are the principle component of biological membranes
- provide an energy reserve when stored as body fat
- are used as hormones in cell signalling
- solubilise and transport other lipids and fat-soluble vitamins

Lipids are derived from the diet and are synthesised de novo. Exact concentrations vary considerably from person to person. When hydrolysed, lipids typically yield fatty acids, complex alcohols or both, which serve as an important substrate for the generation of energy.

Case 4 Tiredness and tingling fingers

Presentation

Rachel Morrison, aged 65 years, visits her general practitioner because she has been tired and generally unwell, with a tingling feeling in her fingers. He requests a number of routine biochemistry blood tests, as well as measurements of urea and electrolytes and thyroid function tests.

Analysis

The most likely cause of her symptoms is hypocalcaemia, a common metabolic cause of tingling in fingers and toes because low calcium causes neuromuscular irritability as it lowers the threshold for membrane depolarisation. Differential diagnoses are vitamin D deficiency, poor nutrition, chronic kidney disease and hypoparathyroidism.

Blood tests are requested to investigate these further. Her very low total 25-hydroxyvitamin D is evidence of severe vitamin D deficiency. Results also show marked hypocalcaemia (low serum calcium) and hypophosphataemia (low serum phosphate). The increased PTH is an appropriate response to hypocalcaemia (secondary hyperparathyroidism). The results for urea and electrolytes and thyroid function are unremarkable.

Blood test results

Concentration	Result	Reference range
Adjusted calcium (mmol/L)	1.75	2.2–2.6
Inorganic phosphate (mmol/L)	0.36	0.7–1.4
Total 25-hydroxyvitamin D (nmol/L)	8	>75
Parathyroid hormone (pmol/L)	36	1.2–6.9
Magnesium (mmol/L)	0.71	0.7–1.0

Table 5.1 Blood test results for a woman presenting with tiredness and tingling fingers

Together, these results suggest vitamin D deficiency has resulted in reduced intestinal calcium and phosphate reabsorption, and that PTH release has increased as a consequence of this to promote calcium reabsorption in the kidney and the formation of 1,25-dihydroxyvitamin D, which is responsible for calcium and phosphate reabsorption in the gut.

Further case

Rachel is referred for a dual-energy X-ray absorptiometry (DEXA) scan. DEXA is an imaging technique that uses X-rays to measure bone density. The results show that her lumbar spine lacks density, with an age-matched T-score of –1.7 (**Figure 5.1**).

Based on the T-score, the diagnosis is osteopenia of the lumbar spine. Rachel is admitted immediately to hospital for intravenous replacement of calcium using calcium gluconate.

Further analysis

The results of a DEXA scan are interpreted as follows.

- Bone mineral density is measured in grams per square centimetre of bone: a score of +1.0 or above is good
- The T-score compares the patient's bone mineral density with that of women in their thirties, the peak years for bone density
  - A T-score between +1 to –1 shows normal bone mineral density
  - A T-score between –1 and –2.5 indicates osteopenia
  - A T-score less than –2.5 indicates osteoporosis
- The Z-score compares the patient's bone mineral density with that of other people of the same gender and age

Case 4 *continued*

Hypocalcaemia: pathophysiology

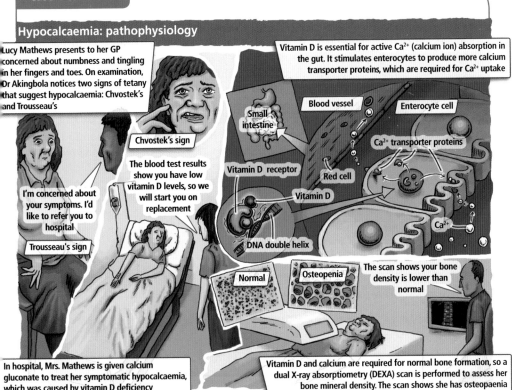

Lucy Mathews presents to her GP concerned about numbness and tingling in her fingers and toes. On examination, Dr Akingbola notices two signs of tetany that suggest hypocalcaemia: Chvostek's and Trousseau's

Chvostek's sign

I'm concerned about your symptoms. I'd like to refer you to hospital

Trousseau's sign

The blood test results show you have low vitamin D levels, so we will start you on replacement

Vitamin D is essential for active Ca^{2+} (calcium ion) absorption in the gut. It stimulates enterocytes to produce more calcium transporter proteins, which are required for Ca^{2+} uptake

Small intestine

Blood vessel

Enterocyte cell

Ca^{2+} transporter proteins

Vitamin D receptor

Red cell

Vitamin D

Ca^{2+}

DNA double helix

Normal

Osteopenia

The scan shows your bone density is lower than normal

In hospital, Mrs. Mathews is given calcium gluconate to treat her symptomatic hypocalcaemia, which was caused by vitamin D deficiency

Vitamin D and calcium are required for normal bone formation, so a dual X-ray absorptiometry (DEXA) scan is performed to assess her bone mineral density. The scan shows she has osteopaenia

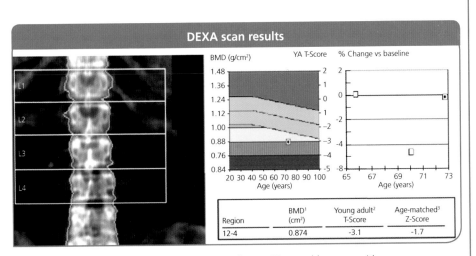

DEXA scan results

BMD (g/cm^2) YA T-Score   % Change vs baseline

Region	BMD[1] (cm^2)	Young adult[2] T-Score	Age-matched[3] Z-Score
12-4	0.874	-3.1	-1.7

Figure 5.1 Dual-energy X-ray absorptiometry scan from a 65-year-old woman with severe hypocalcaemia and hypophosphataemia, as well as low vitamin D levels. BMD, bone mineral density.

Case 4 *continued*

Patients with vitamin D deficiency are generally not given phosphate replacement, because phosphate absorption improves secondary to correction of the vitamin D and therefore the calcitriol 1,25-dihydroxyvitamin D. Rachel is started on oral vitamin D replacement.

Vitamin D is converted in the liver to 25-hydroxyvitamin D and then in the kidneys to its active form, 1,25-dihydroxyvitamin D (**Figure 5.2**). This activated form is responsible for the reabsorption of calcium and phosphate in the gut.

In Rachel's case, the low level of vitamin D stores (25-hydroxyvitamin D) has led to a low level of the activated form of vitamin D, so her body is unable to reabsorb calcium and phosphate in the gut. The vitamin D deficiency has also contributed to her osteoporosis.

> **Vitamin D deficiency affects more than half the population of the UK.** Their vitamin D levels are insufficient because of the limited amount of sunlight and inadequate dietary intake.

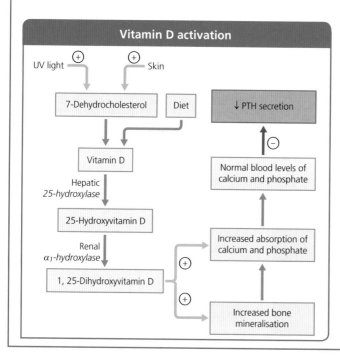

Figure 5.2 Conversion of vitamin D into its activated form, 1,25-dihydroxyvitamin D.

Lipid structures

Lipids are a group of substances with diverse chemical structures and functions. They are categorised as:

- steroids (cholesterol)
- fatty acids (saturated and polyunsaturated)
- storage lipids (acylglycerols)
- membrane lipids (glycerophospholipids and sphingolipids)
- prostaglandins
- terpenes

Steroids

Cholesterol is the major sterol in humans and is present in all body cells and many fluids, mostly in its free form. It is a major component of cell membrane structures, where it is often esterified with a fatty acid. Cholesterol forms the basis of a number of very important molecules, including fat-soluble vitamins (vitamins A, D, E and K) and steroid hormones.

Fatty acids

Fatty acids are hydrocarbon molecules with a carboxylic acid moiety at one end. Those related to human nutrition have a long chain of 12–20 carbons. Fatty acids are classified according to whether they are saturated or not:

- saturated: no double bonds
- monounsaturated: one double bond
- polyunsaturated: multiple double bonds

In the blood, fatty acids are in their free form, bound to albumin or in an esterified form, e.g. triglycerides.

Storage lipids

Acylglycerols (glycerol esters) are storage lipids. They contain a glycerol backbone with a fatty acid attached. The class of acylglycerol is determined by the number of fatty acids attached, e.g. one fatty acid produces monacylglycerol and three triacylglycerol (more commonly known as triglycerides). Triglycerides make up 95% of tissue storage fat and are the main form of glycerol esters found in the plasma.

Membrane lipids

Phospholipids are referred to as membrane lipids because they are the principal component of biological membranes. They are divided into glycerophospholipids and sphingolipids. The fatty acid in glycerophospholipids and sphingolipids usually contains an even number of carbon atoms (14–24). In humans, the fatty acids are unbranched and are saturated or unsaturated.

Sphingolipids are derived from the amino alcohol sphingosine. Ceramide is formed by attaching a fatty acid, containing 18 or more carbon atoms to the amino group through an amide linkage. Ceramide is an important intermediate for the synthesis of sphingomyelin, galactosylceramide and glycosylceramide.

Glycerophospholipids are derived from phosphatidic acid. This basic structure is a phosphatidate, with a glycerol backbone to which two fatty acids and a phosphoric acid are attached as esters.

Prostaglandins

Prostaglandins are derived from fatty acids, mainly arachidonate. They are a series of unsaturated fatty acids containing a cyclopentane ring. Sixteen naturally occurring prostaglandins have been described, but only seven are found frequently in the body (primary prostaglandins).

Terpenes

Terpenes are a polymer of a five carbon isoprene unit. Examples include vitamins A, E and K, and dolichols. Dolichols are key to the glycation of proteins.

Lipolysis

Fats are broken down by lipolysis, which is a form of hydrolysis (see page 29). Lipolysis occurs in adipose and muscle tissue when an increase in energy is required.

The first step in the utilisation of fat as an energy store is the hydrolysis of triglyceride, which forms the principal fat storage molecule in the body. They are a highly concentrated energy source as they are anhydrous and reduced. Lipolysis has three steps:

1. triglyceride hydrolysis by lipases
2. fatty acid linkage to coenzyme A (CoA)
3. transport of long chain fatty acids into the mitochondrial matrix by carnitine

The products of lipolysis are fatty acids and glycerol. Fatty acids undergo fatty acid oxidation in the mitochondria, and glycerol is involved in gluconeogenesis and glycolysis in the liver (see Chapter 4).

Hydrolysis by cyclic AMP–mediated lipases

Triglyceride of adipose tissue is hydrolysed by lipase to yield glycerol and fatty acids (**Figure 5.3**). This in response to fasting, exercise and stress.

Glycerol is then phosphorylated to glycerol 3-phosphate before being oxidised to dihydroxyacetone phosphate. Dihydroxyacetone phosphate, in turn, interconverts to glyceraldehyde 3-phosphate.

> **Triglycerides are present in blood and their measurement is important in the detection and management of disease.** Automated analysers carry out a series of reactions to measure their concentration.
>
> 1. Hydrolysis of triglycerides to glycerol
> 2. Phosphorylation of glycerol to glycerophosphate
> 3. Oxidation of glycerophosphate to dihydroxyacetone phosphate and hydrogen peroxide
> 4. Reaction between the hydrogen peroxide and 4-aminophenazone and 4-chlorophenol, under the catalytic action of peroxidase, to form a red dye
>
> Spectrometry is then used to determine the amount of red dye by measuring absorbance at a wavelength of 505 nm. From this measurement, the concentration of triglycerides is calculated.

Link to glycolysis

Glyceraldehyde-3-phosphate is a key intermediate in the glycolytic pathway and is also a gluconeogenic precursor. This means that it can be converted to either pyruvate or glucose in the liver (see page 103).

Fatty acid linkage to coenzyme A

For fatty acids to be oxidised in the mitochondrial matrix and used to generate energy, they must first be activated; this occurs through the formation of a thioester linkage to co-enzyme A in a two-step reaction:

Step 1: fatty acid + ATP → acyl adenylate + pyrophosphate

Step 2: acyl adenylate + CoASH → acyl CoA + AMP

In the first step the fatty acid reacts with ATP to form acyl adenylate. This is catalysed by acyl CoA synthetase in the outer mitochondrial membrane. In the second step the sulphydryl group of co-enzyme A attacks acyl adenylate to form acyl CoA and adenosine monophosphate (AMP) and CoASH.

The ATP generates a thioester link between a carboxyl group of a fatty acid and the sulfhydryl group of CoA. Acyl CoA synthetase catalyses this reaction in the outer mitochondrial membrane.

During these reactions, two high-energy bonds are consumed and one is formed; this makes the reaction irreversible, because two molecules of ATP are hydrolysed and only one high transfer potential compound is formed. This irreversibility means that acyl-

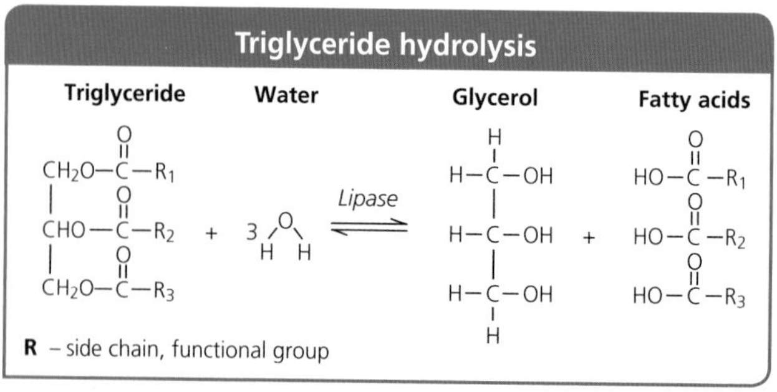

Figure 5.3 Hydrolysis of triglyceride by lipase.

Triglyceride hydrolysis

R – side chain, functional group

CoA can transverse the mitochondrial membrane.

Transport of long chain fatty acids into the mitochondrial matrix

Long chain fatty acids are those with more than 10 carbon atoms. Unlike short- and medium-chain fatty acids, they cannot readily cross the inner mitochondrial membrane to the matrix, where they are oxidised. Therefore a special transport mechanism using the nitrogenous cation carnitine is required (**Figure 5.4**); it has the following steps.

1. Fatty acid activation: free fatty acid in cytosol is bound to CoA to form acyl CoA
2. Transfer: acyl CoA combines with carnitine to form acylcarnitine, in a reaction catalysed by acyltransferase-1
3. Transport: acylcarnitine is transported across the inner mitochondrial membrane by carnitine–acylcarnitine translocase; the acyl group is transferred back to the CoA on the matrix side of the membrane in a reaction catalysed by carnitine acyltransferase-2
4. Reset: carnitine moves from the matrix to the cytosolic side of the mitochondria in exchange for acylcarnitine

This carnitine transporter system across the inner mitochondrial membrane is the rate-limiting step in fatty acid oxidation.

> **Primary carnitine deficiency is a genetic disorder of the cellular carnitine transporter system.** This condition affects 1 in 100,000 newborn babies. Affected individuals cannot utilise fats for energy, especially during fasting.
>
> Primary carnitine deficiency usually manifests itself by 5 years of age with cardiomyopathy, skeletal muscle weakness and hypoglycemia.

Regulation of lipolysis

Lipolysis is regulated through the control of lipase activity.

Lipase is activated by the hormones adrenaline and glucagon.

These hormones activate lipase through a chain of reactions (**Figure 5.5**). They are counter regulatory hormones that are released when there are inadequate energy reserves and during stress.

1. First, they increase adenylate cyclase activity
2. They then increase cyclic adenosine monophosphate (AMP) concentration

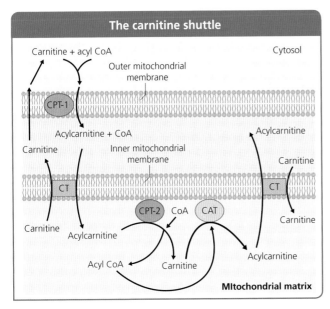

The carnitine shuttle

Carnitine + acyl CoA — Cytosol

Outer mitochondrial membrane

CPT-1

Acylcarnitine + CoA — Acylcarnitine

Carnitine — Inner mitochondrial membrane — Carnitine

CT — CT

CPT-2 CoA CAT — Carnitine

Carnitine — Acylcarnitine

Acyl CoA — Carnitine — Acylcarnitine

MItochondrial matrix

Figure 5.4 The carnitine shuttle: the transmembrane transport of fatty acids into the mitochondrial matrix. CAT, carnitine acyltransferase; CoA, coenzyme A; CPT-1, carnitine acyltransferase-1; CPT-2, carnitine acyltransferase-2; CT, carnitine–acylcarnitine translocase.

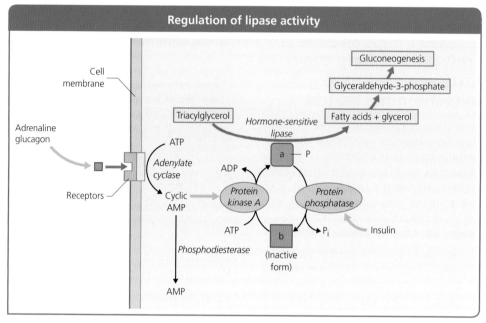

Regulation of lipase activity

Figure 5.5 Regulation of lipase activity.

3. They activate protein kinase A
4. Last, they phosphorylate, and thus activate, lipase

Conversely, lipase is inhibited by insulin, which activates a protein phosphatase enzyme. This dephophorylates the lipoprotein lipase enzyme thus inactivating it. Insulin is released when adequate energy is available from carbohydrate reserves.

β-oxidation

β-Oxidation is a metabolic process in which fatty acids are broken down in the mitochondria to generate acetyl CoA, NADH and $FADH_2$. The former enters the citric acid cycle and the latter act as cofactors in the electron transport chain. It is referred to β-oxidation as oxidation occurs on the β carbon atom. Fatty acids, attached to CoA as acyl CoA, undergo β-oxidation in mitochondria.

This process is a cycle of four reactions (**Figure 5.6**).

1. Oxidation of acyl CoA
2. Hydration of 2-enoyl CoA
3. Oxidation of 3-hydroxy acyl CoA
4. Thiolytic cleavage of 3-keto acyl CoA

The oxidation of acyl CoA to 2-enoyl CoA is catalysed by acyl CoA dehydrogenase and requires flavin adenine dinucleotide in its oxidised form, FAD^+. The reduced form, $FADH_2$, is generated, and the electrons from the prosthetic group of $FADH_2$ are transferred to another flavoprotein, called electron-transferring flavoprotein. This then donates electrons to an electron-transferring flavoprotein called ubiquinone reductase. This leads to the reduction of ubiquinone to ubiquinol and results in the delivery of high-potential electrons to a second proton-pumping site in the respiratory chain. Overall, two ATP are generated per molecule of $FADH_2$.

The hydration of 2-enoyl CoA to 3-hydroxy acyl CoA is catalysed by a stereospecific enzyme called enoyl CoA hydratase, which uses only L-isomers of 2-enoyl CoA as substrates.

The oxidation of 3-hydroxy acyl CoA to 3-keto acyl CoA is catalysed by L-3-hydroxy CoA dehydrogenase. This reaction requires nicotinamide adenine dinucleotide in its oxidised form, NAD^+, and generates the reduced form, NADH. Three molecules of ATP

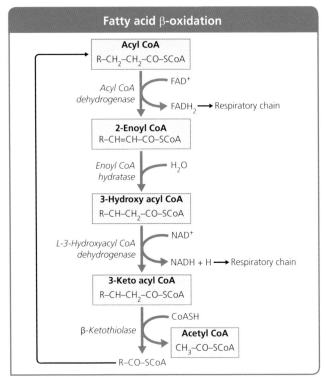

Fatty acid β-oxidation

Figure 5.6 Fatty acid β-oxidation. CoASH, coenzyme A (reduced form); FAD⁺, flavin adenine dinucleotide (oxidised form); FADH₂, flavin adenine dinucleotide (reduced form); NAD⁺, nicotinamide adenine dinucleotide (oxidised form); NADH, nicotinamide adenine dinucleotide (reduced form).

are generated per molecule of NADH, in the electron transport chain in the mitchondria.

Thiolytic cleavage of 3-keto acyl CoA to acetyl CoA is catalysed by β-ketothiolase. This reaction requires CoASH.

In each cycle, the fatty acyl is shortened by two carbon atoms, and FADH₂, NADH and acetyl CoA are generated. Each step in the four-step reaction is catalysed by an enzyme that is specific for the chain length of the acyl CoA. For example, medium-chain acyl CoA dehydrogenase oxidises fatty acyl chains with 4–14 carbons.

> **Saturated fatty acids have no carbon–carbon double bonds; the carbons are 'saturated' with the maximum number of hydrogen atoms.** Monounsaturated fatty acids have one carbon–carbon double bond, and polyunsaturated fatty acids have more than one.

β-oxidation of unsaturated fatty acids

The oxidation of unsaturated fatty acids requires two additional enzymes, an isomerase and a reductase, because they contain double bonds. Monounsaturated fatty acids contain a single carbon–carbon double bond and require an isomerase to shift the position of the double bond so it is a substrate for acyl CoA dehydrogenase. Polyunsaturated fatty acids have multiple double bonds and also require a reducatase enzyme to generate a substrate that can be acted on by enoyl CoA.

Monounsaturated fatty acids

Palmitate is a monounsaturated, 16-carbon fatty acid with a double bond between carbons 9 and 10 (**Figure 5.7**). It is transported into the mitochondria in the same way as saturated fatty acids, and undergoes three cycles of degradation, in the same way that saturated

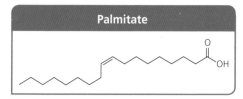

Figure 5.7 Structure of palmitate.

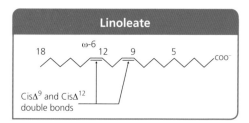

Figure 5.8 Structure of linoleate and the position of double bonds.

fatty acids do. However, in the 3rd round, *cis*-Δ^3-enoyl CoA is formed and is not a substrate for acyl CoA dehydrogenase. An isomerase enzyme resolves this issue, because it converts the *cis*-Δ^3 double bond in a *trans*-Δ^2-enoyl CoA, which is a suitable substrate for acyl CoA dehydrogenase. The reactions following this are the same as those for regular saturated fatty acids.

Polyunsaturated fatty acids

Linoleate is a polyunsaturated fatty acid with *cis*-Δ^9 and *cis*-Δ^{12} double bonds (**Figure 5.8**). After three rounds of β-oxidation, a *cis*-Δ^3 double bond is formed; this is converted to a trans double bond by an isomerase enzyme. The *cis*-Δ^{12} double bond poses an additional problem and after four rounds of β-oxidation forms a *cis*-Δ^4 double bond.

This molecule undergoes dehydrogenation to form a 2,4-dienoyl CoA intermediate. However, this substrate is not compatible with the next enzyme in the β-oxidation pathway. This incompatibility is resolved by the action of a 2,4-dienoyl CoA reductase enzyme. This reduced nicotinamide adenine dinucleotide phosphate (NADPH)-dependent enzyme converts the dienoyl intermediate to a *cis*-Δ^3-enoyl CoA, which is a substrate for the isomerase enzyme discussed earlier. The isomerase enzyme converts this intermediate to the trans form, which allows the substrate to continue through the β-oxidation.

β-oxidation of odd-chain fatty acids

Odd-chain fatty acids are those with an odd number of carbon atoms. Their lipolysis generates one molecule of propionyl CoA and one molecule of acetyl CoA. Normally, two molecules of acetyl CoA are generated.

The propionyl CoA formed enters the citric acid cycle and is converted to succinyl CoA. This is also a metabolite produced when amino acids are oxidised (see page 90).

> **Medium-chain acyl CoA dehydrogenase deficiency is a genetic defect in the enzyme that metabolises medium-chain fatty acids.** It has a prevalence of 1 in 4000–17,000, appears by early childhood and is often triggered by fasting or illness. Symptoms include vomiting, lethargy and hypoketotic hypoglycaemia (a low blood concentration of ketones and glucose). Patients are at risk of seizures, breathing difficulties, liver problems, brain damage, coma and sudden death.

Peroxisomal β-oxidation of fatty acids

As well as occurring in the matrix of mitochondria, fatty acid oxidation occurs in peroxisomes, which are small cellular organelles responsible for the breakdown of very long chain and branched chain fatty acids, polyamines, amino acids and the biosynthesis of plasmalogens. Peroxisomal oxidation occurs when a fat-rich diet is eaten and after the administration of lipid-lowering drugs (e.g. fibrates).

Peroxisomes are responsible for the oxidation of fatty acids that are too long to enter mitochondria, and therefore serve to provide a substrate for beta-oxidation. Once they are oxidised down to the 10-carbon octanoyl CoA, they can move to the mitochondria for further oxidation.

Peroxisomal versus mitochondrial β-oxidation

Peroxisomal oxidation involves specific enzymes present only in peroxisomes. Unlike mitochondrial oxidation, it is not coupled to ATP synthesis. Instead, the high-potential electrons are transferred to oxygen, which generates hydrogen peroxide, a potentially destructive reactive oxygen species. Catalase, an enzyme exclusive to peroxisomes, breaks the hydrogen peroxide down into water and oxygen.

Zellweger's syndrome is one of four rare inherited disorders of peroxisomal biosynthesis. These are caused by defects in any one of the 13 *PEX* genes required for normal peroxisome function. Symptoms include:

- hepatomegaly
- characteristic facial features of high forehead, underdeveloped eyebrow ridges, and wide-set eyes
- intellectual disability
- seizures
- lack of muscle tone in infants; also, they are usually not be able to suck or swallow

Lipogenesis

Lipogenesis is the synthesis of lipids.

Fatty acids synthesis occurs in several tissues, principally in the liver and adipose tissue. Due to today's healthier Western diet fatty acid synthesis is not often required. There are, however, instances where it is essential, for example, embryonic development and during lactation in the mammary gland.

Fatty acid synthesis has four main stages.

1. Formation of acetyl CoA and the citrate shuttle
2. Formation of malonyl CoA
3. Formation of malonyltransferase by fatty acid synthatase using acetyl CoA or malonyl CoA as a substrate
4. The fatty acid elongation cycle

Palmitate is the most common fatty acid in the body. It is also the first fatty acid synthesised during lipogenesis. At physiological pH, it exists as the anion palmitate, dissociated from its H^+ ion.

Formation of acetyl coenzyme A

Fatty acids are synthesised in the cytoplasm from acetyl CoA, which itself is generated from pyruvate by the action of pyruvate dehydrogenase (see page 110), and by mitochondrial β-oxidation of fatty acids. Because synthesis occurs in the cytoplasm, the first step is for acetyl CoA to be transported from mitochondria to the cytoplasm by the citrate shuttle. This consists of three steps:

1. Acetyl CoA reacts with oxaloacetate to form citrate
2. Tricarboxylate translocase transports citrate to the cytosol
3. Citrate is cleaved back to oxaloacetate and acetyl CoA in the cytosol; this reaction is catalysed by an ATP-dependent enzyme called ATP-citrate lyase

One NADPH is generated for every molecule of acetyl CoA transported from a mitochondrion to the cytosol. This means that 8 NADPH are produced to generate one molecule of palmitate. However, the process requires 14 NADPH as reducing agents; the remaining 6 are provided by the pentose phosphate pathway (see page 107).

NADPH is an important cofactor required for biosynthetic (i.e. anabolic) reactions in cells. It is used as a reducing agent, i.e. it reduces chemicals by facilitating the transfer of electrons. It also protects against reactive oxygen species through its role in oxidation-reduction reactions, allowing the regeneration of glutathione. In addition NADPH is responsible for generating free radicals to help destroy pathogens in the immune system.

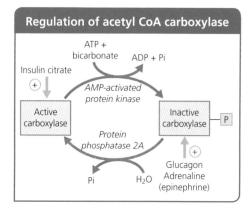

Figure 5.9 Regulation of acetyl coenzyme A carboxylase activity. +, activates; P, phosphate; Pi, inorganic phosphate.

Formation of malonyl coenzyme A

Some acetyl CoA is carboxylated to form malonyl CoA in an irreversible two-step reaction that requires bicarbonate and ATP. It is a commitment step in fatty acid synthesis, because forming fatty acids is the only function of malonyl CoA.

Both steps in the formation of malonyl coenzyme A are catalysed by acetyl CoA carboxylase, a biotin-dependent enzyme.

1. Acetyl CoA is converted to carboxybiotin; one ATP is used
2. The carboxyl group is transferred from the biotin to the acetyl CoA to form malonyl CoA

Biotin is a water soluble B vitamin (B7) and important for carboxylase catalysed reactions.

Regulation of fatty acid metabolism

Fatty acid metabolism is predominately regulated by the action of hormones on acetyl CoA carboxylase, because its activity is affected by hormones (**Figure 5.9**).

■ Adrenaline and glucagon inactivate the acetyl CoA carboxylase activity. This occurs when energy is required
■ Insulin inhibits acetyl CoA carboxylase where there is a not a requirement for energy

Acetyl CoA carboxylase activity is also affected by the availability of citrate, AMP and palmitoyl CoA in the cell. Citrate activates it, whereas AMP and palmitoyl CoA inhibit its activity.

Acetyl coenzyme A carboxylase phosphorylation

The enzyme is controlled by its phosphorylation state: activity is switched off by phosphorylation by an activated AMP protein kinase, and switched on by the removal of the phosphate group by protein phosphatase 2A.

Fibric acid derivatives (fibrates) are used as drugs to lower triglyceride concentration. They:

■ induce gene expression of lipolytic enzymes such as lipoprotein lipase
■ decrease the expression of apolipoprotein C3, a protein that inhibits lipoprotein lipase
■ promote a shift towards larger, more buoyant low-density lipoprotein (LDL) particles that are less susceptible to oxidation and have increased affinity for the LDL receptor

Formation of malonyltransferase

Fatty acid synthetase is a multienzyme protein that synthesises palmitate from either acyl CoA or malonyl CoA. The first step is the formation of malonyltransferase.

This enzyme has three domains.

1. The first domain is where the substrate enters, and contains three enzymes: acetyl transferase, malonyltransferase and β-ketoacyl synthase (collectively referred to as a condensing enzyme)
2. The second domain is the reduction unit, which contains an acyl carrier protein and three enzymes (β-keto acylreductase, dehydratase and enoylreductase)
3. The third domain is the palmitate release unit, which contains the enzyme thioesterase

Fatty acid synthetase activity

Fatty acid biosynthesis begins when the acetyl group of acetyl CoA attaches to the oxygen atom on the side chain of the serine molecule in the active site of acetyl transferase. Malonyl CoA attaches to the active site of malonyltransferase in the same way. These reactions occur in domain 1 of fatty acid synthetase.

The acetyl unit is then transferred to the cysteine sulphur group in the active site of the condensing enzyme. The malonyl group is transferred to the sulphur atom of the phosphopantetheinyl group of the acyl carrier protein of the other chain in the dimer. Both chains in the dimer of domain 1 interact with domains 2 and 3.

The fatty acid elongation cycle

The fatty acid elongation cycle is the last stage of fatty acid synthesis.

Condensation

Elongation begins when the acetyl unit of the condensing enzyme joins to the malonyl unit of the acyl carrier protein in a condensation reaction. Carbon dioxide is produced, and acetoacetyl-S-phosphopantetheinyl is formed on the acyl carrier protein.

Reduction

The active site of the sulfhydryl group on the condensing enzyme is regenerated after this initial reaction and is transported to domain 2, where it undergoes a series of enzymatic reactions. These include a reduction reaction to form a butyryl–acyl carrier protein unit.

This saturated unit then moves from the phosphopantetheinyl sulphur on the acyl carrier protein to the cysteine sulphur on the condensing enzyme. At this stage in the biochemical process, the synthase is ready for another cycle of elongation.

Hydrolysis

The next stage is joining of the butyryl unit on the condensing enzyme with a 2-carbon component of the malonyl unit of acyl carrier protein. This results in the formation of a 6-carbon unit on acyl carrier protein. Five more condensation and reduction reactions produce a palmitoyl unit. The palmitoyl unit is then hydrolysed by thioesterase to palmitate, on domain 3 of the opposite chain.

Further elongation and unsaturation

Palmitate is the starting point for the synthesis of other fatty acids. Longer chain fatty acids are formed by elongation reactions on the cytosolic face of the endoplasmic reticulum. Microsomes add two carbon units to the carbonyl end of saturated and unsaturated fatty acids; elongation of fatty acids is essential for the formation of a number of biological molecules including prostaglandins.

Unsaturation of fatty acids

Microsomal enzyme systems introduce double bonds into, i.e. 'unsaturate', long-chain acyl CoAs, such as in the conversion of stearoyl CoA to oleoyl CoA. The addition of a double bond alters the solubility of the fatty acid. This reaction is catalysed by an oxidase enzyme that introduces a cis-Δ^9 double bond and requires molecular oxygen and NADH. Three membrane-bound proteins catalyse this reaction: NADH cytochrome b_5 reductase, cytochrome b_5 and a desaturase.

The reaction begins when electrons are transferred from NADH to the FAD^{+80} moiety of the enzyme NADH cytochrome b_5 reductase. The next step involves the reduction of the haem iron atom of cytochrome b_5 to the ferrous state. This results in conversion of the non-haem iron atom of the desaturase enzyme from the ferric to the ferrous state. As a result, the ferrous atom interacts with oxygen and the saturated fatty acyl substrate, for example stearoyl CoA. A double bond is formed when two molecules of water are released.

In addition, two electrons from NADH and two from a single bond of the fatty acyl substrate are liberated. When stearoyl CoA is the substrate, oleoyl CoA is formed.

In mammals, unsaturated fatty acids are derived from either palmitoleate (double bond saturation C16:1), oleate (C18:1), linoleate (C18:2) or linolenate (C18:3). Mammals do not have the enzymes to introduce a double bond beyond carbon 9. Consequently, linoleate and linolenate are not be synthesised in mammals and are therefore essential fatty acids.

> **High blood triglyceride levels (hypertriglyceridaemia) can cause inflammation of the pancreas (pancreatitis).** This effect is probably the result of an excess of large, LDL particles called chylomicrons, which can obstruct capillaries and lead to local ischaemia and acidaemia.

Stoichiometry of fatty acid synthesis

There are two main reactions to consider in palmitate synthesis stoichiometry (calculation of the amounts of substances involved).

Reaction 1

The stochiometry of the synthesis of palmitate is:

$$\text{acetyl CoA} + 7\,\text{malonyl CoA} + 14\,\text{NADPH} + 20\text{H}^+$$
$$\downarrow$$
$$\text{palmitate} + 7\,CO_2 + 14\,\text{NADP}^+ + 8\,\text{CoA} + 6\,H_2O$$

Reaction 2

This is the synthesis of malonyl CoA required in reaction 1:

$$7\,\text{acetyl CoA} + 7\,CO_2 + 7\,\text{ATP}$$
$$\downarrow$$
$$7\,\text{malonyl CoA} + 7\,\text{ATP} + 7\,\text{Pi} + 14\,\text{H}^+$$

Overall reaction

The overall stochichiometry for the synthesis of palmitate is:

$$8\,\text{acetyl CoA} + 7\,\text{ATP} + 14\,\text{NADPH} + 6\,\text{H}^+$$
$$\downarrow$$
$$\text{palmitate} + 14\,\text{NADP}^+ + 8\,\text{CoA} + 6\,H_2O$$
$$+ 7\,\text{ADP} + 7\,\text{P}_i$$

The NADPH used in this reaction is derived from the pentose phosphate shunt (see page 107). In contrast, acetyl CoA can come from several reactions:

- fatty acid β-oxidation (see page 132)
- pyruvate dehydrogenase (see page 110)
- catabolism of ketogenic amino acids (see page 90)

Overall the synthesis of palmitate requires 8 molecules of acetyl CoA, 14 molecules of NADPH and 7 molecules of ATP.

Lipogenesis versus fatty acid β-oxidation

Lipogenesis and fatty acid β-oxidation are tightly coordinated but distinct biochemical processes (**Table 5.2**). The former relating to the synthesis of lipids and the latter the breakdown.

Prostaglandin synthesis

Arachidonate is a 20-carbon polyunsaturated fatty acid derived from linoleate. It forms the basis of the prostaglandins: prostacyclins, thromboxanes and leukotrienes (**Figure 5.10**). These locally acting hormones have a short half-life but are vital in stimulating the inflammatory response, regulating blood flow to specific organs, modulating ion transport across membranes and propagating synaptic transmission. The prostaglandins are also involved in the induction of sleep.

> **Aspirin (acetylsalicylate) decreases inflammation by inhibiting the activity of prostaglandin synthase.** It irreversibly inhibits the cyclo-oxygenase activity of this enzyme by acetylating the serine hydroxyl group. It is also an antithrombotic agent, because it blocks the production of prostaglandin A_2, a potent aggregator of blood platelets.

Fatty acid oxidation and synthesis		
Feature	Oxidation	Synthesis
Intracellular location	Mitochondria	Cytoplasm
Initial substrates	Fatty acyl CoA	Acetyl CoA or malonyl CoA
Thioester linkage of intermediates	CoASH	Protein-SH (acyl carrier protein)
Coenzymes	FAD^+ and NAD^+	NADPH
Bicarbonate dependence	No	Yes
Energy state favouring process	High ADP	High ATP
Citrate activation	No	Yes
Acyl CoA inhibition	No	Yes
Highest activity	Fasting or starvation	Fed

ATP, adenosine triphosphate; CoA, coenzyme A; CoASH, Acetyl coenzyme A; FAD^+, flavin adenine dinucleotide (oxidised form); NAD^+, nicotinamide adenine dinucleotide (oxidised form); NADPH, nicotinamide adenine dinucleotide phosphate (reduced form).

Table 5.2 Differences between fatty acid oxidation and synthesis

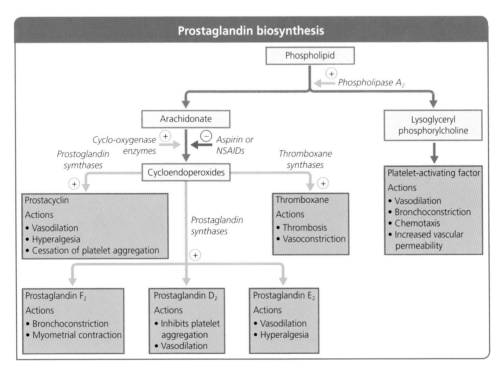

Figure 5.10 Prostaglandin biosynthesis and their actions. +, activates; –, inhibits; NSAID, non-steroidal anti-inflammatory drug.

Ketone body metabolism

Acetyl CoA produced from the β-oxidation of fatty acids has a number of potential fates; if fat and carbohydrate metabolism are balanced, it enters the citric acid cycle. This requires available oxaloacetate for the formation of citrate (see page 111). In a fasting state, oxaloacetate is diverted to facilitate the formation of glucose in the gluconeogenic pathway (see page 119). This causes acetyl CoA to enter another metabolic pathway to produce ketone bodies as an alternative source of fuel to glucose.

Ketone bodies are water soluble molecules produced by the liver from fatty acids during periods of fasting for cells to use as an energy source instead of glucose. The two main ketone bodies are acetoacetate and D-3-hydroxybutyrate.

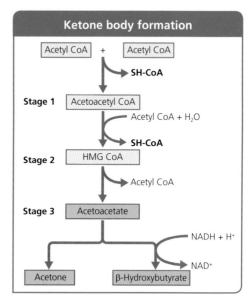

Figure 5.11 Stages of ketone body formation (ketone bodies are shown in green). HMG CoA, 3-hydroxy-3-methylglutaryl CoA.

Ketone body formation

Ketone bodies are formed in the liver in three stages of ketogenesis (**Figure 5.11**). The first stage is the condensation of two molecules of acetyl CoA to form acetoacetyl CoA. This reaction is catalysed by 3-ketothiolase in the reverse reaction to the final step in the β-oxidation pathway.

The second step involves a condensation reaction between acetoacetyl CoA and water and acetyl CoA to form 3-hydroxy-3-methylglutaryl CoA (HMG CoA) and CoA. In the final step, HMG CoA is cleaved to acetyl CoA and acetoacetate by HMG CoA lyase.

D-3-Hydroxybutyrate is formed from the reduction of acetoacetate in the mitochondrial matrix. The equilibrium of this reaction is governed by the ratio of NADH to NAD⁺. If NADH predominates, D-3-hydroxybutyrate will be formed preferentially.

> **Ketotic breath is the smell of acetone in the breath in patients with diabetic or alcoholic ketoacidosis.** It occurs as acetoacetate slowly and spontaneously decarboxylates to acetone, which gives the breath a smell of pear drops.

Ketone energy metabolism

Acetoacetate and D-3-hydroxybutyrate are mainly produced in the liver. They diffuse from the liver into the circulation and make a significant contribution to the energy metabolism of most cells, during fasting or carbohydrate restriction. They play a vital role in cellular respiration as an alternative fuel source to glucose.

Interestingly, acetoacetate is used preferentially to glucose by the heart and renal cortex. During periods of starvation and in diabetes mellitus, the brain adapts to use acetoacetate, and in prolonged starvation the brain derives about 75% of its energy from acetoacetate.

Acetoacetate is a transportable form of acetyl units and also regulates the process of lipolysis. High concentrations of acetoacetate in the blood indicate an abundance of acetyl units and act as a negative feedback mechanism to decrease lipolysis in adipose tissue.

In people with type 1 diabetes, when there is low or no insulin, the body converts to a fasting state to try to increase glucose levels.

■ There is an increase in counter-regulatory hormones, including adrenaline (epinephrine), noradrenaline (norepinephrine), cortisol and glucagon

■ This increases hepatic gluconeogenesis, glycogenolysis, and lipolysis, resulting in severe hyperglycaemia and increased serum concentration of free fatty acids

■ Fatty acids are metabolised by the liver to acidic metabolites, including acetone, D-3-hydroxybutyrate and acetoacetate (diabetic ketoacidosis)

Cholesterol metabolism

Cholesterol is a 27-carbon steroid that gives cell membranes their fluid characteristics, and is the precursor to a number of steroid hormones, including testosterone and cortisol (**Figure 5.12**), vitamin D and bile acids.

Cholesterol is consumed in the diet. It is also synthesised de novo in the liver and intestine. On average, 800 mg of cholesterol is synthesised daily in a person on a low-cholesterol diet.

Cholesterol synthesis

Cholesterol biosynthesis begins with formation of isopentenyl pyrophosphate from acetyl CoA (**Figure 5.13**). This set of reactions starts with the condensation of acetyl CoA with acetoacetyl CoA. The product of the reaction catalysed by HMG CoA reductase is HMG CoA.

Formation of mevalonate

3-Hydroxy-3-methylglutaryl CoA, which is present in the cytosol and mitochondria of the liver, is reduced to mevalonate by HMG CoA reductase. This reaction requires NADPH. The biosynthesis of mevalonate is regarded as the first committed step of cholesterol synthesis, because it is irreversible. Mevalonate is subsequently converted to isopentenyl pyrophosphate in a series of three reactions that require ATP.

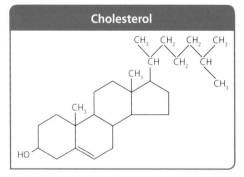

Cholesterol

Figure 5.12 Cholesterol.

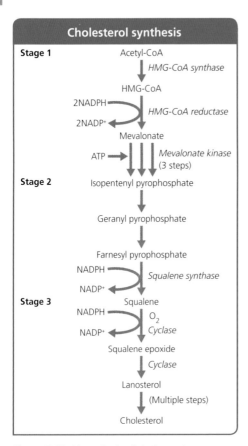

Figure 5.13 Biosynthesis of cholesterol.

Synthesis of squelene

The second stage of cholesterol synthesis is the synthesis of squalene from five molecules of isopentenyl pyrophosphate. This process starts with the isomerisation of isopentenyl pyrophosphate. This results in the formation of dimethylallyl pyrophosphate.

This isomeric compound then condenses to form a 10-carbon molecule, the allylic carbonium ion. The allylic carbonium ion then re-acts with another molecule of isopentenyl pyrophosphate to form geranyl pyrophosphate.

Next, geranyl pyrophosphate is converted to an allylic carbonium ion, which reacts with isopentyl pyrophosphate to form farnesyl pyrophosphate, a 15-carbon molecule. Two molecules of farnesyl pyrophosphate then undergo a reductive condensation, requiring NADPH to form squalene, a 30-carbon molecule.

Formation of squelene epoxide

The third stage of cholesterol biosynthesis begins with the cyclisation of squalene to form squalene epoxide. This reaction requires oxygen and NADPH. Squalene epoxide then undergoes cyclisation to lanosterol in a reaction catalysed by cyclase. Lanosterol is then converted to cholesterol, a 27-carbon molecule, by the removal of three methyl groups and the reduction of a double bond by NADPH.

> **Carbohydrates are the principal energy source for the body.** This is because they are the most efficient body fuel for producing ATP. The order of preference for body fuels is carbohydrate, lipid and finally protein. Protein is used only when carbohydrate and lipid stores have been depleted.

Regulation of cholesterol synthesis

The rate of cholesterol synthesis is closely regulated by the cellular level of cholesterol, through changes in the activity of HMG CoA reductase. Regulation occurs in several ways.

- Sterol regulatory element: this is a transcription factor that markedly inhibits enzyme gene expression in the presence of sterols
- Non-sterol metabolites: these derivatives of mevalonate inhibit enzyme gene expression
- Degradation of reductase enzyme is tightly regulated
- AMP-activated protein kinase: this decreases HMG CoA reductase activity by phosphorylating it, so cholesterol synthesis stops when ATP levels are low

Cholesterol absorption

Most cholesterol in the gut is in its free form, produced from cholesterol esters that are hydrolysed by cholesterol esterases secreted by the pancreas and small intestine. For absorption to proceed, cholesterol must first be made soluble by emulsification; the formation of micelles containing unesterified cholesterol, fatty acids, monoglycerides, phospholipids and conjugated bile acids. Conjugated bile acids act as detergents and are vital for micelle formation.

Most cholesterol is absorbed in the middle jejunum and terminal ileum through the transmembrane transporter protein Niemann–Pick C1 like 1 protein.

Ezetimibe is a potent cholesterol-lowering drug that works by blocking cholesterol absorption mediated by the Niemann–Pick C1 like 1 protein. Statins work by inhibiting HMG CoA reductase, which is the rate-limiting enzyme in cholesterol biosynthesis.

About 30–60% of dietary cholesterol is absorbed daily. Once absorbed into the intestinal mucosa cell, it is packaged into large lipoproteins called chylomicrons.

Familial hypercholesterolaemia is an inherited condition that results in a high concentration of cholesterol in the blood. The disease is inherited in either a heterozygous form (affecting 1 in 500 of the UK population) or a homozygous form (affecting 1 in 1 000 000 of the UK population).

Cholesterol esterification

Cholesterol is esterified in the liver to cholesterol ester by acyl cholesterol acyl transferase, an enzyme that is bound to the membrane of HDL and LDL particles. Esterification is necessary because excessive free cholesterol is cytotoxic, whereas its esters are not. After esterification, cholesterol esters are stored in intracellular lipid drops.

Esterification requires energy-dependent activation of a fatty acid with CoASH to form an acyl CoA. The acyl CoA reacts with a hydroxyl group on cholesterol to form an ester.

Cholesterol esters are also formed in blood by the action of lecithin cholesterol acyl transferase on cholesterol in lipoproteins. This reaction does not require CoASH activity; it occurs because of the transfer of a fatty acid from lecithin.

Cholesterol esters make up 70% of total cholesterol in plasma. Lecithin cholesterol acyl transferase is activated by apolipoprotein A-I, the major apolipoprotein in high-density lipoprotein (HDL) (**Table 5.3**). Cholesterol esters are in the hydrophobic core of the lipoprotein molecule.

Lipoproteins

Lipoproteins are the vesicles of lipid transport. They are spherical particles with non-polar neutral lipids in their core (i.e. triglycerides and cholesterol esters) and more polar amphipathic lipids (i.e. phospholipids

Lipoprotein composition					
Class	Cholesterol (%)	Phospholipids (%)	Apolipoproteins (%)	Triglycerides (%)	Cholesterol esters (%)
Chylomicrons	2	7	2	86	3
Very low density	7	18	8	55	12
Intermediate-density	9	19	19	23	29
Low density	8	22	22	6	42
High density 2	5	33	40	5	17
High density 3	4	25	55	3	13

Table 5.3 Chemical composition of lipoproteins

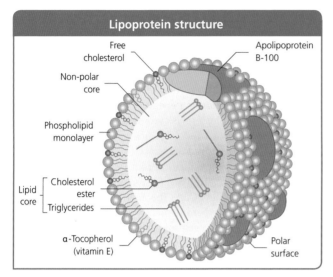

Figure 5.14 Basic structure of a lipoprotein molecule.

and cholesterol) at their surface (**Figure 5.14**). Lipoproteins also contain one or more additional proteins on their surface; these are called apolipoproteins (**Table 5.4**).

Lipoproteins are classified by their physiochemical properties (**Table 5.5**). Generally, larger lipoproteins contain more core lipids, triglycerides and cholesterol esters, and less protein (see **Table 5.3**).

Lipoprotein metabolism

Lipoprotein metabolism has four main pathways with discrete functions in lipid transport.

- the exogenous pathway
- the endogenous pathway
- intracellular cholesterol transport
- reverse cholesterol transport

The exogenous pathway of lipid metabolism

The exogenous lipoprotein pathway transports dietary lipids absorbed by the intestine to the liver and peripheral cells (**Figure 5.15**).

Chylomicrons

The main vesicles of the exogenous pathway are chylomicrons. Chylomicrons are assembled by the microsomal transfer protein in the endoplasmic reticulum of endocytes by combining triglycerides with apolipoprotein B-48 (major lipoprotein in VLDL).

Chylomicron transport

Next, chylomicrons are secreted into the circulation, where they acquire additional lipoproteins (e.g. apolipoproteins E and CI-III) from HDL. Apolipoprotein C-II activates lipoprotein lipase, which is present on the luminal surface of endothelial cells. The lipoprotein lipase then hydrolyses chylomicrons to free fatty acids.

The free fatty acids are either taken up by adipose tissue and stored as triglycerides or taken up by muscle and used as an energy source.

Chylomicron remnant particles

The net result of progressive hydrolysis is that chylomicrons become smaller and are transformed into chylomicron remnant particles, surplus phospholipids and apolipoprotein A-I, are transferred back to HDL. These remnant particles are taken up by the liver through hepatic remnant receptors that recognise apolipoproteins E and B-48. The triglycerides returned to the liver are used to power the biosynthetic activity of the liver, or they are repackaged with apolipoprotein B100 and secreted as very-low-density lipoprotein (VLDL) particles.

Apolipoprotein functions

Apolipoprotein	Function	Lipoprotein carrier(s)
A-I	Cofactor for cholesterol ester transfer protein	CM and HDL
A-II	Unknown	HDL
A-IV	Activation of lecithin cholesterol acyl transferase	CM and HDL
	Secretion of TG from liver-binding protein to LDL receptor	
B-48	Secretion of TG from intestine	VLDL, IDL and LDL
B-100	Secretion of TG from liver-binding protein to LDL receptor	CM
C-I	Activation of lecithin cholesterol acyl transferase	CM, VLDL and HDL
C-II	Cofactor for lipoprotein lipase	CM, VLDL and HDL
C-III	Inhibition of apolipoprotein C-II	CM, VLDL and HDL
	Activation of lipoprotein lipase	
E	Facilitation of uptake of CM and IDL remnants	CM, VLDL and HDL
(a)	Unknown	Lp(a)

CM, chylomicrons; HDL, high-density lipoprotein; IDL, intermediate-density lipoprotein; Lp(a), lipoprotein(a); TG, triglycerides; VLDL, very-low-density lipoprotein.

Table 5.4 Functions of apolipoproteins

Lipoprotein biochemical properties

Variable	CM	VLDL	IDL	LDL	HDL	Lp(a)
Density (g/mL)	<0.95	0.95–1.006	1.006–1.019	1.019–1.063	1.063–1.210	1.040–1.130
Electrophoretic mobility	Origin	Pre-beta	Slow pre-beta	Beta	Alpha	Pre-beta
Molecular weight (Da)	$0.4–30 \times 10^9$	$5–10 \times 10^6$	$3.9–4.8 \times 10^6$	2.75×10^6	$1.8–3.6 \times 10^5$	$2.9–3.7 \times 10^6$
Diameter (nm)	>70	26–70	22–24	19–23	4–10	26–30
Lipid:lipoprotein ratio	99:1	90:10	85:15	80:20	50:50	75:26 to 64:36
Major lipids	Exogenous TG	Endogenous TG	Endogenous TG and CE	CE	PL	CE and PL
Major proteins	A-I	B-100	B-100	B-100	A-I	(a)
	B-48	C-I	E		A-II	B-100
	C-I	C-II				
	C-II	C-III				
	C-III	E				

CE, cholesterol ester; CM, chylomicrons; HDL, high-density lipoprotein; IDL, intermediate-density lipoprotein; LDL, low-density lipoprotein; Lp(a), lipoprotein(a); PL, phospholipid; TG, triglycerides; VLDL, very-low-density lipoprotein.

Table 5.5 Biochemical properties of lipoprotein molecules.

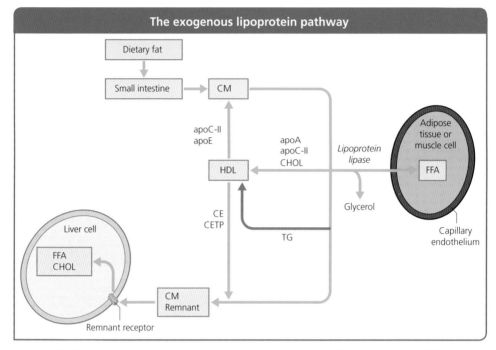

Figure 5.15 The exogenous lipoprotein pathway. apo, apolipoproteins; CE, cholesteryl ester; CETP; cholesteryl ester transfer protein; CHOL; cholesterol; CM, chylomicrons; FFA, free fatty acids; HDL, high-density lipoprotein; IDL, intermediate-density lipoprotein; TG, triglycerides; VLDL, very-low-density lipoprotein

The endogenous pathway of lipid metabolism

This pathway transfers triglycerides synthesised by the liver (or transferred to the liver from the exogenous pathway) to peripheral cells for energy metabolism (**Figure 5.16**).

The main lipoproteins in the endogenous pathway contain apolipoprotein B-100, particularly VLDLs, which also contains apolipoprotein E and apolipoprotein C. The apolipoprotein C-II on the surface of VLDLs activates lipoprotein lipase on the surface of endothelial cells, which leads to the hydrolysis of triglycerides and the release of fatty acids. The progressive hydrolysis of triglycerides in the core of a VLDL particle transforms it into intermediate-density lipoprotein and eventually LDL.

About half of the apolipoprotein B100 particles in the exogenous pathway are removed by hepatic remnant receptors before undergoing complete hydrolysis. The remaining portion is converted to LDL.

The triglyceride on LDL is further depleted by the cholesterol ester transfer protein, which removes triglycerides from LDL in exchange for cholesterol esters from HDL. During the transformation from VLDL to LDL, excess surface phospholipid and lipoproteins (except apolipoprotein B-100) are transferred to HDL.

Most LDL is returned to the liver through the LDL receptor, which recognises the apolipoprotein B-100. Cholesterol returned to the liver has various fates, including:

- secretion of lipoproteins
- synthesis of bile salts
- excretion directly into bile

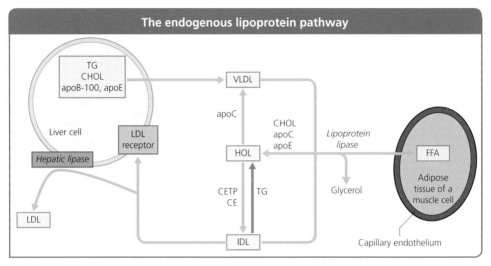

Figure 5.16 The endogenous lipoprotein pathway. apo, apolipoproteins; CE, cholesteryl ester; CETP; cholesteryl ester transfer protein; CHOL; cholesterol; CM, chylomicrons; FFA, free fatty acids; HDL, high-density lipoprotein; IDL, intermediate-density lipoprotein; LDL, low-density lipoprotein; TG, triglycerides; VLDL, very-low-density lipoprotein.

Close observation of Leonardo da Vinci's *Mona Lisa* suggests that she had familial hypercholesterolaemia. She has:

- a yellow, irregular, leather-like spot at the inner end of the left upper eyelid – possibly a xanthelasma
- a well-defined 3-cm swelling on the back of her right hand beneath the index finger – probably a xanthoma

Xanthelasma and xanthoma are both skin lesions of deposited lipids associated with hyperlipidemia.

Intracellular cholesterol transport

The intracellular transport of cholesterol is tightly regulated (**Figure 5.17**), because high cholesterol concentration has serious consequences for the biochemical properties of the cell membrane. For this reason, cholesterol is cytotoxic in excess.

Cellular cholesterol is derived from cellular synthesis, but it is also taken up from extracellular lipoproteins through the LDL receptor. The lipoprotein that binds to the LDL receptor undergoes receptor-mediated endocytosis and is delivered to intracellular lysosomes, where the lipoprotein is degraded.

Apolipoproteins are degraded to small peptides and amino acids. Cholesterol esters are converted to free cholesterol by lysosomal acid lipase. Cholesterol is not catabolised, but it is:

- used for membrane biogenesis
- stored in intracellular lipid drops after re-esterification by acyl cholesterol acyl transferase
- carried from the cell in the reverse cholesterol transport pathway

Regulation

Excess intracellular cholesterol inhibits biosynthesis, because it down-regulates HMG CoA reductase activity at both a transcriptional and a post-translational level. Furthermore, excess cholesterol down-regulates expression of the LDL receptor and induces the synthesis of protein necessary for the reverse cholesterol transport pathway.

Reverse cholesterol transport

The main function of the reverse cholesterol transport pathway (**Figure 5.18**) is to remove excess, and potentially toxic, cellular cholesterol from peripheral cells and return it to the liver for excretion. The main lipoprotein in this pathway is HDL, but there are different mechanisms by which cholesterol is removed from cells.

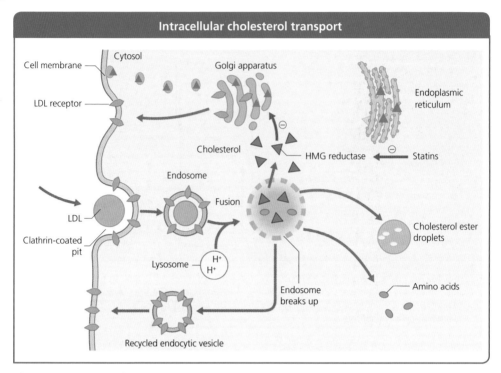

Figure 5.17 Overview of intracellular cholesterol transport. LDL, low-density lipoprotein.

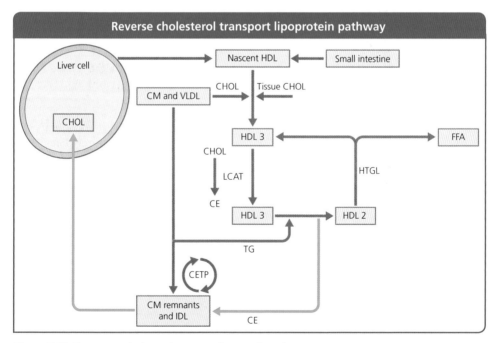

Figure 5.18 The reverse cholesterol transport lipoprotein pathway.

In the 'lipid profile' blood test, the concentrations of cholesterol, HDL cholesterol and triglycerides are measured. The concentration of LDL cholesterol is calculated using the Friedewald equation:

[LDL] (mmol/L) = [total cholesterol] − [HDL cholesterol] − ([triglyceride]/2.2)

The equation is invalid when:

■ chylomicrons are present

■ plasma triglyceride concentration exceeds 4.52 mmol/L

■ the patient has dysbetalipoproteinaemia (type 3 hyperlipoproteinaemia)

ABCA1 transporter

Cholesterol is actively pumped out of cells by the ATP-binding cassette transporter 1 (ABCA1) on to apolipoprotein A-I, which binds to cells to form nascent HDL. Nacent HDL is made in the liver and intestine. The interaction between nascent HDL and ABCA1 in peripheral cells (e.g. in macrophages) results in the removal of cellular cholesterol.

Lecithin cholesterol acyl transferase

This enzyme has a pivotal role in reverse cholesterol transport. This is because cholesterol esters are more hydrophobic than cholesterol and remain trapped in the HDL core until they reach the liver, where they are removed.

Esterification to spherical HDL

The esterification of cholesterol on HDL converts the disc-shaped nascent HDL to spherical HDL, the main form of circulating HDL. The spherical HDL accepts cholesterol that may have been removed from cells by the passive diffusion or the transporter ATP binding cassette transporter G (ATPG1).

Removal by the liver

The next stage of the process is the selective removal by the liver of cholesterol esters from the spherical HDL. This allows lipid-depleted HDL to return to the circulation for subsequent rounds of cholesterol removal from peripheral cells.

The cholesterol ester transfer protein also plays an important part in this pathway, because a large portion of cholesterol removed from HDL is transferred on to LDL as cholesterol esters. These cholesterol esters are removed from the circulation by hepatic LDL receptors.

Increasing HDL ('good') cholesterol has been proposed as a way to reduce cardiovascular risk. HDL concentration is increased by exercise, taking nicotinic acid (Vitamin B3), consuming alcohol in moderation, losing weight and stopping smoking.

Metabolic fate of cholesterol

As well as being a core constituent of all cell membranes, cholesterol is a precursor of steroid hormones and vitamin D.

Steroid hormones

Cholesterol is the precursor for five major classes of steroid hormone (**Figure 5.19**):

■ prostagens (e.g. progesterone)
■ glucocorticoids (e.g. cortisol)
■ mineralocorticoids (e.g. aldosterone)
■ androgens (e.g. testosterone)
■ oestrogens (e.g. oestrogen)

Each of these classes of steroid has a specific function (**Table 5.6**).

Vitamin D

Cholesterol is also the precursor of vitamin D, which plays a pivotal role in maintaining serum calcium and phosphate metabolism. **Figure 5.2** details the synthesis of vitamin D from 7-dehydrocholesterol, which is present in the skin. This product is photolysed by ultraviolet light to previtamin D3, which spontaneously isomerises to vitamin D3.

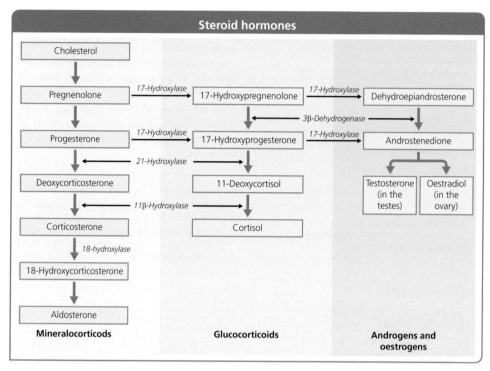

Figure 5.19 Steroid hormones.

Functions of major steroids		
Steroid group	Example steroid	Examples of biological functions
Glucocorticoids	Cortisol	Modulates carbohydrate metabolism
		Inhibits uptake and utilisation of glucose
		Enhances gluconeogenesis
		Increases gluconeogenic enzymes
		Produces immunosuppression by inhibiting lipocortin activity
		Increases free water excretion
Mineralocorticoids	Aldosterone	Increases sodium reabsorption (and therefore blood pressure) in the kidney, colon and sweat glands
		Increases potassium and hydrogen ion excretion in the cortical collecting ducts of the kidneys
Androgens	Testosterone	Produces secondary sex characteristics (e.g. growth of pubic hair and penis)
Oestrogens	Oestrogen	Stimulates endometrial and uterine growth
		Promotes secondary sexual characteristics in females
		Enhances bone formation
		Promotes protein synthesis
		Decreases low-density lipoprotein and increases high-density lipoprotein cholesterol
Progestogen	Progesterone	Stimulates release of oocytes and prepares uterus for implantation
		Promotes breast development
		Increases bone mass and prevents bone loss

Table 5.6 Functions of the major steroids

Answers to starter questions

1. LDL particles transport cholesterol into the artery wall where it is retained by proteoglycans. The cholesterol attracts macrophages, which engulf the LDL particles. With an excess of LDL, macrophages are overwhelmed by excessive lipid and form foam cells. Later, scar tissue and cholesterol deposits are seen in the plaque. As plaques grow there is an increasing risk of rupture. This in turn promotes blood clotting and arterial stenosis. If severe enough this can cause a heart attack, stroke, or result in peripheral vascular disease.

2. Saturated fat is composed of triglycerides containing only saturated fatty acids, i.e. those with no double bonds present along the length of the carbon chain between the individual carbon atoms. In other words, the carbon atoms are fully "saturated" with hydrogen atoms. A diet high in saturated fatty acids is believed to be associated with an increased risk of cardiovascular disease and cancer.

3. Oxidation of carbohydrates and lipids provides the majority of the energy required by the human body. Carbohydrates provide a readily available source of energy, ultimately as glucose, whereas lipids are an energy store for use when carbohydrate stores – in the form of glycogen - run low. The amount of lipid energy stored far exceeds the energy stored as glycogen since the human body is limited in glycogen storage capacity compared with lipids. Lipid reserves in a 70kg male contain 100,000 kcal of energy; enough for 30–40 days without food. Comparatively, free glucose only provides energy for minutes; 40 kcal.

4. All cell membranes are a lipid bilayer; a structure based on the hydrophobic properties of lipids. This separates aqueous compartments from their surroundings, allowing the separation of molecules and ions to where they are required. Lipid bilayers are ideally suited to this role because they are impermeable to hydrophilic molecules (water-soluble molecules). As lipid bilayers are particularly impermeable to ions, cells regulate salt concentrations and pH by various transport mechanisms that enable movement of ions across their membranes.

5. Steroids make good hormones because they are hydrophobic (i.e. fat-soluble). This is advantageous because cell membranes are composed of a phospholipid bilayer, which is also hydrophobic. This means steroids diffuse through the cell membrane of a target cell. Fat-insoluble (i.e. hydrophilic) molecules are unable to transverse the cell membrane. Once inside the cell the steroid hormone binds with a specific receptor found only in the cytoplasm of the target cell where it increases or decreases gene expression of target genes.

Chapter 6
Haemoglobin metabolism

Starter questions

Answers to the following questions are on page 176.

1. Why do competitive athletes train at altitude?
2. How are the colour of blood and faeces related?
3. Why is anaemia a huge global problem?
4. Why is orange juice better for iron absorption than tea or coffee?
5. Why do bruises turn yellow?

Introduction

Haemoglobin is a protein in red blood cells. It transports, stores and removes oxygen and carbon dioxide from the body. These processes are necessary because:

- oxygen is essential for the effective and efficient metabolism of fuels such as carbohydrate, fat and protein
- the carbon dioxide produced during metabolism of these fuels is toxic and therefore needs to be eliminated from the body

Most of the body's carbon dioxide (70%) is dissolved, in the form of bicarbonate, in plasma.

However, only 1% of the body's oxygen (1%) is carried in its dissolved form; the vast majority (99%) is transported bound to haemoglobin. Haemoglobin enables the effective movement and storage of these gases by increasing their gas solubility and interacting reversibly in gas exchange.

This chapter focuses on haemoglobin structure, metabolism and function. It also provides a brief overview of haemopoiesis (the formation of platelets and blood cells generally) and erythropoiesis (the formation of red blood cells specifically).

Case 5 Chest pain

Presentation

A 24-year-old African–Caribbean woman, Anna Henderson, presents with chest pain. She has a known history of sickle cell anaemia, and has had several similar episodes in the past.

Anna usually has moderate anaemia, with a haemoglobin concentration of 80–100 g/L (normal range, 118–148 g/L). On this occasion, she became unwell 2 days ago with a cough and fever. The next day, pain started in the right side of her chest and has gradually become more severe. She now grades it as 9 on a scale of 0 (no pain) to 10 (worst possible pain).

Analysis

The normal structure of adult haemoglobin is a tetramer comprising two α chains and two β chains (see page 159). A point mutation in the DNA encoding this molecule can cause the 6th amino acid of the β chain, glutamic acid, to be substituted by valine.

Different types of sickle cell disease arise from this error (**Table 6.1**).

- Patients with sickle cell anaemia are homozygous for this mutation; >75% of their haemoglobin is sickle haemoglobin (HbS), with two α chains plus two mutant β chains

- Patients with sickle cell trait are heterozygotes; their haemoglobin has only one mutant β chain and they are asymptomatic
- Patients with other types of sickle cell disease, which present a similar clinical picture to that of sickle cell anaemia, have one sickle allele paired with another abnormal allele for the β chain, which carries a different type of mutation

In its deoxygenated configuration, HbS polymerises, leading to a distortion of red blood cells called sickling (**Figure 6.1**), increased red blood cell breakdown and blockage of capillaries. The resulting interruption to the microcirculation further

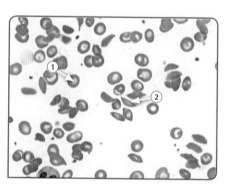

Figure 6.1 Blood film showing (1) normal red blood cells and (2) sickled red blood cells.

Sickle cell diseases		
Type	Genes encoding β chains of haemoglobin	Clinical picture
HbSS	Two copies of *HbS* gene	Sickle cell anaemia
HbSC	One *HbS* and one *HbC* gene	Similar to that of sickle cell anaemia but usually milder
HbS/β° Thal	One *HbS* and one β° Thal gene (no β chain produced)	Similar to that of sickle cell anaemia
HbS/β+Thal	One *HbS* and one *β+Thal* gene (reduced production of β chain)	Variable severity
HbC, haemoglobin C; HbS, sickle haemoglobin.		

Table 6.1 Sickle cell diseases caused by abnormal haemoglobin

Case 5 *continued*

Sickle cell crisis: pathophysiology and treatment

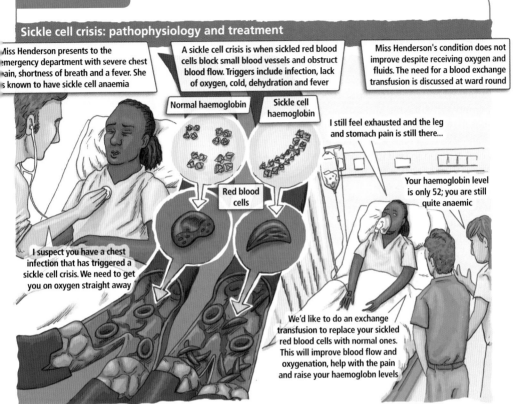

Miss Henderson presents to the emergency department with severe chest pain, shortness of breath and a fever. She is known to have sickle cell anaemia

A sickle cell crisis is when sickled red blood cells block small blood vessels and obstruct blood flow. Triggers include infection, lack of oxygen, cold, dehydration and fever

Miss Henderson's condition does not improve despite receiving oxygen and fluids. The need for a blood exchange transfusion is discussed at ward round

Normal haemoglobin

Sickle cell haemoglobin

Red blood cells

I still feel exhausted and the leg and stomach pain is still there...

Your haemoglobin level is only 52; you are still quite anaemic

I suspect you have a chest infection that has triggered a sickle cell crisis. We need to get you on oxygen straight away

We'd like to do an exchange transfusion to replace your sickled red blood cells with normal ones. This will improve blood flow and oxygenation, help with the pain and raise your haemoglobn levels

reduces tissue oxygenation, which produces more deoxygenated HbS and thus exacerbates the sickling process.

Further case

Anna is in severe pain and has signs of a chest infection. Her temperature is 38.5°C, and she appears dehydrated, with hypotension and reduced skin turgor.

A full blood count reveals that she is severely anaemic, with a haemoglobin concentration of 52 g/L. Initial treatment consists of pain relief, antibiotics to treat her chest infection and intravenous fluids to rehydrate and restore circulation. Supplemental oxygen is given to help reverse red cell sickling. However, her condition continues to deteriorate, so an exchange transfusion is carried out: her blood is partially replaced with blood from a donor with normal haemoglobin. Anna makes a slow but steady recovery.

Blood cells

About 7–8% of total body weight is blood, which is vital for transport of nutrients and materials to and from cells, protection against infections, and regulation of temperature, pH and blood pressure. Blood is largely composed of plasma and three other components: red blood cells, white blood cells and platelets. Red cells, white cells and platelets constitute up to half of the circulating blood volume in health; the other half is plasma. Blood:

- transports oxygen from the lungs to the tissues for the generation of energy
- transports carbon dioxide from the tissues to the lungs for removal
- takes nutrients from the digestive tract to storage locations (e.g. liver)
- carries waste products from the muscle and liver to the kidney for excretion in urine
- transports hormones from endocrine glands to their target cells
- produces clotting at sites of blood vessel damage
- carries antibodies and white blood cells to fight infections
- regulates core body temperature
- regulates pH and water balance

White blood cells

White blood cells (leucocytes) make up about 1% of the total blood volume of a healthy adult. They are key players in the immune response, and have a half-life in the circulation, ranging from hours to several days.

There are five types of white blood cell. All derive from haemopoietic stem cells (page 173), but they have different structures and functions. The two predominant types of white blood cell are neutrophils and lymphocytes.

- Neutrophils are the most common type (55–70% of the total white blood cell count); they have a half-life of < 1 day, so they are constantly being produced to protect the body by fighting infections
- Lymphocytes are the second most common type (20–50% of the total white blood cell count) and are sub-divided into T and B cells:
  - T cells directly attack infected cells and also regulate the function of other immune cells
  - B cells make antibodies to specifically target foreign materials

The other three types of white cells are basophils (1% of total and involved in immune response to parasites); monocytes (2–10% of the total which are the precursors of macrophages which digest bacteria) and eosinophils (1–6% of total with a role in digesting antigen-antibody complexes and in mechanisms associated with allergy and asthma).

Platelets

Platelets (thrombocytes) have a lifespan of 5–9 days and make blood clot. They are considered fragments of cells, because they lack the nucleus and many of the organelles present in most cells. However, they do contain numerous growth factors, such as platelet-derived growth factor and transforming growth factor-β, and these hormones have significant roles in the repair and regeneration of connective tissues.

Red blood cells

Red blood cells (erythrocytes) are the most abundant cells in plasma (44–45% of plasma volume). Their volume is expressed as a percentage of the overall blood volume; this is called the haemocrit and is part of a full blood count profile.

The main function of red blood cells is to transport oxygen to tissues and remove carbon dioxide from them. Therefore their structure, a biconcave disc with a flattened centre, provides a large surface area to facilitate gas exchange. Red blood cells also have a flexible cell membrane that enables movement through small capillaries.

Another function of red blood cells is the buffering of hydrogen ions through the 'chloride shift' mechanism (see page 173).

Despite their name, red blood cells are technically not cells, because they lack subcellular organelles, for example a nucleus and mitochondria. Red blood cells have an average lifespan of 120 days.

> **A full blood count is a range of blood tests that provide information about circulating blood cells.** This information includes the proportion of red blood cells, white blood cells and platelets; the concentration of haemoglobin; and the size of red blood cells. The full blood count is useful for indicating many disease states, including anaemia, infections and haematological malignancies.

Haemopoiesis

Haemopoiesis is the production of blood cells and platelets from pluripotent stem cells (haemopoietic stem cells) (**Figure 6.2**). From birth, the main site of haemopoiesis is the medullary cavity of the bone marrow. However, during gestation, extramedullary haemopoiesis also occurs in the fetal liver and spleen (**Figure 6.3**).

Various growth factors (e.g. glycoproteins, such as interleukins) regulate stem cell differentiation by binding cell surface receptors to trigger replication or differentiation, or to activate cell function. A constant supply of blood cells is maintained by a balance of cell differentiation and programmed cell death (apoptosis). In certain pathological conditions, such as haemoglobinopathies (blood disorders resulting from mutations of the gene encoding haemoglobin), myeloproliferative disorders and neoplasms involving the bone marrow, haemopoiesis can switch back to the spleen and liver as the bone marrow environment becomes unsuitable for haemopoiesis.

Erythropoiesis

Red blood cell production (erythropoiesis) occurs entirely in the red bone marrow; yellow marrow consists of fat). Red marrow is present mainly in the flat bones, such as the sternum, cranium, pelvis, ribs and vertebrae, as well as at the ends of the long bones (the epiphyseal ends), such as the humerus and femur. At birth, all bone marrow is red, but as we age, this is replaced by fatty yellow marrow.

> **In cases of severe blood loss,** the yellow marrow of long bones is able to convert back to red marrow, as haemopoietic activity increases.

To maintain a sufficient number of functioning red blood cells, their synthesis is switched on by low oxygen levels. Low oxygen is detected by the highly vascular kidneys, which produce the hormone erythropoietin in response. Erythropoietin then triggers the undifferentiated cells in the red bone marrow to produce mature red blood cells, each containing millions of haemoglobin molecules.

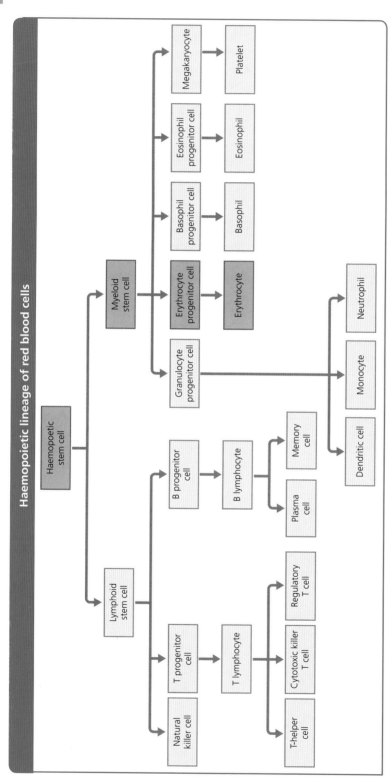

Figure 6.2 Hierarchy highlighting the haemopoietic lineage of red blood cells. All blood cells are derived from pluripotent stem cells.

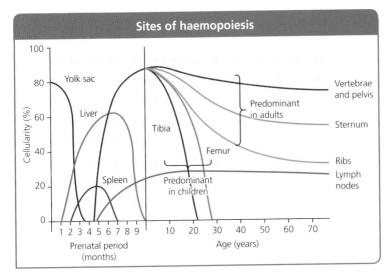

Figure 6.3 Sites of haemopoiesis during gestation and throughout life.

Haemoglobin structure

Haemoglobin is a tetramer; it has four sub-units (**Figure 6.4**). It contains two sets of two identical globin (protein) chains, two α-like and two β-like, which are held together by non-covalent interactions to produce the haemoglobin molecule. Each of the four globin chains is folded to produce a hydrophobic pocket, which accommodates a haem group.

The haem groups are covalently attached to the globin chains (one haem per globin). Each haem group is able to bind one oxygen molecule. Haemoglobin bound to oxygen is called oxyhaemoglobin. Haemoglobin that has relinquished its oxygen is deoxyhaemoglobin.

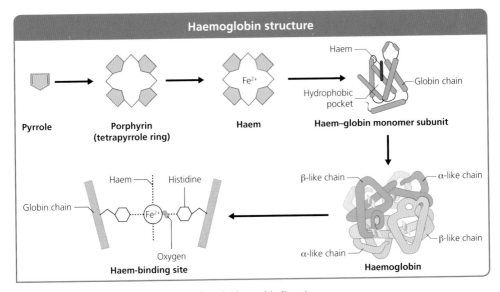

Figure 6.4 Haemoglobin structure, including the haem-binding site.

The haem group

The haem group comprises a porphyrin (tetrapyrrole) ring containing a central iron (ferrous, Fe^{2+}) atom. Porphyrin compounds are able to absorb light, and it is the haem group that gives haemoglobin, and therefore blood, its red colour. Haem is a component of a number of important biomolecules, including myoglobin (the oxygen storage protein) and the cytochrome P450 enzymes .

In haemoglobin, one oxygen molecule binds to the central Fe^{2+} atom in each haem group. Histidine molecules in the hydrophobic pocket of the globin chain also associate with the iron and oxygen atoms, thus preventing the bound oxygen molecule from oxidising Fe^{2+} to the ferric Fe^{3+} state. Fe^{3+} is unable to bind oxygen, therefore the histidine molecules enable haemoglobin to bind oxygen without becoming permanently oxidised, and it is this property of haemoglobin that permits continuous cycles of oxygen binding and release.

Oxidised haemoglobin, methaemoglobin, in which the iron in some of the haem molecules is oxidised to the Fe^{3+} state, has reduced affinity for oxygen (see page 172).

Effect of oxygen binding

The binding of an oxygen molecule to a haem group slightly alters the structure of the haemoglobin molecule, giving it a more open, relaxed structure (termed 'R'). The R structure allows oxygen easier access to its binding site, thus facilitating its binding and release. In contrast, deoxyhaemoglobin has a closed, tense structure (termed 'T'). Its oxygen-binding side is less accessible, so it has a lower affinity for oxygen. This means it is easier for subsequent oxygen molecules to bind haemoglobin once the first oxygen is bound (see page 170).

Myoglobin is an oxygen storage protein in the cytosol of muscle cells. It is similar to haemoglobin but has just one globin chain with a single haem group. Oxygen released by haemoglobin in the muscle tissue capillaries diffuses across the cellular membranes into the muscle cell cytosol, where it binds to myoglobin.

Haemoglobin synthesis

Haemoglobin is synthesised in progenitors of red blood cells called normoblasts and reticulocytes. Synthesis stops before the red blood cell is mature, and the completed haemoglobin molecules then remain in the cytosol throughout its lifetime. Haem and globin are made separately within the cell before their assembly into the final haemoglobin molecule.

Mature red blood cells have no organelles. Therefore they are unable to synthesise haemoglobin.

Haem synthesis

Haem is synthesised from the precursors glycine and succinyl coenzyme A by a series of eight reactions (**Figure 6.5**). Each of these reactions is catalysed by a different enzyme (**Table 6.2**). Four of these enzymes are in the mitochondria, where synthesis begins and ends, and the other four are in the cytosol.

The porphyrias (Greek: porphyros, 'purple') are inherited or acquired diseases of the haem synthetic pathway. They are caused by a partial deficiency of one of the enzymes in the pathway, which leads to an accumulation of precursors. Deficiencies in seven of the eight enzymes of the pathway have been identified. The symptoms that develop depend on the enzyme affected, and therefore the precursors that accumulate.

Globin synthesis

Globin is synthesised on ribosomes in the cytosol of immature red blood cells. As with all proteins, the primary structure (i.e. sequence of amino acids) of the globin chains is determined by the nucleotide sequences in the globin genes.

In humans, there are two α-like globin and five β-like globin chains, which differ in amino acid sequence and are each designated by a different Greek letter (α, β, γ_1, γ_2, δ, ε and ζ).

A different gene encodes each of the different globin chains. All the β-chain genes are on chromosome 11, and the α-chain genes are on chromosome 16. One copy of each gene is present on each chromosome, except for the α gene, which has two copies (**Figure 6.6**).

Assembly of haemoglobin

Haemoglobin assembly occurs in the cytosol once the globin chain is released from the ribosome. Haem molecules diffuse from the mitochondria into the cytosol, and the globin chain folds around the haem molecule to produce one subunit of haemoglobin. This subunit then interacts with another subunit to form a dimer. Finally, two dimer molecules come together to form the haemoglobin tetramer.

The correct formation of haemoglobin depends on the availability of haem and globin in the cytosol, as well as the relative proportions of each globin chain. Haemoglobin is formed through the coordinated regulation of haem and globin synthesis, by a mechanism that has yet to be fully elucidated.

Haem synthesis is regulated by the negative feedback of haem on the first enzyme in

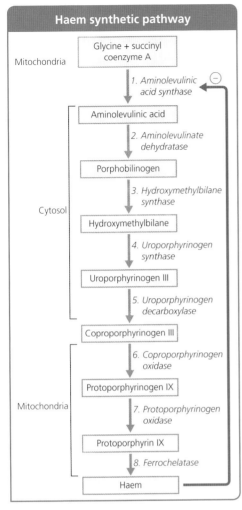

Figure 6.5 Synthetic pathway for haem, showing the negative feedback for haem production.

Haem synthesis

Step(s)	Process
1 and 2	Formation of a pyrrole molecule, a compound containing four carbon atoms and one nitrogen atom joined in a ring structure
3	Linkage of four pyrrole molecules to form a linear tetramer
4	Formation of the porphyrin (tetrapyrrole) ring
5–7	Decarboxylation and oxidation
8	Incorporation of the iron atom

Table 6.2 Steps in haem synthesis

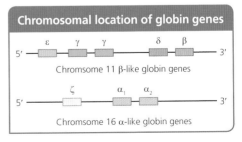

Figure 6.6 Location of the globin genes on chromosomes 11 and 16.

the pathway, aminolevulinic acid synthase. This feedback prevents excessive haem production. Globin synthesis is also partly regulated by haem, because it has a positive feedback effect on the translation of globin messenger RNA. This ensures that when haem is in short supply, the synthesis of globin is down-regulated, and when haem is available, globin synthesis is increased.

Types of haemoglobin

The different α-like and β-like globin chains (α, β, γ_1, γ_2, δ, ε and ζ) are expressed at different stages of human development, i.e. embryonic, fetal and adult (**Figure 6.7**). This differential expression gives rise to several types of haemoglobin (**Table 6.3**).

- Embryonic haemoglobins are expressed only by red blood cell precursors in the yolk sac for up to 8 weeks, after which haemoglobin production by the fetus takes over
- Fetal haemoglobin is normally expressed up to the 1st year of life but occasionally persists into adulthood; this type of haemoglobin has a higher affinity for oxygen than that of adult haemoglobin, and this property ensures the efficient transfer of oxygen from the mother to the developing fetus
- Adult haemoglobin makes up most (about 96%) of haemoglobin in adults; about 6% of adult haemoglobin is HbA_1 (adult haemoglobin to which sugar residues

have been attached to the globin chains non-enzymatically). HbA_2 and fetal haemoglobin each count for about 2% of the total haemoglobin

> **Haemoglobin A1c is haemoglobin with one glucose molecule attached to the N terminal of each β-like globin chain.** This type of haemoglobin has a role in the monitoring of diabetes mellitus. The rate of haemoglobin A1c formation is proportional to blood glucose concentration over the lifetime of the red blood cell. Therefore the haemoglobin A1c value provides an estimate of long-term glucose control, for example over the previous 3 months.

Types of haemoglobin		
Stage of development	Type	Globin chains
Embryonic	Hb Gower 1	$\zeta_2\varepsilon_2$
	Hb Gower 2	$\alpha_2\varepsilon_2$
	Hb Portland	$\zeta_2\gamma_2$
Fetal	HbF	$\alpha_2\gamma_2$
Adult	HbA	$\alpha_2\beta_2$
	HbA_2	$\alpha_2\delta_2$
	HbF	$\alpha_2\gamma_2$

Hb, haemoglobin; HbA, adult haemoglobin; HbF, fetal haemoglobin.

Table 6.3 The different types of haemoglobin expressed at each stage of development.

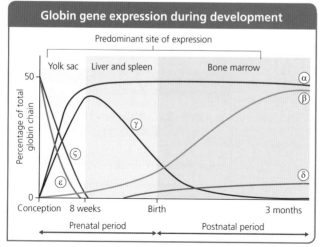

Globin gene expression during development

Figure 6.7 Differential expression of globin genes throughout the stages of human development.

Haemoglobin breakdown

Old red blood cells are removed from circulation once they become senescent (significantly deteriorated). This typically occurs around 120 days after maturation, or when cells become abnormal in size or shape. They are removed by macrophages of the reticuloendothelial system in the spleen, liver and bone marrow. A small proportion (about 10%) haemolyse (burst) in circulation, and the fragments of these cells are engulfed by circulating macrophages.

Haemoglobin released from degraded red blood cells is broken down into haem and globin chains by lysosomal enzymes in macrophages. Haem released as a result of this process accounts for 80% of free haem in the body. The other 20% is derived from the degradation of other haem-containing proteins, such as catalase, peroxidase and the cytochromes.

Haem breakdown

Haem is broken down into biliverdin by haem oxygenase in macrophages in a reaction that requires oxygen and the reducing agent nicotinamide–adenine dinucleotide phosphate (reduced form, NADPH) (**Figure 6.8**). Iron and carbon monoxide are released during this reaction.

Biliverdin is then reduced to bilirubin by a cytosolic enzyme called biliverdin reductase, which requires nicotinamide–adenine dinucleotide or NADPH for its action. Bilirubin is a yellow pigment that is non-toxic when produced at normal concentrations. In a typical adult, 425–685 μmol of bilirubin is produced every day.

Bilirubin excretion and metabolism

Free bilirubin, being insoluble in water, binds to albumin and is transported in the blood from the macrophage to the liver (**Figure 6.9**). When the bilirubin–albumin complex reaches the liver, the bilirubin dissociates from albumin and is taken up through facilitated diffusion into the hepatocyte. Once in the hepatocyte, bilirubin binds to glutathione s-transferase proteins (e.g. ligandin) until it is conjugated with glucuronic acid, forming a water-soluble compound that is more efficiently excreted in bile.

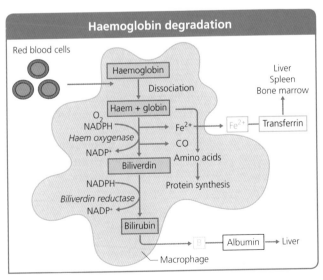

Figure 6.8 Haemoglobin metabolism to bilirubin. B, bilirubin; CO, carbon monoxide; Fe^{2+}, iron; NADP, nicotinamide–adenine dinucleotide phosphate; NADPH, nicotinamide–adenine dinucleotide phosphate (reduced form).

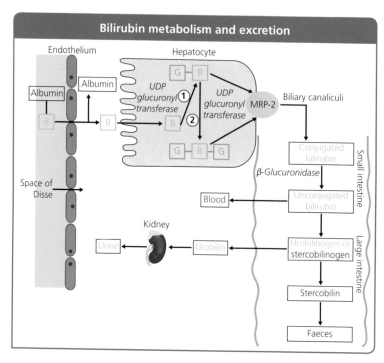

Figure 6.9 Bilirubin metabolism and excretion. ①, 1st glucuronidation step; ②, 2nd glucuronidation step. B, bilirubin; B-G, bilirubin monoglucoronide; B-GG, bilirubin diglucuronide; MRP-2, multidrug-resistant–like protein-2 transporter; UDP, uridine diphosphate.

Jaundice develops when the concentration of bilirubin in the blood is markedly increased, due to the failure in conjugation and/or elimination of bilirubin from the blood. Clinically, this condition is apparent as yellow discoloration of the sclera when blood bilirubin reaches a concentration of about 40 µmol/L (twice the upper limit of the reference range). Jaundice suggests a biliary or liver disease ranging in severity from trivial to life-threatening.

Bilirubin conjugation

The conjugation of bilirubin and glucuronic acid, mediated by one or more isoforms of uridine diphosphosphate glucuronyl transferase, produces two water-soluble forms of bilirubin: mono- and dibilirubin glucuronide. This process occurs through two separate glucuronidation steps (see **Figure 6.9**). Conjugated bilirubin is then secreted through the multidrug-resistant–like

protein-2 transporter, against a concentration gradient, into bile.

Having passed into the small intestine through the biliary tree, conjugated bilirubin is deconjugated through the action of intestinal bacteria with glucuronidase activity. A small fraction of the unconjugated bilirubin is reabsorbed from the intestine through the reticuloendothelial system and subsequently excreted in bile.

Most of the unconjugated bilirubin is reduced by intestinal anaerobes to urobilinogen and stercobilinogen.

- A small fraction of urobilinogen spontaneously oxidises to urobilin, which contributes to the colour of normal urine
- Stercobilinogen also spontaneously oxidises to stercobilin, which contributes to the normal colour of faeces

Iron release

Iron released during the degradation of haem is transported by transferrin (the iron transport protein) from macrophages to the liver and spleen. Here, it is stored as ferritin (the iron storage protein). Transferrin also transports iron to red bone marrow for the synthesis of haemoglobin.

Globin breakdown

The globin chains released from the degradation of haemoglobin are broken down into amino acids. These are then either metabolised or recycled for use in the synthesis of new proteins.

A premature neonate born at 35 weeks' gestation is noticed to be clinically jaundiced, with yellow sclera. Liver function tests are requested, and the results are as follows.

- Bilirubin: 100 μmol/L (reference range, <21 μmol/L)
- Alkaline phosphatase: 250 U/L (reference range, 30–300 U/L)
- Alanine aminotransferase: 20 U/L (reference range, < 35U/L)
- Protein: 68 g/L (reference range, 60–80 g/L)
- Albumin: 36 g/L (reference range, 35–50 g/L)

The increased bilirubin concentration is consistent with the clinical jaundice. This is a common condition in premature babies; it is caused by immature liver enzyme activity and usually resolves with time and phototherapy.

Iron homeostasis

Iron is an essential component of haemoglobin (see page 159), which contains two thirds of total body iron, and myoglobin. Iron is also essential for the function of many enzymes, such as ribonucleotide reductase, which is responsible for catalysing the formation of deoxyribonucleotides from ribonucleotides.

Free iron is toxic, so it is stored in the body bound to the intracellular protein ferritin. Although present in all cells, most iron is stored in the reticuloendothelial system.

Iron is transported in the blood by transferrin, a carrier protein that is able to carry up to two atoms at a time. Transferrin receptors on the surface of some cells, e.g. hepatocytes and enterocytes, allow them to take up iron depending upon their requirements.

Iron homeostasis is summarised in **Figure 6.10**. Four types of cell have key roles in this process:

- duodenal enterocytes
- hepatocytes
- reticuloendothelial macrophages
- red blood cells

Low haemoglobin concentration requires investigation with a range of laboratory tests.

- White blood cell count: for evidence of inflammation, infection and cancers (cell count can increase or decrease dependent on the disease, e.g. with infection and inflammation they increase)
- Platelet count: to assess clotting abnormalities
- Reticulocyte (young red blood cell) count: to assess marrow activity
- Blood film: to check cell morphology (e.g. sickle cells) and determine if more than one pathology is present
- Serum iron, transferrin and ferritin: to detect iron deficiency
- Serum vitamin B12 and folate: deficiencies cause anaemia

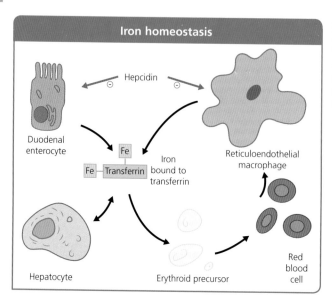

Figure 6.10 Overview of iron homeostasis, showing the four types of cell that metabolise iron: duodenal enterocytes (which absorb iron from the diet), hepatocytes, reticuloendothelial macrophages and red blood cells.

Iron metabolism in duodenal enterocytes

After ingestion, iron is reduced by the action of ferric reductase in the brush border of duodenal enterocytes (**Figure 6.11**). It is then transported across the cell membrane and into the enterocyte through the divalent metal iron transporter-1. Iron is stored in the cell as ferritin, and the remainder is transported across the basolateral membrane and out of the cell through the iron exporter ferroportin-1.

Iron metabolism in hepatocytes

Exported iron is then loaded on to apotransferrin (transferrin with no bound iron) to produce holotransferrin (transferrin with bound iron). At the hepatocyte, holotransferrin binds to the transferrin receptor (**Figure 6.12**). The resulting complex localises to clathrin-coated pits, where they turn inside out to initiate endocytosis.

Specialised endosomes form and are acidified by the intake of hydrogen ions through proton pumps in their membrane. The acidification of the endosomes causes conformational changes in transferrin that cause it to release its iron. Acidification also facilitates proton-coupled

iron transport out of the endosomes through the activity of the divalent metal iron transporter-1. After these events, apotransferrin and the transferrin receptor return to the cell surface and dissociate.

Iron is stored, bound to ferritin, in hepatocytes. Alternatively, it is exported through ferroportin-1. Exported iron then binds to transferrin to form holotransferrin, which transports the iron to where it is required, such as with the erythroid precursors in the red marrow.

Iron metabolism in reticuloendothelial macrophages

Reticuloendothelial macrophages clear senescent red blood cells from circulation. These cells release iron from haem for export to the circulation or they store it in ferritin.

Role of hepcidin

Hepcidin, a peptide hormone produced by the liver, is a key regulator of iron homeostasis. It blocks the release of iron from enterocytes and reticuloendothelial macrophages by degrading the iron exporter (membrane protein) ferroportin-1.

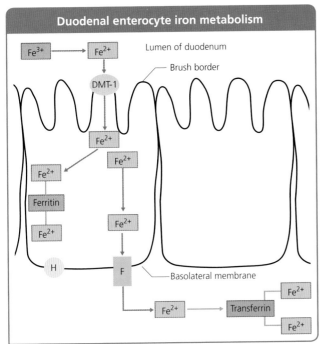

Figure 6.11 Iron metabolism by the duodenal enterocyte. DMT-1, divalent metal iron transporter-1; F, ferroportin 1; Fe^{2+}, ferrous iron; Fe^{3+}, ferric iron; H, hephaestin.

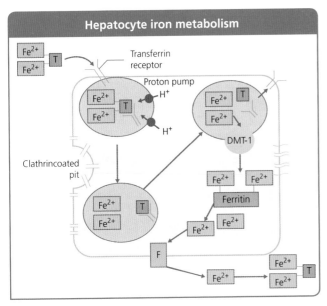

Figure 6.12 Iron metabolism by the hepatocyte. DMT-1, divalent metal iron transporter-1; F, ferroportin 1; Fe^{2+} ferrous iron, Fe^{3+}, ferric iron T, transferrin.

- In iron deficiency states, hepcidin levels are low, therefore the transport protein ferroportin-1 allows the entry of iron from duodenal enterocytes into the blood, as well as the recirculation of iron from macrophages into the plasma

- In states of iron excess, hepcidin levels are high, promoting the internalisation and degradation of ferroportin-1; this response decreases iron absorption from the gut as well as iron release from macrophages

Disorders of iron homeostasis

Disorders of iron homeostasis can be categorised as states of iron deficiency or iron excess.

Iron deficiency is the most common cause of anaemia worldwide. The condition may be associated with:

- glossitis (inflammation of the tongue)
- angular stomatitis (redness and maceration of the skin around the angle of the mouth)
- koilonychias (spoon-shaped nails)

> Slowly developing anaemia, such as that of chronic disease e.g. cancer, is often asymptomatic, because compensatory mechanisms enhance the oxygen-carrying capacity of the blood. In particular, an increase in 2,3-bisphosphoglycerate (see page 171) causes the oxyhaemoglobin dissociation curve to shift to the right (a Bohr shift), so that oxygen is more readily released to the tissues.

Iron excess can occur acutely, or chronically, usually as a result of haemochromatosis. Iron overload rarely occurs as a result of excessive iron intake, but this can happen in people with alcoholic liver disease. Causes of iron deficiency and excess are summarised in **Table 6.4**.

Anaemia

Anaemia is the decreased concentration of haemoglobin in the blood, below the reference range for the age and sex of the individual person. In healthy men and women, normal ranges are 133–167 g/L and 118–148 g/L, respectively. The clinical features of anaemia are shown in **Table 6.5**.

Haemoglobin concentration is affected by changes in plasma volume. Therefore anaemia is also classified by mean cell volume, the normal reference range for which is 80–100 fL.

Anaemia is categorised into three major types by mean cell volume (**Figure 6.13**):

- hypochromic microcytic anaemia (low mean cell volume)

Causes of iron deficiency and excess	
Deficiency	**Excess**
Blood loss (e.g. from blood donation or trauma)	Hereditary haemochromatosis (HH)
	HFE related HH
	Non–HFE related HH
	Juvenile haemochromatosis (haemojuvelin or hepcidin related)
	Transferrin receptor-2 related HH
	Ferroportin related HH
Malabsorption (e.g. from coeliac disease or after gastric surgery)	Iron-loading anaemia (e.g. thalassaemia major or sideroblastic anaemia)
Infancy (increased iron requirement)	Parenteral (e.g. multiple blood transfusions)
Pregnancy (increased iron requirement)	Metabolic syndrome
Heavy menstruation	Chronic liver disease (e.g. hepatitis C, alcoholic liver disease or non-alcoholic steatohepatitis)
Gastrointestinal bleed (e.g. from NSAID use or cancer)	African iron overload (increased iron intake from cooking in iron pans)
Chronic kidney disease	Acaeruloplasminaemia (absence of the transport protein caeruloplasmin)
	Atransferrinaemia (absence of the iron transport protein)
	Neonatal iron overload

HFE, human haemochromatosis protein; NSAID, non-steroidal anti-inflammatory drug.

Table 6.4 Causes of iron deficiency and iron excess.

Anaemia: signs and symptoms		
Non-specific symptoms	Non-specific signs	Specific signs
Fatigue	Pale skin colour	Koilonychia (in iron deficiency anaemia)
Headaches and faintness	Tachycardia	Jaundice in cases of haemolytic anaemia
Breathlessness	Systolic flow murmur	Bone deformities are often present in patients with thalassaemia major
Angina	Cardiac failure	
Intermittent claudication		
Palpitations		

Table 6.5 Clinical signs and symptoms of anaemia.

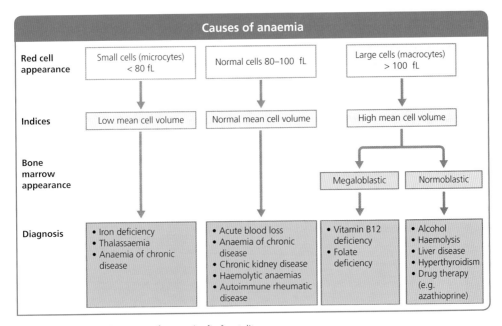

Figure 6.13 The main causes of anaemia. fL, femtolitre.

- normochromic normocytic anaemia (normal mean cell volume)
- macrocytic anaemia (high mean cell volume)

Remember that anaemia is a sign, (**Table 6.5**) not a diagnosis. Therefore its underlying cause must be identified and treated.

Haemoglobin function

The primary function of haemoglobin is to bind oxygen in the lungs and release it to body tissues. Haemoglobin also transports carbon monoxide, carbon dioxide, nitric oxide and can act as an anti-oxidant and a regulator of iron metabolism.

Haemoglobin binds carbon monoxide as well as oxygen. Its affinity for carbon monoxide is 245 times greater than its affinity for oxygen. Therefore when both gases are present, haemoglobin preferentially reacts with carbon monoxide to form carboxyhaemoglobin.

The presence of enough carbon monoxide can lead to decreased oxygen in the blood, the consequence of which is hypoxia (reduced oxygen supply to body tissues).

Pulse oximetry is a non-invasive method for monitoring haemoglobin oxygen saturation in arterial blood. The sensor, placed on a fingertip, passes light of two wavelengths , red light (600–750 nm) and infra-red (850–1000 nm) through the bloodstream. Light of differing wavelength differentiates between oxyhaemoglobin and deoxyhaemoglobin. Oxygenated blood absorbs more infrared light and allows red to pass through; deoxygenated haemoglobin the opposite. By subtracting the first reading before the pulse from the second after it, the oxygen saturation (SaO_2) is estimated.

Oxygen transport

The haemoglobin molecule has four haem groups, each with an iron group able to bind one oxygen atom. Oxygen saturation refers to the percentage of haemoglobin-binding sites in the circulation that are occupied by oxygen.

Haemoglobin is not always fully saturated, and it is the partial pressure of oxygen (pO_2) to which the haemoglobin is exposed that determines how much oxygen binds. The lungs have a high pO_2, so their oxygen readily binds to haemoglobin. As blood circulates, oxygen is released to the tissues, because their pO_2 is lower. The amount of oxygen in the blood depends on both the haemoglobin concentration and the percentage saturation.

Partial pressure describes the contribution of one gas in a gas mixture to the total pressure. Oxygen comprises 21% of air, so its pO_2 is 21% (about 21 kPa). In contrast, the partial pressure of carbon dioxide (pCO_2) of inspired air is negligible.

Oxyhaemoglobin dissociation curve

The binding of oxygen to haemoglobin is driven by pO_2, as is made evident by the oxyhaemoglobin dissociation curve (**Figure 6.14**). This shows the relationship between pO_2 (x-axis) and the percentage oxygen saturation (y-axis). The binding of oxygen by haemoglobin is cooperative, meaning that the binding of one molecule facilitates the binding of the next, thus increasing the affinity of haemoglobin for oxygen. This is reflected in the sigmoidal nature of the curve. Haemoglobin's affinity for the 4th oxygen molecule is about 300 times that for the 1st, and the curve then reaches the plateau stage as the haemoglobin becomes saturated.

The oxyhaemoglobin dissociation curve shows the key properties of oxygen transport by haemoglobin.

- At a concentration of 14 kPa, the percentage saturation of haemoglobin is near maximal
- In the capillaries of resting tissues, pO_2 is nearer 5 kPa, and the percentage saturation is about 70%
- The difference between the saturation levels is the amount of oxygen released from the haemoglobin to the tissues

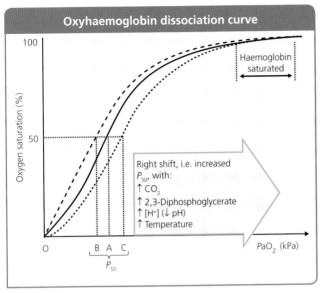

Figure 6.14 The oxyhaemoglobin dissociation curve for the binding of oxygen to haemoglobin. (B) Reference curve; (A) haemoglobin has an increased affinity (relinquishes oxygen less readily but binds it more easily); (C) haemoglobin has a decreased affinity (relinquishes oxygen more readily but requires a high partial pressure to achieve the same % oxygen saturation).

- More active tissues use more oxygen thereby lowering the capillary pO_2 and causing haemoglobin to release more oxygen

Atmospheric pO_2 is 21 kPa. However, the pO_2 in the lungs is only 14 kPa, because:

- air is humidified by the upper airway, so the partial pressure of water vapour reduces the pO_2
- gas exchange is a dynamic process, with continual carbon dioxide diffusion out of the capillaries and into the alveoli, and reciprocal oxygen uptake

P$_{50}$

The pO_2 at which haemoglobin is 50% saturated is the P_{50}. This value is used to compare the relative affinities of different haemoglobins for oxygen.

- An increased P_{50} indicates a 'shift to the right' of the oxyhaemoglobin dissociation curve, meaning that a higher pO_2 is required to maintain haemoglobin at 50% oxygen saturation, i.e. a decreased affinity
- Conversely, a lower P_{50} shifts the curve to the left, indicating a higher affinity

Normal adult haemoglobin has a P_{50} of 3.5 kPa, whereas fetal haemoglobin has a P_{50} of 2.7 kPa; this reflects the fact that fetal blood has a higher oxygen affinity than its mother's blood. In contrast, HbS, present in patients with sickle cell anaemia, has a considerably higher P_{50} of 4.5 kPa.

Factors influencing haemoglobin oxygen-affinity

The affinity of haemoglobin for oxygen is influenced by many factors and also varies with different types of haemoglobin. The result is to shift the oxyhaemoglobin dissociation curve either to the right (representing a lower affinity for oxygen) or to the left (an increased affinity for oxygen). When haemoglobin has an increased affinity for oxygen (being tightly bound), it is less likely to release its oxygen to the tissues and tissue hypoxia could occur despite adequate oxygen in the blood.

pH and carbon dioxide: the Bohr effect

The Bohr effect concerns the effect of pH on the oxygen affinity of haemoglobin. In acidic conditions, (lower pH, i.e. increased [H$^+$]), the curve shifts to the right, so haemoglobin has a lower affinity for oxygen. This effect occurs in tissue capillaries, where more oxygen is released in the acidic conditions generated by metabolism.

In exercising tissues, pCO_2 is high and pH is low because of the formation of carbonic acid (see page 201). With continuous strenuous exercise, anaerobic metabolism produces lactate in muscles, which further decreases pH. This increase in pCO_2 and decrease in pH shifts the dissociation curve to the right, releasing more oxygen to the tissues.

In the lungs, pCO_2 is low and pH high (i.e. low $[H^+]$), which shifts the dissociation curve to the left. Therefore oxygen uptake is enhanced and haemoglobin becomes highly saturated.

Temperature

Compared with changes in pH, pCO_2 and pO_2, changes in temperature have a less dramatic effect on haemoglobin oxygen affinity. An increase in temperature, which occurs in exercising tissues, shifts the dissociation curve to the right, causing oxygen release. Conversely, hypothermia shifts the curve to the left, enhancing oxygen uptake. Temperature affects protein structure, enzyme activity and binding.

2,3-Diphosphoglycerate

This is a by-product of energy production by red blood cells. The Luebering-Rapoport Shunt branches from glycolysis (page 116) to produce 2,3-diphosphoglycerate from 1,3-bisphosphoglycerate (**Figure 6.15**). The presence of 2,3-diphosphoglycerate lowers the oxygen affinity of haemoglobin, because it binds specifically to the deoxygenated (not the oxygenated) form. Thus 2,3-diphosphoglycerate facilitates the unloading of oxygen at the tissues; this is termed a heteroallosteric effect.

Production of 2,3-diphosphoglycerate is an adaptive mechanism by which cells signal the reduced oxygen availability of a tissue.

- In conditions such as hypoxemia (low oxygen levels), anaemia, congestive heart failure and chronic lung disease, increased levels of 2,3-diphosphoglycerate shift the curve to the right
- Septic shock can lead to low levels of 2,3-diphosphoglycerate in states of septic shock leads to an increased affinity for oxygen, shifting the curve to the left. The decreased 2,3-diphosphoglycerate is reported to be due to increased basal metabolic rate in sepsis which drives glycolysis

Iron oxidation state

In a healthy person, 1–2% of haemoglobin is present as methaemoglobin. Methaemoglobin has a reduced oxygen-carrying capacity, therefore it shifts the curve to the left and does not give up oxygen as easily as haemoglobin does. The reduced capacity is due to iron present in the ferric (Fe^{3+}) state rather than

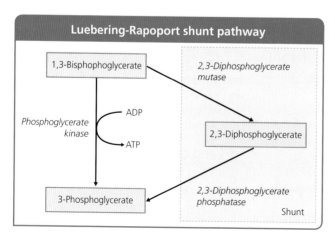

Figure 6.15 Luebering-Rapoport shunt pathway.

Luebering-Rapoport shunt pathway

1,3-Bisphophoglycerate

2,3-Diphosphoglycerate mutase

Phosphoglycerate kinase

ADP

ATP

2,3-Diphosphoglycerate

3-Phosphoglycerate

2,3-Diphosphoglycerate phosphatase

Shunt

ferrous (Fe^{2+}) state, so it is unable to carry oxygen. The concentration of methaemoglobin is increased by exposure to environmental chemicals, such as nitrates and chlorobenzenes, as well as to various pharmaceutical compounds (local anesthetic agents), including amyl nitrates (used to treat cyanide poisoning and also as a recreational drug) and nitroprusside. Some genetic conditions, e.g. a deficiency of NADH methemoglobin reductase or pyruvate kinase deficiency, also increase methaemoglobin concentration.

Type of haemoglobin

Fetal arterial oxygen pressures are lower than those of an adult. Therefore fetal haemoglobin has a higher affinity for oxygen at lower partial pressures, thus prioritising oxygen delivery from mother to fetus through the placenta. This is evident in the oxygen dissociation curve for fetal haemoglobin, which is displaced to the left relative to adult haemoglobin. In adults, fetal haemoglobin can be reactivated pharmacologically as seen in trials with hydroxyurea in sickle cells disease, where increased fetal haemoglobin reduced the number of sickle cell crises such as in the treatment of sickle cell disease.

Transport of carbon dioxide

Haemoglobin also transports carbon dioxide, the toxic end product of cellular energy production in mitochondria. The amount produced depends on the rate of metabolism and the relative amounts of carbohydrate, fat and protein metabolised. Carbon dioxide diffuses out of the cells and is transported in the blood to the lungs, where it is removed by exhalation. The pCO_2 is 5.5–6.8 kPa in venous blood and 4.7–6.0 kPa in arterial blood.

Carbon dioxide is transported in the blood by three mechanisms:

1. 70–80% is transported as bicarbonate in the plasma
2. 10–20% is carried as carbamino groups on haemoglobin after it has diffused into the red blood cells
3. 5–10% is dissolved in plasma, i.e. it is weakly soluble

Bicarbonate

Bicarbonate is a key buffer in blood. The ability to enter and exit red blood cells helps balance the extracellular and extracellular pH and carbon dioxide concentration. In red blood cells, carbon dioxide reacts with a water molecule to generate carbonic acid, which in turn dissociates into hydrogen and bicarbonate ions:

$$CO_2 + H_2O \rightleftharpoons H_2CO_3 \rightleftharpoons H^+ + HCO_3^-$$

In plasma, this reaction occurs without any enzymatic enhancement. However, in red blood cells the reaction is accelerated by the enzyme carbonic anhydrase (see page 183). For each molecule of carbon dioxide converted, a bicarbonate and a hydrogen ion are produced. The bicarbonate diffuses out of the cell down the concentration gradient into plasma. However, to maintain electroneutrality, a negative ion must move into the cell. Therefore the bicarbonate ion is exchanged for a chloride ion, a mechanism referred to as the chloride shift (**Figure 6.16**).

The hydrogen ion is unable to exit the cell to maintain neutrality, because it is buffered by haemoglobin. All cellular membranes are relatively impermeable to hydrogen ions, because their level (pH) needs to be tightly regulated to prevent fluctuations.

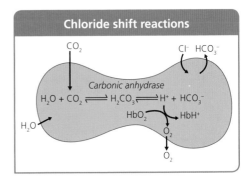

Chloride shift reactions

Figure 6.16 Reactions in the chloride shift, in which a bicarbonate ion is swapped for a chloride ion to enable transportation of carbon dioxide and maintain the electroneutrality of the cell.

Carbamino compounds

Carbamino compounds, such as carbaminohaemoglobin, are proteins that contain carbon dioxide with a free amino group. A carbamino group lowers haemoglobin's affinity for oxygen through the Bohr effect (see page 171).

After haemoglobin releases oxygen in the tissues, it then has increased affinity for carbon dioxide. This is known as the Haldane effect. The nature of the binding and the number of molecules it binds is not yet known. The carbon dioxide is then transported back to the lungs in venous blood, which is given its blue appearance by carbaminohaemoglobin.

Disorders of haemoglobin

There are two groups of haemoglobin disorders: haemoglobinopathies and thalassemias. Both are caused by mutations in the globin genes. Haemoglobinopathies are caused by abnormal forms of globin, whereas thalassemias are the result of reduced amounts of normal globin.

Haemoglobinopathies

These disorders are caused by mutations that result in an amino acid substitution in the globin chain. This change results in haemoglobin with:

- increased or decreased oxygen affinity
- reduced stability, causing increased breakdown
- reduced solubility

Haemoglobins containing the variant (abnormal) globin chains are named using letters of the alphabet, e.g. HbC and HbD. Other than HbS (for sickle haemoglobin), the letter does not stand for anything. Some haemoglobins are further named depending on where they were discovered (e.g. HbD$_{punjab}$) or by the name of the person who identified them (e.g. Hb$_{lepore}$). More than several hundred globin variants have been identified; however, only a few alter the structure or function of the haemoglobin molecule and thus give rise to clinically significant disease.

Sickle cell disease

Sickle cell disease is caused by haemoglobin variants such as HbS, HbC and HbD that have reduced solubility. HbS has reduced solubility because, in its deoxygenated form, it aggregates to form long polymers called tactoids. These distort the red blood cell into an elongated, rigid sickle shape, which often become trapped in the smaller blood vessels to cause ischaemia and tissue damage.

Initially, this distortion is a reversible process once the HbS binds another oxygen molecule. However, after several sickling episodes the red blood cells remain irreversibly sickled.

The presence of other forms of haemoglobin prevents HbS from polymerising. Consequently, sickle cell disease manifests when a person has two alleles that both encode the faulty HbS (i.e. the homozygous state). However, the haemoglobin variants HbC and HbD also cause sickle cell disease if paired with HbS in compound heterozygotes.

Interestingly, having a normal haemoglobin allele paired with a HbS allele confers some protection against malaria. This provides an evolutionary reason for why HbS is maintained in populations where malaria is endemic, such as Africa and parts of Asia, India and the Mediterranean.

Cyanosis

Haemoglobin variants with reduced oxygen affinity, such as HbM, cause cyanosis (blue discoloration of skin caused by increased carbaminohaemoglobin). These variants are unable to keep the iron atom in haem in its reduced Fe^{2+} state, resulting in increased amounts of methaemoglobin.

Methaemoglobin, because of its ferric (Fe^{3+}) state, is unable to bind oxygen. The amount of methaemoglobin is expressed as the percentage of the total haemoglobin.

■ Normally, only 1–2% of haemoglobin is methaemoglobin

■ A methaemoglobin percentage of 50–70% causes acidosis, arrhythmias, seizures or coma

■ A methaemoglobin percentage >70% is often fatal

Drugs that cause methaemoglobinaemia include amyl nitrite, chloroquine and sulfonamides.

Erythrocytosis

Haemoglobin variants with increased oxygen affinity are associated with erythrocytosis (increased red blood cell mass) and increased haemoglobin concentration. The increased affinity for oxygen reduces the release of oxygen to body tissues, causing a hypoxia that stimulates red blood cell production. The resulting increased haematocrit increases the risk of thrombosis. More than 40 structural variants with increased oxygen affinity are known.

Haemolytic anaemia

This is a type of anaemia caused by red blood cell breakdown (haemolysis). Haemolytic anaemia is associated with haemoglobin variants with reduced stability. More than a hundred variants cause reduced stability of the globin chain, resulting in a shortened red blood cell lifespan and premature destruction in the spleen.

Thalassemias

Thalassemias are a group of genetic disorders caused by a reduction in globin chain synthesis. They are classified according to the globin chain affected: α-thalassemias are associated with reduced α-globin synthesis, and β-thalassemias with reduced β-globin chain synthesis. Different mutations cause this by:

■ deletion of a whole globin gene
■ synthesis of a shortened, non-functional chain
■ disabling transcription or translation of the gene
■ incorrect splicing of the messenger RNA

The thalassemias range in clinical severity from mild anaemia (thalassemia minor) to severe anaemia, growth retardation and bone malformations (thalassemia major). The severity depends on whether the globin chain is completely or partially absent, and whether the individual is homozygous or heterozygous for the mutation. Heterozygotes for a partial deficiency (thalassemia trait) are usually asymptomatic, whereas the most severe forms (e.g. in which there is no α-globin production) are incompatible with life (**Table 6.6**).

The symptoms of α-thalassemias usually occur only when three or more copies of the four α-globin genes are affected. Reduction in the expression of one globin chain causes a relative excess of the unaffected chain in the cytosol, resulting in abnormal formation of the haemoglobin tetramer. An example is haemoglobin H (haemoglobin with four β-globin chains). These abnormal haemoglobin aggregates cause anaemia by reducing red blood cell life.

To provide the haemoglobin that the body needs, β thalassaemia major is treated with blood transfusions every 2–4 weeks. Patients also receive chelation therapy, which binds the excess iron and aids its excretion in urine. A cure is possible only by bone marrow transplantation or cord blood transplantation, where blood-producing stem cells from a newborn's umbilical cord are injected into the patient's marrow.

Thalassemias		
Disorder	Genotype	Signs and symptoms
β-thalassemia major	Homozygous (β⁰β⁰ or β⁺β⁺) or compound homozygous (β⁰β⁺)	Severe anaemia, jaundice, failure to thrive, bone abnormalities and hepatospleenomegaly presenting at about 6 months
β-thalassemia intermedia	Various	Moderate anaemia
β-thalassemia minor or trait	Heterozygous (ββ⁰, ββ⁺)	Asymptomatic or mild anaemia $$Increased haemoglobin A_2$$
Silent carrier	Three copies of normal α gene	Asymptomatic
α-thalassemia trait	Two copies of normal α gene	Asymptomatic Possible slightly low haemoglobin
Haemoglobin H disease	One copy of normal α gene	Production of haemoglobin H (β_4) Haemolytic anaemia
Bart's disease	No copies of normal α gene	Production of Bart's haemoglobin (γ_4) Hydrops fetalis Fetal death in utero unless diagnosed early and treated with aggressive transfusions

β⁰, mutation causing complete absence of β globin; β⁺, mutation causing partial deficiency of β globin.

Table 6.6 Thalassemic disorders and their symptoms

Answers to starter questions

1. At higher altitudes, the air contains less oxygen. Therefore pO_2 is reduced, which shifts the points on the oxyhaemoglobin dissociation curve to the left. The haematological response to this change is to increase the amount of haemoglobin and the number of red blood cells (and thus the haematocrit).The production of red blood cells is stimulated by erythropoietin, a hormone produced by the kidney in response to low pO_2. An increase in 2,3-diphosphoglycerate also occurs, stimulated by an increase in intracellular pH which regulates the activity of the enzyme bisphophoglyceromutase (Figure 6.15). In muscles, the 2,3-diphosphoglycerate causes the oxyhaemoglobin dissocation curve to shift to the right, so that more oxygen is unloaded in these tissues. With continual altitude exposure and training, the body physiologically acclimatises by, for example, increasing skeletal muscle vascularity and tissue myoglobin to improve blood and cellular oxygen transport, respectively.

2. The normal brown colour of faeces is a consequence of the oxidation of stercobilinogen, a colourless product of haemoglobin degradation by gut bacteria, to stercobilin, which appears brown. Oxidation results in the loss of an electron from the outer electron shell of the stercobilinogen molecule, which alters its electron structure. This structural change alters the wavelength at which the molecule emits absorbed light, and therefore the colour it appears. If stools become pale, this indicates a blockage of the flow of bile into the intestine.

Answers *continued*

3. About a third of the world's population, 2 billion people, are anaemic. Most cases of anaemia are caused by iron deficiency, which is a consequence of inadequate diet and the most common nutrient deficiency globally. Anaemia is a particular problem in poorer areas affected by endemic infections that precipitate and perpetuate anaemia: malaria, HIV, tuberculosis and chronic helminthiasis (infection by parasitic worms).

4. Juices rich in vitamin C, such as those from citrus, berries and guava, aid iron absorption. They do this by converting iron to its non-oxidised state (Fe^{2+}), which is more easily absorbed by enterocytes in the duodenum. In contrast, tea, coffee and some herbal teas contain antioxidant polyphenols, which form complexes with iron in the gut lumen and thus prevent its absorption.

5. Bruises result from capillary damage, which causes blood to leak into interstitial spaces. The gradual change in the colour of a bruise is the result of the breakdown of haemoglobin in the leaked blood. In this process, the central iron atom of the haem group is oxidised in the following sequence of reactions: red-blue haemoglobin to green biliverdin, biliverdin to orange-yellow bilirubin, and bilirubin to yellow-brown haemosiderin. The bruise fades as the constituents of the leaked blood are degraded and reabsorbed.

Chapter 7
Body fluid homeostasis

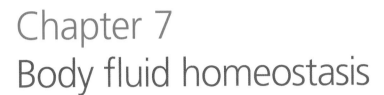

Starter questions

Answers to the following questions are on page 201.

1. Why is acidosis more common than alkalosis?
2. How can increased plasma potassium concentration (>7.0 mmol/L) cause the heart to stop?
3. What are the biochemical functions of water?
4. Why is pH regulation important for the body?
5. Why is chronic hyponatraemia less likely than acute hyponatraemia to cause neurological symptoms?

Introduction

Within the body there are different types of bodily fluids. These are found in the intra- and extracellular fluid compartments. The focus of this chapter is on fluids found in the extracellular fluid compartment, which is broken down into vascular and extra-vascular. The vascular compartment includes plasma. The extravascular compartment includes interstitial (including lymphatic), cerebrospinal, pleural, pericardial and gastrointestinal fluids. All bodily fluids have important roles, including the delivery of oxygen and nutrients to tissues and the removal of metabolic waste. In addition, they provide an environment for biochemical reactions to occur. In clinical practice bodily fluids are analysed to assess if electrolyte and hormone abnormalities are present.

Case 6 Injuries sustained in a traffic collision

Presentation

A 15-year-old girl presents to the emergency department after being hurt in a road traffic collision. She is hypotensive (blood pressure, 90/60 mmHg) and tachycardic (heart rate, 110 beats/min). Her Glasgow coma score is reduced (8 out of 15). She has lost a significant amount of blood (2 L). The evaluation of this patient includes an arterial blood gas analysis to assess her acid base status.

Analysis

The results of the arterial blood gas analysis show a severe increased-anion-gap metabolic acidosis (low bicarbonate, large negative base excess and increased lactate and anion gap), as well as hyperkalaemia (increased potassium) (**Table 7.1**). The increased-anion-gap acidosis is caused by lactic acid accumulation, which is a result of tissue hypoxia (type A lactic acidosis) and ischaemia. The presenting signs are consistent with these results: the patient is hypotensive as a consequence of blood loss, and the physiological response to hypotension is to increase heart rate to improve tissue perfusion.

The blood gas analysis results show little evidence of respiratory compensation for the acidosis, because $Paco_2$ is within normal limits; compensation would decrease $Paco_2$, because faster breathing decreases carbon dioxide in the blood. The cause of the hyperkalaemia is probably multifactorial, with acidosis and trauma injury promoting the leakage of potassium from cells.

Further case

A blood sample is sent to the laboratory for measurement of urea and electrolytes.

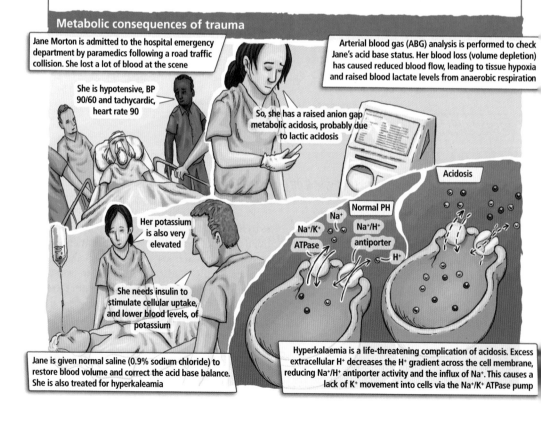

Metabolic consequences of trauma

Jane Morton is admitted to the hospital emergency department by paramedics following a road traffic collision. She lost a lot of blood at the scene

She is hypotensive, BP 90/60 and tachycardic, heart rate 90

Arterial blood gas (ABG) analysis is performed to check Jane's acid base status. Her blood loss (volume depletion) has caused reduced blood flow, leading to tissue hypoxia and raised blood lactate levels from anaerobic respiration

So, she has a raised anion gap metabolic acidosis, probably due to lactic acidosis

Acidosis

Normal PH

Na⁺

Na⁺/K⁺ ATPase

Na⁺/H⁺ antiporter

H⁺

Her potassium is also very elevated

She needs insulin to stimulate cellular uptake, and lower blood levels, of potassium

Jane is given normal saline (0.9% sodium chloride) to restore blood volume and correct the acid base balance. She is also treated for hyperkalaemia

Hyperkalaemia is a life-threatening complication of acidosis. Excess extracellular H⁺ decreases the H⁺ gradient across the cell membrane, reducing Na⁺/H⁺ antiporter activity and the influx of Na⁺. This causes a lack of K⁺ movement into cells via the Na⁺/K⁺ ATPase pump

Case 6 *continued*

Arterial blood gas analysis results		
Component	Result	Reference range
pH	7.05	7.35-7.45
Carbon dioxide, Pa_{CO_2} (kPa)	5.1	4.5-6.0
Oxygen, Pa_{O_2} (kPa)	13.7	11.0–14.0
Bicarbonate (mmol/L)	10	22–29
Base excess	−19.0	± 2.5
Anion gap (mmol/L)	26	6–16
Potassium (mmol/L)	6.3	3.5-5.3
Sodium (mmol/L)	140	135–145
Lactate (mmol/L)	10.2	< 1.9
Chloride (mmol/L)	100	99–109

Table 7.1 Results of arterial blood gas analysis for a 15-year-old girl injured in a traffic collision

The results confirm the presence of hyperkalaemia and show that the patient also has an increased concentration of urea.

Further analysis

The increased urea is consistent with blood loss and intravascular volume contraction; this is referred to as prerenal uraemia.

The patient is initially treated with insulin and normal saline (0.9%) to reduce potassium (insulin stimulates cellular potassium uptake) and improve renal perfusion. This treatment causes the acid–base disturbance to resolve as the excess acid load is buffered by phosphate and passes into the urine, and the lactate is recycled in the Cori cycle (lactic acid cycle). The patient is also given calcium gluconate to stabilise the myocardium and thus protect it from the arrhythmias associated with hyperkalaemia. The biochemical focus is calcium gluconate - securing the airway is the overall priority.

> **Hyperkalaemia is a medical emergency when potassium concentration exceeds 7.0 mmol/L.** At this concentration, cardiac arrhythmias usually occur. Treatment options to reduce potassium include intravenous insulin and dextrose, nebulised salbutamol and haemodialysis.

pH

Every day, biochemical reactions in the body produce large quantities of acid (**Table 7.2**). These reactions lead to the net formation of 40-80 mmol of hydrogen ions in a 24-h period. These ions mainly result from the oxidation of sulphur-containing amino acids (see page 182).

Excess acid is disposed of through the kidneys into the urine (see page 185). It is also buffered by the proteins within the body.

pH is a measure of the acidity (i.e. hydrogen ion concentration) of an aqueous solution such as blood and other body fluids. It is measured in arterial blood gas analysis, using a sample of blood taken from the radial artery.

The lower the pH, the more hydrogen ions are present, and the more acidic the arterial blood. Conversely, a higher pH indicates a basic solution. pH must remain within narrow limits (7.35-7.45) in biological systems because the majority of enzymes and biochemical processes within the body work optimally close to pH 7.

Calculating pH

pH is calculated from the negative logarithm of the hydrogen ion concentration:

$$pH = -\log [H^+]$$

Acid generation by physiological processes				
Type of acid	Production	Rate of production (mmol/24 h)	Disposal	Rate of disposal (mmol/24 h)
Carbon dioxide	Tissue respiration	20,000	Excretion by lungs	20,000
Lactate	Glycolysis	1300	Gluconeogenesis	1300
Fatty acids	Lipolysis	600	Re-esterification and oxidation	600
Ketoacids	Ketogenesis	400	Oxidation	400
H^+ from urea synthesis	Ureagenesis	1100	Oxidation of amino acids	1100
Sulphuric acid	Metabolism of amino acids	40	Renal excretion	40

Table 7.2 Acid generation by normal physiological processes

pH has no units. It varies in a reciprocal and non-linear fashion with hydrogen ion concentration.

Because pH is based on a logarithmic scale (**Figure 7.1**), it is often difficult to appreciate how the concentration of hydrogen ions in the blood has changed. The normal pH of blood is 7.35–7.45 (equivalent to hydrogen ion concentration 35-45 nmol/L).

- If the pH of the patient's blood decreases to < 7.35, they have an acidaemia
- If pH increases to >7.45, they have an alkalaemia

Strictly, the term acidosis describes a pathological disturbance that can result in acidaemia but may not do so because of the existence of a simultaneous disturbance (i.e. a compensatory process having the opposite effect). Similarly, alkalosis does not always result in alkalaemia.

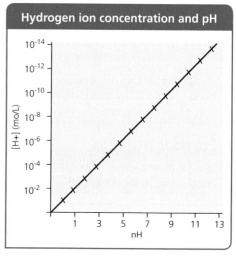

Figure 7.1 Logarithmic relationship between hydrogen ion concentration and pH

Systems that maintain acid–base homeostasis

A buffer limits the extent to which hydrogen ion concentration changes the pH of physiological fluids in situations that cause a tendency to change. Buffering plays an essential role in maintaining the pH of blood, intracellular fluid and extracellular fluid.

The body has four buffer systems (**Table 7.3**). A buffer is a solution containing a weak acid, i.e. one that only partially dissociates into hydrogen ions and its conjugate base (anion). Therefore the addition of strong acid or base to such a solution does not greatly alter its pH. The equilibrium of the reaction is represented as follows:

$$H^+ + A^- \rightleftharpoons HA$$

hydrogen ion + conjugate base $\rightleftharpoons$ weak acid

- When an acid is added to a buffer system, base anions react to form a weak acid, shifting the equilibrium right
- When a base is added, the weak acid dissociates, shifting the equilibrium left

The dissociation of the weak acid varies according to the acidity of the environment, thereby stabilising the amount of hydrogen ions present, i.e. the pH.

Bicarbonate–carbonic acid buffer system

The major buffer system in the body is the bicarbonate–carbonic acid system. Carbonic acid is a weak acid that dissociates into bicarbonate and a hydrogen ion:

$$H_2CO_3 \rightleftharpoons HCO_3^- + H^+$$

carbonic acid $\rightleftharpoons$ bicarbonate + hydrogen ion

- If hydrogen ions are added to this system, they react with the bicarbonate to form carbonic acid (i.e. the equilibrium shifts left), thus the concentration of hydrogen ions in the solution is limited by the formation of carbonic acid at the expense of bicarbonate
- Conversely, removal of hydrogen ions causes the reverse reaction (i.e. the equilibrium shifts right), resulting in the formation of hydrogen ions and bicarbonate

Systems that maintain acid–base homeostasis			
Buffer system	Mechanism	Location	Importance
Bicarbonate–carbonic acid	Carbonic acid is a weak acid H$^+$ combines with bicarbonate to form carbonic acid via carbonic anhydrase	Blood	Major extracellular buffer in blood
Phosphate	Mono- and di-hydrogen phosphate combine with H$^+$ to enable efficient buffering of H$^+$ in urine Present in very low concentrations in blood to be effective	Urine	Major buffer in urine
Proteins	Contain weak acidic and basic groups and therefore can buffer H$^+$	Blood	Minor extracellular buffer in blood Major intracellular and tissue buffer
Bone	H$^+$ is buffered by proteins within bone matrix Increased H$^+$ stimulates bone resorption and alkaline minerals act as buffers	Blood	Extracellular buffer Particularly important in chronic acidosis (e.g. chronic kidney disease)
Ammonia	Ammonium is a weak acid and is a route for H$^+$ disposal	Urine	Minor urinary buffer has a role in H$^+$ elimination in severe chronic acidosis

Table 7.3 Systems that maintain acid–base homeostasis

For a buffer to maintain pH within the normal limits in situations in which there is an equal tendency for the amount of hydrogen ions to increase or decrease, the concentration of hydrogen ions and conjugate base must be equal.

The carbonic acid formed by the bicarbonate–carbonic acid system dissociates into carbon dioxide and water in a reaction catalysed by the enzyme carbonic anhydrase. The carbon dioxide is then removed by the lungs. The dissociation of carbonic acid is governed by the equilibrium constant K_a:

$$H_2CO_3 \rightleftharpoons CO_2 + H_2O$$
$$\text{carbonic acid} \rightleftharpoons \text{carbon dioxide} + \text{water}$$

The bicarbonate–carbonic acid buffer system is described by the Henderson-Hasselbalch equation, which combines the previous two equations to give:

$$CO_2 + H_2O \rightleftharpoons H_2CO_3 \rightleftharpoons HCO_3^- + H^+$$
$$\text{carbon dioxide} + \text{water} \rightleftharpoons \text{carbonic acid} \rightleftharpoons$$
$$\text{bicarbonate} + \text{hydrogen ion}$$

The Hendersen-Hasselbalch equation is then used to derive the pH of blood:

$$pH = pK_a + \log[\text{bicarbonate}]/0.225 \times [P\text{aco}_2]$$

In this equation, pK_a is the dissociation constant (6.1 in this system), 0.225 is Bunsen's coefficient and $P\text{aco}_2$ is the partial pressure of carbon dioxide in kilopascals (kPa). In health, the ratio of bicarbonate to $P\text{aco}_2$ is 20:1. The body will compensate for changes in this ratio.

Phosphate buffer system

Monohydrogen phosphate and dihydrogen phosphate are present in blood. In theory they would be a highly effective buffer, but their low concentrations limit their buffering capacity. In contrast, urinary monohydrogen phosphate serves as a highly effective buffer.

Urine is acidified by active secretion of hydrogen ions by the intercalated cells of the distal tubules of the proximal collecting duct. The maximum amount of acid excreted into urine is 38 μmol/L (pH = 4.5). Hydrogen ions are buffered by phosphate, so a significant proportion of them are excreted.

Monohydrogen phosphate is titrated to dihydrogen phosphate ($H_2PO_4^-$) in the cortical collecting tubules of the kidneys for urinary excretion (**Figure 7.2**). Aldosterone stimulates the secretion of hydrogen ions when it enters the principal cell, where it promotes the opening of sodium channels and increases Na^+-K^+-ATPase activity. The consequent movement of sodium ions generates a negative potential in the tubule lumen, causing potassium ions to move into it along the electrochemical gradient.

Aldosterone also stimulates the Na^+-K^+-ATPase in the intercalated cell, thus enhancing hydrogen ion secretion. Titratable acid secreted as hydrogen ions binds to the conjugate anions (monohydrogen phosphate) and is excreted in the urine. The hydrogen ions secreted arise from the reaction between water and carbon dioxide in the presence of carbonic anhydrase.

The bicarbonate regenerated in this process is then able to contribute to the restoration of buffering capacity (**Figure 7.3**). Filtered bicarbonate combines with secreted hydrogen ions to form carbonic acid. Carbonic acid subsequently dissociates into carbon dioxide and water in a reaction catalysed by carbonic anhydrase.

Carbonic anhydrase is present in the brush border of renal tubular cells. Carbon dioxide diffuses into the tubular cell down a concentration gradient. Inside the cell, it reacts with water to form carbonic acid; this reaction is also catalysed by carbonic anhydrase. Carbonic acid further dissociates to bicarbonate and hydrogen ions. Bicarbonate moves into the bloodstream, and hydrogen ions pass back into the tubular fluid in exchange for sodium.

This mechanism of hydrogen ion excretion is highly effective. However, it is insufficient to remove the daily burden of hydrogen ions produced by intermediary metabolism.

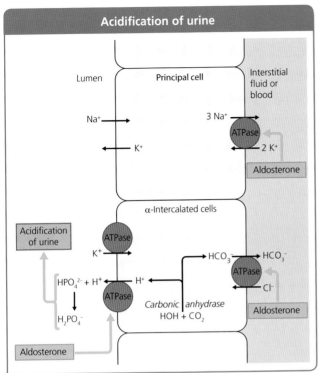

Figure 7.2 Acidification of urine by titration of monohydrogen phosphate (HPO_4^{2-}) to dihydrogen phosphate ($H_2PO_4^-$) in the cortical collecting tubule.

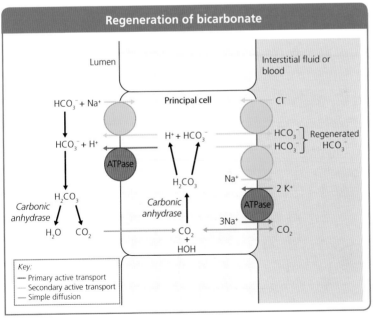

Figure 7.3 Regeneration of bicarbonate in the renal tubular cells. Filtered bicarbonate (HCO_3^-) combines with secreted hydrogen ions to form carbonic acid (H_2CO_3), which then dissociates into carbon dioxide and water in a reaction catalysed by carbonic anhydrase.

The body's buffer systems have huge buffering capacity and a practically immediate effect. Therefore the body is able to resist large changes in the concentration of hydrogen ions. This ability is essential, because dynamic metabolic systems require many reactions that would otherwise cause significant changes in acid–base balance.

Proteins

All proteins are able to buffer hydrogen ions, albeit to varying extents. A protein's buffering ability greatly depends on the number of polar amino acids in its structure.

Haemoglobin is an essential buffer in red blood cells; each molecule is able to accept a several hydrogen ions. Haemoglobin is a particularly effective buffer in its deoxygenated state (see page 173), therefore its buffering ability is facilitated by oxygen release through the Bohr effect (see page 171).

Plasma proteins such as albumin buffer hydrogen ions. However, their molar concentration is lower than that of haemoglobin, and therefore their buffering capacity is less.

Intracellular proteins contribute to buffering, particularly in chronic acidosis (e.g. chronic kidney disease). In chronic acidosis, these proteins contribute up to one third of the total buffering capacity of the body. The remainder is achieved by oral bicarbonate replacement therapy.

Bone

In patients with chronic kidney disease (associated with irreversible kidney damage and reduced glomerular filtration), bone provides a vital buffer because it serves as a large reservoir of phosphate and bicarbonate. However, prolonged buffering by bone contributes to combined chronic kidney disease–metabolic bone disease, also known as renal osteodystrophy.

Ammonia

Ammonia is not a buffer, but it has a critical role in the maintenance of acid–base homeostasis. Ammonia provides a route for ammonium disposal that, unlike urea synthesis, does not generate hydrogen ions (**Figure 7.4**).

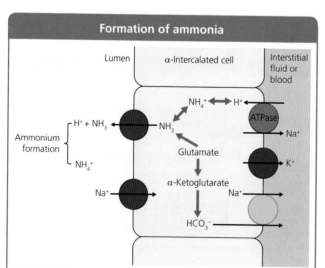

Formation of ammonia

Figure 7.4 Formation of ammonium (NH_4^+) from ammonia (NH_3) in the distal tubule of the kidney. The ammonia used to buffer hydrogen ions is synthesised, mainly from glutamate, in the proximal convoluted tubule. Glutamate is broken down into bicarbonate, which is secreted into peritubular fluid at the sodium–bicarbonate (Na^+-HCO_3^-) cotransporter.

Acid–base balance

The four main components to the pathophys-iology of an acid disturbance are:

- generation of the disturbance
- buffering disturbance
- compensation
- correction

Types of acid–base disturbance

There are numerous causes of acid–base dis-turbances. These causes can be divided into four states:

- metabolic acidosis (**Table 7.4**)
- metabolic alkalosis (**Table 7.5**)
- respiratory acidosis (**Table 7.6**)
- respiratory alkalosis (**Table 7.7**)

These disturbances do not always occur in isolation; often, more than one disturbance occurs simultaneously to produce a mixed acid–base disturbance with metabolic com-ponents, respiratory components or both (see **Tables 7.4–7.7**).

Compensation

The body has two main compensatory mech-anisms for acid–base disturbances: respira-tory and metabolic.

- In a single acid–base disturbance when the primary disturbance is metabolic, the compensatory mechanism will be respiratory
- If the primary disturbance is respiratory, the compensatory mechanism will be metabolic

Metabolic acidosis: causes	
Increased anion gap	**Normal anion gap**
Ketoacidosis	**Renal causes**
Diabetes	Renal tubular acidosis
Alcoholism	Use of carbonic anhydrase inhibitors
Starvation	
Lactic acidosis	**Gastrointestinal causes**
Type A (impaired perfusion)	Severe diarrhoea
Type B (impaired carbohydrate metabolism)	Ureteroenterostomy or obstructed ileal conduit
Renal failure	Drainage of pancreatic or biliary secretions
Uraemic acidosis	Small bowel fistula
Acidosis with acute kidney injury	**Other causes**
Toxins	Recovery from ketoacidosis
Ethylene glycol	Ammonium chloride loading test
Ethanol or methanol	
Salicylates	

Table 7.4 Causes of metabolic acidosis

Metabolic alkalosis: causes	
Metabolic alkalosis: causes	
Addition of base to extracellular fluid	**Potassium depletion**
Milk alkali syndrome	Primary hyperaldosteronism
Excessive intake of sodium bicarbonate	Cushing's syndrome
Recovery phase after organic acidosis	Secondary hyperaldosteronism
Massive blood transfusion (caused by citrate metabolism)	Use of certain drugs (e.g. carbenoxolone)
Chloride depletion	Use of potassium-losing diuretics
Loss of acidic gastric juice	Excessive liquorice (contains glycyrrhizic acid) intake
Use of diuretics	Bartter's syndrome
After hypercapnia	Severe potassium depletion
Excess faecal loss (e.g. in cases of villous adenoma)	**Other disorders**
	Laxative abuse
	Severe hypoalbuminaemia

Table 7.5 Causes of metabolic alkalosis

Respiratory acidosis: causes	
Central nervous system disorders	**Lung or chest wall defects**
Depression of respiratory centre (e.g. through use of opiates, sedatives and anaesthetics)	Chronic obstructive airways disease
	Chest trauma (e.g. pneumothorax)
Central nervous system trauma, infarct, haemorrhage or tumour	Diaphragmatic paralysis or splinting
	Pulmonary oedema
Hypoventilation of obesity (e.g. Pickwickian syndrome)	Acute respiratory distress syndrome
Cervical cord trauma or lesions	Restrictive lung disease
High central neural blockade	Aspiration
Poliomyelitis	**Airway disorders**
Tetanus	Upper airway obstruction
Cardiac arrest with cerebral hypoxia	Laryngospasm
Nerve or muscle disorders	Bronchospasm or asthma
Guillain–Barré syndrome	**External factors**
Myasthenia gravis	Inadequate mechanical ventilation
Use of muscle relaxant drugs	
Toxins (e.g. organophosphates and snake venom)	

Table 7.6 Causes of respiratory acidosis

Respiratory alkalosis: causes	
Central causes (direct action on respiratory centre)	**Hypoxaemia**
Head injury	Respiratory stimulation through action on peripheral chemoreceptors
Stroke	
Anxiety hyperventilation syndrome	Pulmonary causes (through action on intrapulmonary receptors)
'Supratentorial' causes (e.g. pain)	
Use of certain drugs (e.g. analeptic agents)	Pulmonary embolism
Endogenous compounds (e.g. progesterone during pregnancy, cytokines during sepsis and toxins in patients with chronic liver disease)	Pneumonia
	Asthma
	Pulmonary oedema (all types) (through direct action on ventilation)
	Overventilation

Table 7.7 Causes of respiratory alkalosis

Respiratory compensation is faster than metabolic compensation. This is because it takes longer for the kidney to regenerate or excrete bicarbonate than it does to change the rate of the respiratory drive to increase or decrease the elimination of carbon dioxide through the lungs.

The aim of the compensatory mechanisms is to maintain the ratio of bicarbonate to carbon dioxide at the normal ratio of 20:1.

■ An acid–base disturbance is fully compensated only when the pH is back within its normal reference range
■ A disturbance is partially compensated when there is evidence that the body has attempted to adapt to the acid–base disturbance but the pH has not returned to a value within the normal reference range

Correction

The acid–base disturbance is fully corrected when the pH, carbon dioxide and bicarbonate are within the reference range (7.35–7.45).

Interpreting blood gas results

Investigation of acid–base disturbances requires evaluation of the metabolic and respiratory components that affect this balance. Useful approaches to the evaluation of patients with acidaemia or alkalaemia are shown in **Figures 7.5** and **7.6**, respectively.

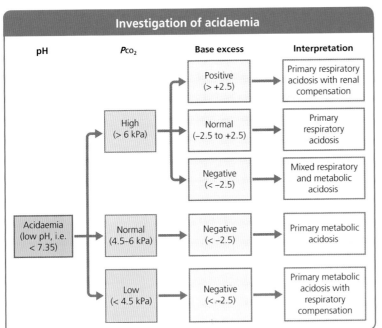

Figure 7.5
Algorithm for
investigation of
acidaemia.

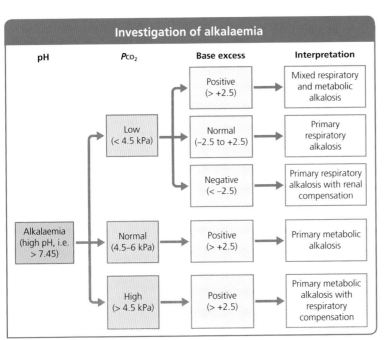

Figure 7.6
Algorithm for
investigation of
alkalaemia.

These algorithms can be used to interpret arterial blood gas results.

The starting point for the interpretation of blood gas results is to establish if the pH shows that the patient has an acidaemia or an alkalaemia.

- Acidaemia: pH < 7.35
- Alkalaemia: pH > 7.45

The next step is to determine if this disturbance is a metabolic disorder, a respiratory disorder or a mixed metabolic–respiratory disorder.

- A metabolic disorder is indicated by an increase or decrease in bicarbonate and base excess
- A respiratory disorder is indicated by an increase or decrease in the partial pressure of carbon dioxide

Base excess is a calculated value that helps confirm whether a disorder is metabolic or respiratory.

- Negative base excess supports the presence of a metabolic acidosis; it is a measure of how much alkali would have to be added to the blood to bring the pH into the normal reference range
- Positive base excess supports a metabolic alkalosis; it is a measure of how much

acid would have to be added to the blood to bring the pH into the normal reference range

Anion gap

The anion gap is the difference between the major cations (**positively charged ions**) and anions (negatively charged ions) measured in the extracellular fluid:

$$\text{anion gap} = ([Na^+] + [K^+]) - ([Cl^-] + [HCO_3^-])$$

The reference range for anion gap is 6–16 mmol/L. This difference is caused by the presence of negatively charged proteins, mainly albumin. This is because the body is charge neutral; albumin is negatively charged and therefore contributes to the negatively-charged pool of anions that maintain a neutral charge. It is, however, not considered in the formula, creating an apparent anion gap.

The clinical utility of the anion gap is often overlooked, because not all laboratories measure chloride and bicarbonate, due to cost considerations and difficulties in measurement. These measurements would determine whether a patient has a normal or an increased anion gap, information that helps narrow down the cause of the acid–base disorder (see **Tables 7.4–7.7** for examples).

Maintenance of fluid balance

The body contains numerous types of fluid, for example serum, sweat, bile, saliva and tears. These fluids comprise water (the main component), dissolved ions (electrolytes) and water-soluble molecules such as glucose and proteins. The amount and distribution of water in the body differs with age and sex (**Table 7.8**).

The volume and composition of body fluids must be maintained for cells and organs to function normally.

Distinct clinical signs can be detected in cases of disturbance of fluid balance (**Figure 7.7**):

- excess fluid volume (hypervolaemia)
- reduced fluid volume (hypovolaemia)

Distribution of water in the body			
	Infant (1 year old)	Man (40 years old)	Woman (40 years old)
Weight (kg)	7	70	60
Total body water (L)	4.9	42	30
Intracellular volume (L)	3.15	28	18
Extracellular fluid volume (L)	1.75	14	12
Intravascular volume (L)	0.35	2.8	2.4

Table 7.8 Distribution of water in the body

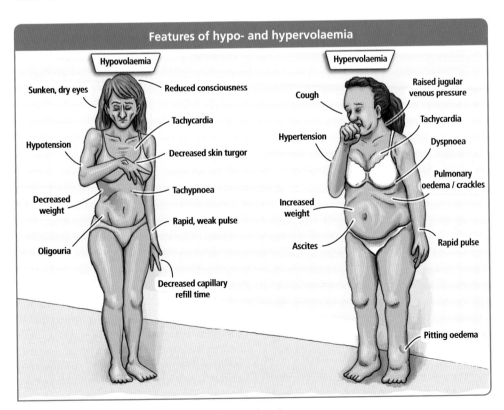

Figure 7.7 Key features of hypovolaemia and hypervolaemia.

Fluid distribution in the body

Body fluid is in two main compartments: the intracellular fluid space and the extracellular fluid space (**Figure 7.8**). **Table** 7.8 shows the amount of water in these compartments. The extracellular fluid space is further subdivided into the:

- intravascular space (plasma volume)
- interstitial space (includes lymph)
- transcellular fluid

Transcellular fluid is formed by the transport activity of cells and includes pleural, pericardial, cerebrospinal, gastrointestinal and peritoneal fluids.

The composition of the intracellular fluid is very different from that of the extracellular fluid (**Table 7.9**). The predominant electrolyte is potassium in the intracellular fluid and sodium in the extracellular fluid. The distribution of these electrolytes is maintained by an energy-dependent pump on the cell membrane: the Na⁺–K⁺–ATPase pump.

Composition of intracellular and extracellular fluid		
Electrolyte	Concentration in intracellular fluid (mmol/L)	Concentration in extracellular fluid (mmol/L)
Sodium	10	140
Potassium	140	4.0
Chloride	10	100
Bicarbonate	10	25
Calcium	0.0001	1.0
Phosphate	50	1.0
Magnesium	2.7	0.5

Table 7.9 Electrolyte composition of intracellular and extracellular fluid. Concentrations refer to the ionised fraction (i.e. biologically active)

Solute concentrations: osmolality, osmolarity and tonicity

Osmolality, osmolarity and tonicity are distinct terms of solute concentration that often create confusion.

- Osmolarity is a measure of solute concentration; it is the number of osmoles of solute per litre of solution
- Osmolality is the measure of solute concentration; it is the number of osmoles of solute per kilogram of solvent. This measurement is used in clinical practice because it is independent of temperature (solvent is measured per kg of solvent and not per litre of solution; volume varies with temperature, mass does not)
- Tonicity is a measure of the effective osmotic pressure gradient, defined by the water potential (potential energy of water that influences the tendency of water to move from one area to another due to osmosis), of two solutions separated by a semipermeable membrane

There are three classes of tonicity: hypertonic, hypotonic and isotonic. A hypertonic solution has a higher concentration of solute(s), a hypotonic solution has a lower concentration of solute(s), and an isotonic solution is one in which the osmole concentration is the same on both sides of the membrane.

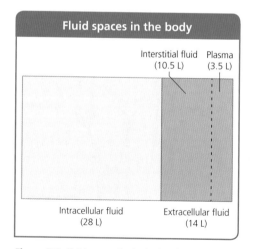

Fluid spaces in the body

Interstitial fluid (10.5 L)   Plasma (3.5 L)

Intracellular fluid (28 L)   Extracellular fluid (14 L)

Figure 7.8 Fluid spaces in the body of a 70-kg man.

Intravenous fluid replacement is a common hospital treatment to increase blood pressure and rehydrate patients. The most common fluids used for this treatment are:

- normal saline (0.9% sodium chloride)
- dextrose (5%)
- Hartmann's physiological solution (0.6% sodium chloride, 0.32% sodium lactate, 0.04% potassium chloride and 0.027% calcium chloride)

If 1L of dextrose is infused into a patient, only one ninth will stay in the extracellular fluid compartment. In contrast, if 1L of normal saline is infused, one third will stay in the extracellular fluid. Because extracellular fluid volume is essential for maintaining blood pressure, low blood pressure is treated with saline.

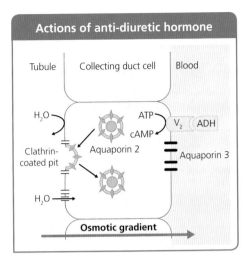

Actions of anti-diuretic hormone

Figure 7.9 Action of antidiuretic hormone (ADH) in the kidney. ADH binds to the V_2 receptor on the basolateral membrane, which results in the formation of cyclic adenosine monophosphate (cAMP) from adenosine triphosphate (ATP). This reaction leads to fusion of aquaporin 2 vesicles with the impermeable apical membrane. Water is also drawn across the cell and taken up by the blood through aquaporin 3 channels along the medullary osmotic gradient.

Regulation of fluid homeostasis

Maintenance of the volume and pressure of body fluids is essential for perfusion of organs and tissues, adequate delivery of oxygen and nutrients, and removal of metabolic waste.

Fluid pressures

Fluid homeostasis is governed by three pressures: osmotic, oncotic and hydrostatic.

Osmotic pressure

The movement of water (solvent) through the body occurs through protein channels in cell membranes; these channels are called aquaporins (**Figure 7.9**). This movement is predominantly influenced by osmotic pressure from dissolved particles (solute) in the extracellular fluid and intracellular fluid on either side of the cell membrane.

Osmosis is the movement (diffusion) of water across a semipermeable membrane, such as a cell membrane, from the side of low solvent concentration to the side of high solute concentration. The osmotic pressure is the difference in total solute concentrations between the two compartments; the side with the lower solute concentration has the higher osmotic pressure.

The water content of body spaces depends on the solute concentration (also referred to as osmolality) in the respective body spaces. This is true for most cells in the body; the exceptions are cells with highly specialised cell membranes (e.g. nephrons and sweat gland cells).

Oncotic pressure

The other major factor controlling the movement of water is oncotic pressure (also known as colloid osmotic pressure). Oncotic pressure is the consequence of the difference in extracellular fluid protein content between the plasma and the interstitial fluid. In health, albumin is the major protein contributing to colloid oncotic pressure.

Hydrostatic pressure

This is the result of the contractile force of the heart across the afferent capillary membranes, which creates a counterforce to oncotic pressure. The changing oncotic and hydrostatic pressure across gradients across the capillary bed is called Starling's force.

> **Ascites is the accumulation of extracellular fluid in the peritoneal cavity.** Over 30 L of fluid can accumulate in severe cases. The most common causes of ascites are liver cirrhosis (advanced irreversible liver disease) and metastatic disease (neoplastic disease that has spread).

Monitors of plasma volume

Several mechanisms monitor the effective plasma volume. These include intrathoracic volume receptors (e.g. arterial stretch receptors), hepatic volume receptors, arterial baroreceptors, intrarenal baroreceptors and tissue receptors. All these control mechanisms fine-tune the renal conservation of water as they can influence the hormonal regulation of fluid balance.

Control of fluid balance

Water output from the body is controlled by the actions on the kidney of a hormone called antidiuretic hormone (ADH also called arginine vasopressin) (see **Figure 7.9**). ADH is released in response to increased extracellular fluid osmolality. In contrast, hydration suppresses secretion of ADH.

ADH is a nonapeptide synthesised in the magnocellular neurones in the hypothalamus as preproantidiuretic hormone (its precursor peptide). It is stored in neurosecretory granules in the posterior pituitary gland as proantidiuretic hormone, and is released into the circulation as ADH.

The thirst centre in the hypothalamus also contributes to regulating fluid balance. The activity of the thirst centre is governed by the shrinking and swelling of osmoreceptor cells (cells that detect changes in osmolality) in response to changes in extracellular osmolality.

> **A cause of hyponatraemia is the syndrome of inappropriate antidiuretic hormone (i.e. ADH).** In this hormonal imbalance, ADH is produced when a patient is euvolaemic (has normal body volume), thus a clinical picture of dilutional hyponatraemia (too much water retention) is produced.

Maintenance of electrolyte balance

The major extracellular cations and anions are sodium and potassium, and chloride and bicarbonate, respectively. Sodium is the dominant extracellular cation and potassium the intracellular cation. The fundamental differences in electrolyte composition are maintained by energy requiring cell membrane transport pumps (Na^+ – K^+ – ATPase). The distribution of electrolytes is such that there is no difference in charge or osmolality between the extra and intracellular fluid compartments. Electrolyte homeostasis is essential in maintaining cellular fluid distribution and regulating cellular membrane potentials. Other important electrolytes present at lower concentrations include calcium and magnesium (cations) and chloride and phosphate (anions).

> **Osmolality can be measured or calculated, and the difference between them is the osmolal gap.** An increased gap indicates the presence of an osmotically active substance that has not been considered in the calculation, for example ethanol or mannitol.
>
> Calculated osmolality = 2 [Na^+] + [K^+] + [glucose] + [urea] (all in mmol/L)
>
> Osmolal gap = measured osmolality - calculated osmolality (reference range < 10 mmol/L)

Sodium

Sodium is the major extracellular cation that has a important role in maintaining extracellular volume. In health, its plasma concentration ranges from 133 to 146 mmol/L. The daily intake of sodium varies greatly, depending on a person's diet. The body has sophisticated control mechanisms to maintain sodium concentration.

Renal control of sodium

The kidney is pivotal in maintaining sodium balance. It can conserve 99.9% of its filtered load, resulting in a urinary sodium excretion rate of <1 mmol/L. Conversely, in cases of excessive sodium intake, the kidney has the capacity to excrete up to 300 mmol/L in urine.

The proximal renal tubule normally reabsorbs 80% of sodium in the glomerular filtrate. The volume of fluid reabsorbed with sodium in the proximal tubule is facilitated by the protein concentration of blood in the postglomerular peritubular capillary bed, because it exerts an oncotic effect.

The fine-tuning of sodium reabsorption and excretion is regulated by hormones (**Figure 7.10**).

- Aldosterone promotes sodium reabsorption
- The naturetic peptides, atrial natriuretic peptide and brain natriuretic peptide, promote sodium excretion

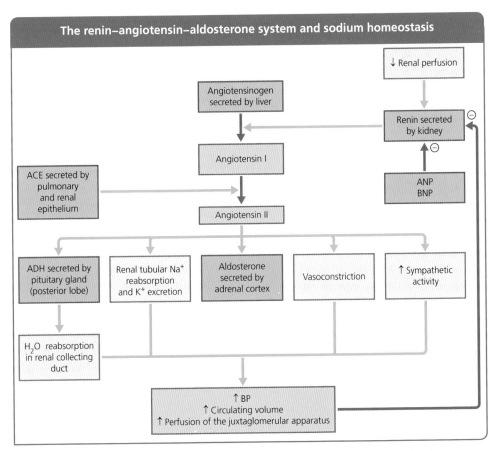

Figure 7.10 The renin–angiotensin–aldosterone system and its role in sodium homeostasis. ACE, angiotensin-converting enzyme; ADH, antidiuretic hormone; ANP, atrial natriuretic peptide; BNP, brain natriuretic peptide.

Aldosterone

This hormone is synthesised in the zona glomerulosa of the adrenal cortex in response to low plasma sodium concentration, extracellular fluid volume contraction and decreased renal perfusate pressure. It is formed in the final step of the renin–angiotensin–aldosterone system. Aldosterone stimulates the reabsorption of sodium in the distal convoluted tubule, in exchange for potassium or hydrogen ions.

Atrial natriuretic peptide and brain natriuretic peptide

These peptides antagonise the actions of aldosterone. They are secreted in response to stretching of the cardiac wall.

Atrial and brain natriuretic peptide increase the rate of glomerular filtration in the kidney and the consequent excretion of sodium in the urine. They also reduce renin secretion from the juxtaglomerular apparatus, and decrease aldosterone secretion in the adrenal cortex to promote vasodilation of the peripheral vasculature (see **Figure 7.10**).

> **N-terminal pro–brain natriuretic peptide is measured to screen patients for heart failure.** A significant increase in the concentration of N-terminal pro–brain natriuretic peptide indicates that there is increased ventricular stretch. Urgent referral for echocardiography is warranted if the concentration is > 2000 pg/mL.

Hyponatraemia and hypernatraemia

The main causes of hyponatraemia (plasma sodium concentration < 125 mmol/L) and hypernatraemia (plasma sodium concentration typically > 145 mmol/L) are summarised in **Figures** 7.11 and 7.12, respectively. These conditions are categorised according to whether the patient's intravascular volume is low (hypovolaemia), normal (euvolaemia) or increased (hypervolaemia), and whether their urinary sodium excretion is low or high.

> **Hyponatraemia is a common electrolyte disorder in hospitalised patients.** The cause is often multifactorial; common causes include inappropriate fluid therapy, the use of certain medications, e.g. diuretics. The management of hyponatraemia is complex, because the electrolyte disturbance is related to the volume status of the patient. Therefore treatment depends on the underlying cause being corrected.

Potassium

Potassium has several functions in the body. These include:

■ generation of the electrical potentials that conduct nerve impulses

> **A patient attends an endocrine surgery clinic after identification of an incidental mass in the adrenal gland (so-called adrenal incidentaloma) on a computerised tomography scan.** To assess if the mass is functional (i.e. producing hormone), various hormones and urea and electrolytes are measured. All results are normal except for the following.
>
> ■ Renin: < 0.2 ng/mL/h (supine reference range, 0.2–2.8 ng/mL/h)
>
> ■ Aldosterone: 2000 pmol/L (supine reference range, 140–850 pmol/L)
>
> ■ Serum sodium: 148 mmol/L (reference range, 133–146 mmol/L)
>
> ■ Serum potassium: 2.8 mmol/L (reference range, 3.5–5.3 mmol/L)
>
> These results suggest the incidental mass is functional, and they confirm that the patient has Conn's syndrome (primary hyperaldosteronism). The excess aldosterone is responsible for the hypernatraemia and hypokalaemia. Potassium replacement is started, and the patient is booked for elective surgery to remove the adrenal mass.

■ promotion of skeletal and smooth muscle contraction (so potassium is essential for normal digestive and muscular function)

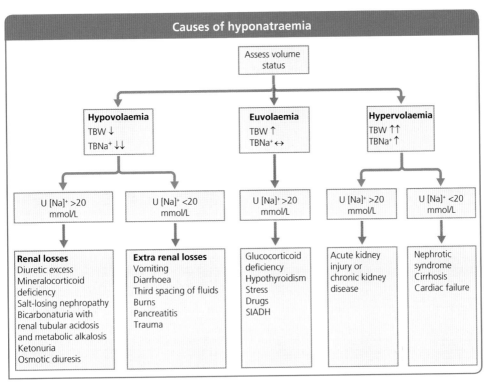

Figure 7.11 Causes of hyponatraemia. SIADH, syndrome of inappropriate antidiuretic hormone; TBNa+, total body sodium; TBW, total body water; U[Na+], urinary sodium concentration.

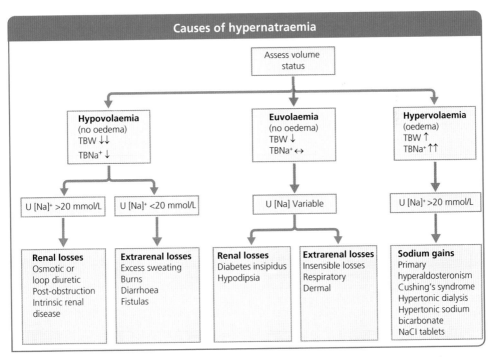

Figure 7.12 Causes of hypernatraemia. TBNa+, total body sodium; TBW, total body water; U[Na+], urinary sodium concentration.

- roles in cardiac muscle contractility and function

Potassium is present in the plasma at much lower concentrations than sodium (see **Table 7.9),** and represents about 2% of total body stores.

Hypokalaemia and hyperkalaemia have various causes (**Table 7.10**).

Na+-K+-ATPase pump

Several factors influence the extracellular fluid concentration of potassium. Central to this is the Na+-K+-ATPase pump on the cell membrane, because its activity affects the distribution of potassium between the extracellular fluid and intracellular fluid.

The activity of this pump is influenced by acid–base status. Therefore there is an association between:

- hypokalaemia (low plasma potassium concentration) and alkalosis

- hyperkalaemia (high plasma potassium concentration) and acidosis

The latter is worse in the presence of inorganic acid (e.g. hydrochloric acid) rather than organic acid (e.g. lactic acid) as organic acids are cleared from the body faster.

Other factors influencing the Na+-K+-ATPase pump include insulin, which acts directly on it to stimulate the movement of potassium into the intracellular fluid. Catecholamines alter the distribution of potassium through their α-and β-adrenergic actions. The former promote hyperkalaemia by decreasing cellular uptake, and the latter promote hypokalaemia by increasing cellular uptake.

Potassium and hydrogen ions (blood acidity)

Potassium directly stimulates the secretion of aldosterone in the adrenal cortex as it activates the renin-angiotensin-aldosterone system.

Causes of hypokalaemia and hyperkalaemia	
Hypokalaemia	**Hyperkalaemia**
Inadequate intake	**Increased intake**
Fasting	**Intravenous potassium replacement**
Anorexia	**Increased retention**
During rapid cell synthesis	Decreased glomerular filtration rate
Increased loss	Potassium-sparing diuretics (e.g. amiloride)
	Addison's disease (i.e. hypoaldosteronism)
Excessive sweating	Increased post-tubular reabsorption after surgical urinary
Magnesium deficiency	diversion
Gastrointestinal losses (e.g. fistula, diarrhoea)	
Renal tubular acidosis types 1 and 2	**Redistribution (in vitro)**
Use of loop and thiazide diuretics	Haemolysis of red blood cells
Primary hyperaldosteronism (i.e. Conn's syndrome)	Storage of whole blood at low temperature
Secondary hyperaldosteronism	Release from platelets or white blood cells
Glucocorticoid excess	**Redistribution (in vivo)**
Drug-related potassium loss (e.g. with penicillin and cisplatin use)	Acidosis
Redistribution (in vitro)	Insulin deficiency
	Use of certain drugs (e.g. beta-blockers)
Uptake by white cells	
Uptake by red cells after insulin administration	
Redistribution (in vivo)	
Alkalosis	
Insulin administration	
Use of adrenergic agonists	
Toxic chemicals (e.g. barium and toluene)	

Table 7.10 Causes of hypokalaemia and hyperkalaemia

- An increased plasma potassium concentration stimulates aldosterone secretion
- A low plasma potassium concentration suppresses aldosterone secretion

Aldosterone promotes the exchange of potassium and hydrogen ions for sodium in the kidney. Consequently, the relative proportions of potassium and hydrogen ions in the distal convoluted tubule of the kidney, and the body's ability to secrete hydrogen ions, determine the effect of systemic acidosis or alkalosis on potassium excretion. Generally, acidosis promotes potassium retention and alkalosis potassium excretion.

> Hypokalaemia and hyperkalaemia have a broad spectrum of clinical features, reflecting the breadth of function of potassium.
>
> - Hypokalaemia can cause muscle weakness, polyuria (increased urine output) and paralytic gut ileus (reduced movement of gastrointestinal tract)
> - Hyperkalaemia can cause paraesthesia and flaccid paralysis
>
> Both conditions can cause serious cardiac arrhythmias (detected by electrocardiography).

Calcium

The main roles of calcium in the body are divided into structural and metabolic. The body contains about 1 kg of calcium; 99% of which is in the skeleton. In health, the total concentration of calcium in the extracellular fluid is between 2.2 and 2.6 mmol/L. About half of this calcium is ionised and therefore biologically active. The remainder is inactive and bound to proteins and complexes (e.g. citrate, phosphate and sulphate).

Calcium homeostasis is principally regulated by three organs: the gastrointestinal tract, the kidneys and bone (**Figure 7.13**). The causes of hypocalcaemia and hypercalcaemia are shown in **Table 7.11**.

Gastrointestinal regulation of calcium

The gastrointestinal absorption of calcium is regulated by active and passive processes. The active process is mediated by 1,25-dihydroxyvitamin D (calcitriol). 1,25-Dihydroxyvitamin D stimulates the synthesis of calbindin-D (a vitamin D transport protein), which facilitates the absorption of calcium in the duodenum and upper jejunum.

Calcium is also absorbed passively by the small intestine and in the colon. The presence

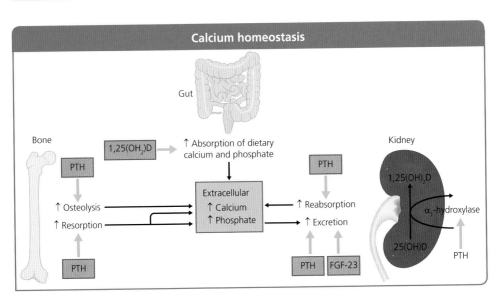

Figure 7.13 Calcium homeostasis. 1,25-(OH)$_2$D, 1,25-dihydroxyvitamin D; 25-(OH)D, 25-hydroxyvitamin D; FGF-23, fibroblast growth factor 23; PTH, parathyroid hormone.

Causes of hypocalcaemia and hypercalcaemia	
Hypocalcaemia	**Hypercalcaemia**
Hypoparathyroidism	**Common (about 90%)**
■ Magnesium deficiency	**Primary hyperparathyroidism**
■ Post-surgical damage or neck irradiation (to thyroid or parathyroid gland)	**Malignant disease**
■ Infiltrative (e.g. haemochromatosis, Wilson's disease and metastases)	■ Metastases and myeloma
	■ Parathyroid hormone–related peptide–secreting tumour
■ Genetic (e.g. DiGeorge's syndrome)	■ Lymphoma (cells containing α_1-hydroxylase)
Parathyroid hormone resistance	■ Parathyroid hormone–secreting (exceptionally rare)
■ Pseudohypoparathyroidism	**Uncommon (about 10%)**
Abnormalities of vitamin D metabolism	**Vitamin D excess**
■ Vitamin D deficiency	**Exogenous (therapeutic use of 1,25-dihydroxyvitamin D)**
Deficient α_1-hydroxylase enzyme activity	
■ Chronic kidney disease	**Endogenous (e.g. sarcoidosis and tuberculosis)**
■ Acidosis	**Thiazides**
■ Vitamin D-dependent rickets type 1	
Vitamin D resistance	**Lithium**
■ Vitamin D-dependent rickets type 2	**Oestrogen excess**
Other causes	**Addison's disease**
■ Spurious (e.g. haemolysis and EDTA contamination)	**Tertiary hyperparathyroidism**
■ Acute pancreatitis	**Hyperthyroidism**
■ Hyperphosphataemia	**Familial benign hypocalciuric hypercalcaemia**
■ Blood transfusion	
■ Sepsis	
■ Hungry bone syndrome	
■ Rhabdomyolysis	
■ Bisphosphonate therapy	

EDTA, ethylenediaminetetra-acetic acid.

Table 7.11 Causes of hypocalcaemia and hypercalcaemia

in the gut of phosphate, oxalate (from green vegetables) and phytate (from unrefined cereals) decreases the absorption of calcium.

Renal regulation of calcium

About 98% of calcium filtered by the kidney is reabsorbed in the proximal tubules. This process does not require energy; it occurs between the intracellular space between cells (the paracellular route) and is linked to the movement of sodium via passive diffusion.

The fine-tuning of calcium reabsorption is an active process that occurs against an electrochemical gradient. Calcium is reabsorbed at the distal convoluted tubules and the initial portion of the collecting duct. This active

process starts at the luminal membrane of the tubule through the transporter channels TRPV5 and TRPV6. Calcium then diffuses bound to calcium-binding proteins (called calbindins) through the cytosol and is actively extruded across the opposite basolateral membrane through a sodium–calcium exchanger called NCX1 and a calcium-ATPase called PCMA1b.

Parathyroid hormone and bone calcium

The active reabsorption of calcium is under the hormonal regulation of parathyroid hormone. Parathyroid hormone is an 84–amino acid peptide synthesised by the chief cells of the parathyroid gland.

Calcium-sensing membrane receptors in the parathyroid gland monitor the concentration of ionised ('free') calcium in the extracellular fluid. Low ionised calcium concentrations increase the synthesis of parathyroid hormone, and high concentrations inhibit it. Parathyroid hormone:

- stimulates the active reabsorption of calcium at the distal tubule and collecting duct of the kidney
- stimulates the synthesis of the α1-hydroxylase enzyme in the kidney, which promotes the conversion of 25-hydroxyvitamin D to its active form, 1,25-dihydroxyvitamin D; this, in turn, promotes calcium and phosphate reabsorption in the gastrointestinal tract
- reduces proximal tubular reabsorption of phosphate and bicarbonate
- stimulates osteoclasts (indirectly) to release calcium from bone

The process of bone resorption begins when parathyroid hormone binds to osteoblasts, the cells responsible for creating bone. Binding stimulates osteoblasts to increase their expression of receptor-activated nuclear kappa-B ligand (RANKL). It also inhibits their expression of a decoy receptor called osteoprotegerin.

Primary hyperparathyroidism and malignancy account for 90% of cases of hypercalcaemia (plasma calcium > 2.6 mmol/L). Therefore investigation of hypercalcaemia includes measurement of parathyroid hormone concentration; if it is high, a parathyroid cause is suggested.

Osteoprotegerin normally binds to RANKL, thus blocking it from interacting with receptor-activated nuclear kappa (RANK), a receptor for RANKL. The decreased amount of osteoprotegerin available for binding the excess RANKL means that RANKL binds to RANK. This stimulates osteoclast precursors to fuse, forming new osteoclasts. The formation of new osteoclasts promotes bone resorption.

Calcitonin

An additional hormonal influence on calcium homeostasis is calcitonin. This hormone is produced by the parafollicular cells of the thyroid gland. Although its physiological role is poorly defined, it is known to reduce plasma calcium concentration.

Answers to starter questions

1. Acidosis is more common than alkalosis because metabolic processes generally generate acid (see **Table 7.2**). This is because metabolic energy is produced by oxidation-type reactions, culminating in acid formation. Consequently, humans have a number of adaptive mechanisms to deal with acid production.

2. Increased potassium concentration causes depolarisation of cardiac cell membranes. This effect causes voltage-controlled sodium channels to open, but not enough to start an action potential and thereby cause a wave of heart muscle contraction. Within milliseconds, these channels inactivate and become refractory. The reduction in the number of active sodium channels means that more depolarisation is needed to reach the threshold for triggering an action potential and making the heart contract.

   This mechanism underlies the neuromuscular, cardiac and gastrointestinal organ dysfunctions associated with hyperkalaemia. The most serious is cardiomyocyte dysfunction, which increases the risk of ventricular fibrillation (arrhythmic contraction of the ventricles) and asystole (the heart stopping).

Answers *continued*

3. Water-containing fluid spaces in the body constitute 40–70% of body weight. Water has several essential biological roles, including acting as a solvent, transporting metabolites and helping to maintain a constant temperature.

   - The water molecule is polar, therefore other polar molecules, such as salts, sugars and amino acids, readily dissolve in water, enabling their transport in solutions
   - Non-polar molecules such as lipids do not dissolve in water but are carried by it
   - The high specific heat capacity of water means that it does not change temperature very easily; this property helps it to maintain temperature homeostasis
   - Its high latent heat of vaporisation means that sweating cools the body

4. pH regulation in the body is critical for normal function.

   - Most energy in the form of ATP is generated in the mitochondrial electron transport system, dependent on the H^+ gradient across the inner mitochondrial membranes
   - pH changes alter the surface changes and physical conformation of proteins, thereby affecting their function
   - pH determines the degree of ionisation of weak acids and bases, therefore it can affect the deposition of these substances

5. Acute symptomatic hyponatraemia develops in < 48 h. When serum sodium concentration decreases below 125 mmol/L, neuronal swelling can cause neurological symptoms. This effect is less likely in chronic hyponatraemia, because cells have time to adapt to changes in sodium concentration.

   a. The initial cerebral oedema increases interstitial hydraulic pressure, forcing fluid out of the brain and into the cerebrospinal fluid
   b. Neurons lose solutes (e.g. Na^+ and K^+), leading to the osmotic movement of water out of the cells and thus decreasing brain swelling

Chapter 8
Nutrition

Starter questions

Answers to the following questions are on page 234.

1. How does deficiency in vitamin B1 result in neurological disorders?
2. What are the main fuels which supply blood glucose during the fed and fasting states?
3. Why does fatty food taste good?
4. What is hunger?
5. Why is blood clotting affected by blockage in the bile ducts?
6. What is the metabolic syndrome?
7. What is the basal metabolic rate and how is it determined?
8. Are vitamin supplements necessary?

Introduction

Adequate nutrition is essential for development, growth and normal body functions. These require the ingestion of nutrients: essential dietary compounds that are unable to be synthesised by the body in adequate amounts or at a sufficient rate. There are six major classes of nutrient:

- carbohydrates
- fats (including essential fatty acids)
- proteins (including essential amino acids)
- water
- minerals
- vitamins

These classes are divided into macronutrients or micronutrients. Macronutrients are required in large amounts (carbohydrates, fats, proteins and water). Micronutrients (minerals and vitamins) are required in smaller amounts relative to the macronutrients. A deficiency in each of the vitamins causes specific clinical effects (**Figure 8.1**).

Carbohydrates, fats and proteins have been discussed in Chapters 3–5. This chapter

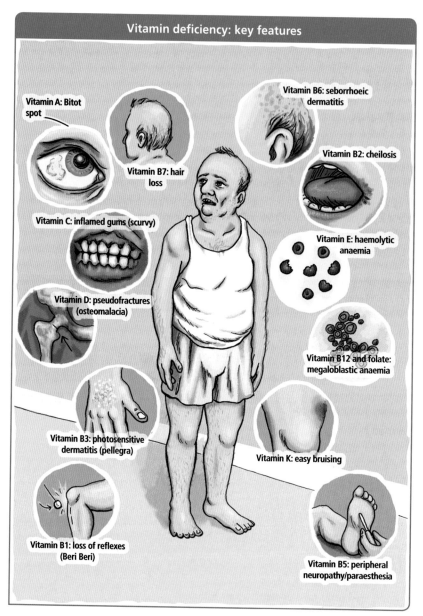

Vitamin deficiency: key features

Vitamin A: Bitot spot

Vitamin B6: seborrhoeic dermatitis

Vitamin B7: hair loss

Vitamin B2: cheilosis

Vitamin C: inflamed gums (scurvy)

Vitamin E: haemolytic anaemia

Vitamin D: pseudofractures (osteomalacia)

Vitamin B12 and folate: megaloblastic anaemia

Vitamin B3: photosensitive dermatitis (pellegra)

Vitamin K: easy bruising

Vitamin B1: loss of reflexes (Beri Beri)

Vitamin B5: peripheral neuropathy/paraesthesia

Figure 8.1
Key features of vitamin deficiencies.

focuses on vitamins, minerals, essential amino acids and essential fatty acids, as well as the balance of nutrition.

Nutrition may be inadequate because of insufficient food intake, impaired digestion and absorption or inability to process the component nutrients. Excessive nutritional intake leads to substantial health problems, namely obesity and the coronary heart disease, hypertension and cancer with which it is associated.

Nutrition must be balanced in patients with clinical conditions such as diabetes, renal disease and many inherited metabolic disorders. A balanced diet consists of plenty of fruit, vegetables and starchy foods; some protein and dairy products with a small amount of fats and sugar.

Case 7 Yellow skin and diarrhoea

Presentation

Jeff Brown, a 32-year-old man, presents to his general practitioner (GP) with visibly yellow skin, abdominal pain and diarrhoea of 3 days' duration. He has no history of alcoholism, foreign travel or drug misuse. Physical examination is unremarkable apart from a slight tremor, abdominal tenderness and distension in the upper right quadrant. The GP thinks that the patient is suffering from depression. Routine bloods are requested.

Analysis

The patient is jaundiced; the yellowing of his skin is caused by accumulation of bilirubin in the body. His blood results are shown in **Table 8.1**. The urea and elec-

trolyte profile is unremarkable, and the results of the thyroid function tests show

Blood test results		
Concentration	Result	Reference range
Bilirubin (µmol/L)	109	<21
Alkaline phosphatase (U/L)	155	30–130
Alanine transaminase (U/L)	150	<35
Albumin (g/L)	41	35–50
Protein (g/L)	91	60–80
C-reactive protein (mg/L)	42	<5

Table 8.1 Results of blood tests for a man presenting with yellow skin and diarrhoea

Wilson's disease: presentation and cause

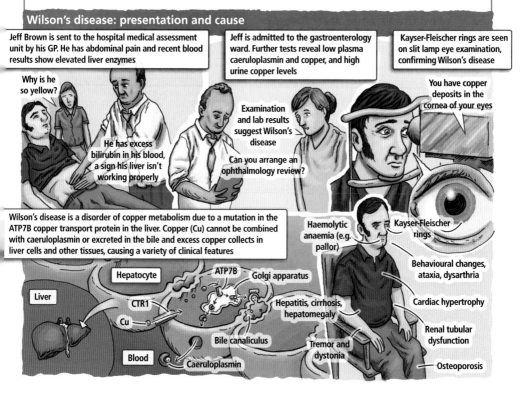

Jeff Brown is sent to the hospital medical assessment unit by his GP. He has abdominal pain and recent blood results show elevated liver enzymes

Jeff is admitted to the gastroenterology ward. Further tests reveal low plasma caeruloplasmin and copper, and high urine copper levels

Kayser-Fleischer rings are seen on slit lamp eye examination, confirming Wilson's disease

Why is he so yellow?

He has excess bilirubin in his blood, a sign his liver isn't working properly

Examination and lab results suggest Wilson's disease

Can you arrange an ophthalmology review?

You have copper deposits in the cornea of your eyes

Wilson's disease is a disorder of copper metabolism due to a mutation in the ATP7B copper transport protein in the liver. Copper (Cu) cannot be combined with caeruloplasmin or excreted in the bile and excess copper collects in liver cells and other tissues, causing a variety of clinical features

Hepatocyte

ATP7B

Golgi apparatus

Liver

CTR1

Cu

Hepatitis, cirrhosis, hepatomegaly

Bile canaliculus

Blood

Caeruloplasmin

Haemolytic anaemia (e.g. pallor)

Kayser-Fleischer rings

Behavioural changes, ataxia, dysarthria

Cardiac hypertrophy

Renal tubular dysfunction

Tremor and dystonia

Osteoporosis

Case 7 *continued*

that the patient is euthyroid (normal thyroid function).

Further case

The patient's abdominal pain is ongoing, so he is admitted to hospital. A liver specialist requests a clotting screen (increased clotting time) and a specialist liver screen. Clotting screens measure the components of the clotting pathway. More commonly a prothrombin time (PT) is determined which measures the rate at which prothrombin is converted to thrombin in the presence of activated clotting factors (calcium and thromboplastin). This checks for deficiencies in factors VII, V, X, prothrombin and fibrinogen (extrinsic and common pathway factors).

The results of these additional tests show a decreased concentration of the copper-carrying protein caeruloplasmin (0.11 g/L; reference range, 0.18–0.34 g/L) and serum copper (10 μmol/L; reference range, 12–25 μmol/L). Caeruloplasmin is a positive acute phase protein. However, the concentration is low despite increased C-reactive protein. A raised CRP suggests inflammation or infection as it is the classic acute phase protein, released to activate the complement system promoting phagocytosis to remove bacteria. With a low caeruloplasmin, a 24-h urine copper test is the next appropriate test, as well as an ophthalmic examination.

The results of the 24-h copper test show a urinary copper output of 3.8 μmol/24 h. A result of < 1.0 is normal, and > 1.6 suggests Wilson's disease (a genetic disorder causing a build-up of copper in the body).

The ophthalmic examination finds copper deposits in the cornea (Kayser–Fleischer rings).

Further analysis

Liver biopsy is the gold standard for confirming a diagnosis of Wilson's disease. However, in this case the procedure is contraindicated because of the patient's clotting impairment. Instead, he undergoes a penicillamine challenge: penicillamine is used to chelate the copper, which enables its excretion in urine. A subsequent 24-h urine copper test gives a result of 8.4 μmol/24 h. Together, these results confirm excess copper and its release into the urine. Thus the diagnosis of Wilson's disease is confirmed.

> **Wilson's disease is an autosomal recessive disease in which the liver is unable to transport and store copper.** Therefore copper is deposited in the eyes, liver, basal ganglia and other tissues. Patients usually present in the 1st decade of life with liver disease, or in the 3rd decade with neuropsychiatric symptoms. Serum copper concentration is usually low, because >90% of the body's copper is bound to caeruloplasmin.

The presenting hepatitis (inflammation of the liver) resolves, along with the jaundice, and the patient is discharged on lifelong chelation therapy (trientine). At subsequent follow-up appointments, the patient reports that he has not had any recurrence of the presenting symptoms.

Energy balance

The body requires energy to maintain metabolic processes, to enable physical activity and to grow. In a resting state, energy is required for thermoregulation, active movement of ions across membranes, cell division and basal functioning of the cardiorespiratory system.

Energy requirements for each person vary in both the physically active state and the resting state. The energy needed depends on body size, body composition, gender, age, nutritional status and environment. Furthermore, people have different energy requirements particularly in short-term situations, such as illness, pregnancy and environmental changes. Energy requirement is greatest in infants and young children, when body tissue is developing rapidly. However, the energy needed per kilogram of body weight gradually declines as adults grow older, from their twenties into old age.

> **The law of thermodynamics states energy cannot be created or destroyed, but moved from one form to another.**
>
> Energy intake = energy output (basal metabolic rate) + thermogenesis + physical activity

Energy expenditure (encompassing output, activity and thermogenesis) and energy intake are not always equal. A sustained period of energy utilisation, or lack of intake, leads to consumption of body stores, including protein, glycogen and fat. If energy is not ingested or otherwise aided by nutrition, these stores become depleted and a state of malnutrition develops. Conversely, if energy intake is greater than energy expenditure, obesity results.

Dietary energy is largely obtained through carbohydrate and fat, with each accounting for 40–50% of a western diet. Protein provides a source of amino acids for protein production and will also provide energy when carbohydrate and fat intake is inadequate. Alcohol accounts for 5–8% of average energy intake in adults who drink regularly.

> **Homeostasis is the term for the metabolic regulatory mechanisms required to keep the body in a constant condition with respect to physiological function and reserves of energy and nutrients.** Homeorhesis refers to the regulatory mechanisms that allow the body to change from one homeostatic condition to another, for example during growth in childhood.

Food energy

Food energy is energy derived from food through the process of cellular respiration. In simple terms, it was originally calculated by burning foodstuffs in a measured amount of water and calculating the temperature increase. The amount of energy needed to cause that temperature rise could then be calculated.

$$\text{Total energy} = \text{digestible energy} + \text{non-digestible energy}$$

Digestible energy is the amount of energy that is available to be absorbed from food. In a person eating an average western diet, digestible energy accounts for about 95% of the energy, because the diet is largely carbohydrate and fat. Non-digestible energy is the energy from food that is unable to be broken down so is excreted through the gut in faeces. **Figure 8.2** shows the fate of the digestible energy.

Table 8.2 shows that protein has higher energy content per gram than carbohydrate. However protein oxidation is not as efficient as that of carbohydrate, and the process requires adenosine triphosphate (ATP) to form the end product, urea. This results in only about 4 kcal/g or 16.8 kjoules/g being available for the body to use as energy.

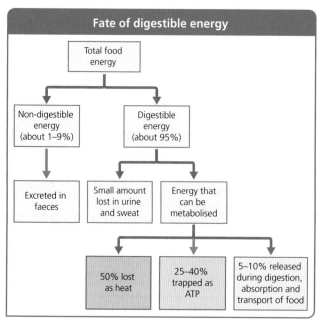

Figure 8.2 Fate of digestible energy. ATP, adenosine triphosphate.

Major dietary sources of energy		
Source	Total energy (kcal/g)	Total energy (kJ/g)
Carbohydrate	4.0	16.8
Fat	9.0	37.8
Protein	4.0	16.8
Alcohol	7.0	29.4

Table 8.2 Major sources of energy in the diet and the total energy released on oxidation

Energy requirements

Energy is used by the body for three main processes.

- Basal metabolic rate: energy used to carry out normal body functions (e.g. breathing and circulation)
- Thermic effect of food: energy required for digestion and absorption of food
- Physical activity: the energy consumed depends on the intensity and duration of the activity

A minimum requirement is necessary to sustain these processes and to provide sufficient energy for extra physical activity. Energy requirements are affected by:

- environmental temperature
- pregnancy and lactation
- age (**Figure 8.3**)
- growth

Body composition

A man of average build (weighing about 72 kg) is typically composed of 85% fat-free mass and 15% fat. The fat-free mass, also known as lean body mass, is 72% water, 20% protein and 8% bone mineral. Women tend to have a higher percentage of fat, typically 18–20%, compared with men with 10–15%. It is thought this is an evolutionary phenomena for pregnancy and nurturing offspring. In both sexes, fat content tends to increase with age.

Body fat is measured by anthropometry (Greek: 'measurement of man'). Anthropometry is a series of body measurements, and the values are applied against a defined population average. In defining body composition, various measurements are used (**Table 8.3**).

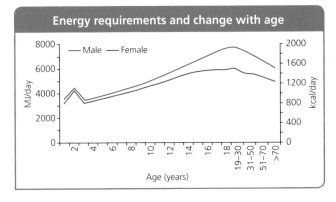

Figure 8.3 Energy requirements and change with age. Data is the estimated basic energy requirements per day and takes no account of activity level. Over 18 years of age, the figures are for men (1.8 m, 70 kg) and women (1.6 m, 56 kg) with a of BMI 22.

Measurement of body composition		
Measurement	**Method**	**Comments**
Height and weight	Body mass index calculation: weight (kg)/ height (m)^2	Not an accurate indicator of body fat, because people with large muscle mass have high body mass index but not high body fat
Upper arm measurements – Upper arm length – Triceps skin fold – Mid-upper arm circumference	Calculation of the upper arm muscle area and the upper arm fat area, which allows the percentage of the arm that is fat to be determined and the value compared with data in reference tables	The formula used assumes negligible bone content and circular cross section with uniform cutaneous fat; neither of which is correct. Bone contributes 18% (men) and 17% (women) to the cross-sectional area.
Skin fold thickness	Use of callipers to pinch the skin at various standardised points on the body	Measures only subcutaneous fat, so used mostly for repeat measurements to determine change
Bioelectrical impedance analysis	Measurement of resistance between a pair of conductors when a small current is sent through the body; fat is anhydrous, so it is a poor conductor of electrical current	The amount of resistance provides a measure of body fat, but hydration can cause errors, and fat is distributed differently between males and females; also, electrodes at different sites can provide different readings (e.g. when stood on or held)

Table 8.3 Measurements and tools used to define body composition

Vitamins

Vitamins are organic (carbon-containing) compounds that are required by the body in small, limited amounts. The body cannot synthesise vitamins in sufficient quantities, so they are considered an essential dietary requirement.

Classically, vitamins are classified into those that are fat-soluble and those that are water-soluble.

- Vitamins A, D, E and K are fat-soluble
- Members of the vitamin B family and vitamin C are water-soluble

The vitamins have diverse functions, with differing bodily requirements, body storage levels, deficiency rates and effects.

Fat-soluble vitamins are absorbed through the gastrointestinal tract in a process that requires bile acids and micelle formation in the gut lumen. Fat-soluble vitamins are more likely to accumulate in the body and lead to hypervitaminosis as excess is stored in adipose tissue.

Water-soluble vitamins are not readily stored, because as they are soluble, any excess is excreted through the kidneys, into urine. through the kidneys. Therefore regular intake of water-soluble vitamins is required to prevent deficiency, but excess in less likely than with fat-soluble vitamins. Although referred to in the singular term as 'vitamin', each vitamin encompasses a group of compounds, as detailed below.

pose tissue, and they are not easily absorbed or excreted. **Table 8.4** summarises the key characteristics of the fat-soluble vitamins. Treatment of deficiency is by pharmaceutical replacement and excess, cessation of supplementation and management of the signs and symptoms. **Table 8.5** summarises how fat soluble vitamins are processed.

Fat-soluble vitamins

The fat-soluble vitamins, A, D, E and K, are all structurally different. However, they are all non-polar, water-insoluble compounds. Collectively, they are stored in the liver and adi-

Vitamin A

Vitamin A has many functions. It is an unsaturated long-chain alcohol attached to a β-ionone ring (**Figure 8.4**). Vitamin A occurs in three main forms:

Characteristics of fat-soluble vitamins		
Vitamin	Sources	Key functions
A	Dairy products, fish and liver, carrots, pumpkin	Helps eyes respond to light changes
		Bone growth, cell division, gene expression, reproduction, regulation of immune system
		Maintenance of moist membranes in eyes, nose, throat and skin.
D	Dairy products, oily fish, cod liver oil, sunlight (via skin)	Calcium and phosphate homeostasis
		Linked to other homeostatic mechanisms involved with immune system regulation, cardiovascular homeostasis and muscle function. Increased vitamin D concentration is linked to a reduced risk of certain cancers e.g. breast and bowel
E	Vegetable oil, fruit and vegetables, grains and nuts	Antioxidant, protects lipids including cell membranes from oxidative damage
K	Gut bacteria	Blood clotting, dependent factor for proteins e.g. osteocalcin,

Table 8.4 Characteristics of fat-soluble vitamins

Regulation of fat soluble vitamins		
Process	Tissue	Comment
Absorption	Small intestine	Requires dietary fat, therefore malabsorption conditions (e.g. Crohn's disease) result in deficiency.
		Levels in food not reduced by cooking (compared to water-soluble vitamins)
		Vitamin K and vitamin B7 produced in the gut
		Vitamin D produced in skin via ultraviolet B
Storage	Adipose tissue, liver	Stored for later use
Excretion	Kidney	Slower than water-soluble vitamins because preferentially stored in fat tissue rather than excreted
Toxicity	Adipose tissue, liver	Pharmaceutical ingestions can cause toxicity as they are readily stored and not excreted; vitamin A and D toxicity is more frequent than vitamin E and K due to availability of supplements in large doses, e.g. excess stored vitamin K can prevent normal blood clotting

Table 8.5 Processing of fat soluble vitamins

Vitamin A structure

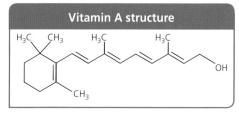

Figure 8.4 Structure of vitamin A.

- retinoic acid
- 11-*cis*-retinal
- β-carotene

Because of its long polyene chain, vitamin A exists in many geometric isomers as a result of a *cis* or *trans* configuration of four of the five double carbon bonds. Polyenes are polyunsaturated organic compounds containing one or more sequences of alternating double and single carbon–carbon bonds.

The most common sources of vitamin A are liver and fish liver oils. It is also present in dairy products such as butter and margarine. β-Carotene is in plants and fruits, such as carrots, squashes and sweet potato and is converted in the body to active vitamin A.

Retinoic acid

This acts as a steroid hormone. The primary function of retinoic acid is to increase epi-thelial cell turnover through the retinoic acid receptor. When bound to chromatin, retinoic acid increases the synthesis of proteins controlling the growth and differentiation of epithelial cells. Retinoic acid is present in small amounts in food, and it is also synthesised by the body from ingested vitamin A.

11-Cis-retinal

The 11-*cis*-retinal form of retinol is a component of the visual pigment rhodopsin. The 11-*cis*-retinal binds to opsin protein to form rhodopsin, which enables the eye to adapt to darkness (**Figure 8.5**). Light stimulation triggers changes in membrane potential that are transmitted to the brain cortex and perceived as light. The rhodopsin is then split into opsin and all-*trans*-retinal (another form of vitamin A). Regeneration is by isomerisation of *trans*-retinal back to *cis*-retinal and recombination with opsin. The whole cycle takes about 45 min.

> **Nyctalopia or night blindness is one of the first signs of vitamin A deficiency.** Vitamin A is required for synthesis of rhodopsin, the visual pigment needed to see in low light conditions. Zinc is also required for effective vitamin A action.

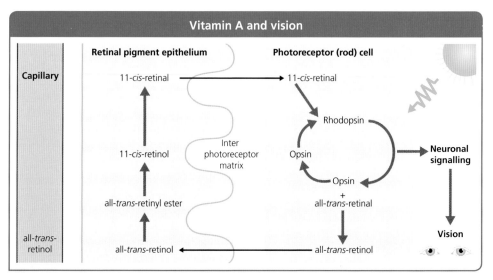

Figure 8.5 Role of vitamin A in vision.

β-Carotene

This is an antioxidant and the red-orange pigment abundant in vegetables and fruits. It is a precursor of vitamin A and is the major dietary source of provitamin A.

One molecule of β-carotene is cleaved into two molecules of vitamin A. However, the yield of vitamin A from β-carotene hydrolysis is less than this depending on enzyme activation and the availability of the cofactor, iron in vivo.

Vitamin A deficiency

This deficiency is rarely seen in high-income countries, because the amount stored in the liver is usually enough to last 3–4 years. However, vitamin A deficiency is common in low- and middle-income countries, particularly in children, and is considered one of the most common preventable causes of blindness.

Deficiency is caused not only by inadequate intake but also by malabsorption, in particular fat malabsorption. Symptoms include impaired light adaptation and night blindness, which are reversible. Vitamin A deficiency also leads to abnormal functioning of the mucus-secreting epithelia in the eyes. Consequently, the eyes become dry and unable to produce tears (xerophthalmia). This eventually leads to thickening of the epithelium and keratin accumulation in the conjunctiva (Bitot's spots).

If the keratinisation is left untreated, opaque scar tissue forms, resulting in blindness. The general effects of vitamin A deficiency on the epithelium lead to thickened, dry skin and impaired mucosal functioning.

Vitamin A excess

Hypervitaminosis A is a serious condition and leads to dry and itchy skin, hair loss and hepatomegaly (an enlarged liver). Other manifestations include thinning of the bones, increased risk of fractures and increased resorption.

Excess from dietary intake is possible only from ingestion of preformed vitamin A, such as that in liver and fish oils. Toxicity is difficult from pro forms of vitamin A, such as β-carotene, because conversion to active vitamin A is tightly regulated.

Vitamin D

Vitamin D is a family of fat-soluble vitamins. In humans, vitamin D2 (ergocalciferol) and vitamin D3 (cholecalciferol) are the most important being responsible for the absorption of calcium from the gastrointestinal tract. Structurally, vitamin D is a derivative of cholesterol and therefore not present in plants. Vitamin D3 synthesised in the skin using UV-B exposure from sunlight, is its natural source (**Figure 8.6**).

Although always referred to as vitamin D, the parent compound is not the active form but a prohormone. The active forms of vitamin D are:

- 1,25-dihydroxyvitamin D3 (1,25-dihydroxycholecalciferol)
- 1,25-dihydroxyvitamin D2 (1,25-dihydroxyergocalciferol)

Activation starts with hydroxylation to a 25-hydroxy form in the liver; 25-hydroxyvitamin D is the major circulating form. Additional 1-α-hydroxylation by the kidney produces the active form.

> **Total serum 25-hydroxyvitamin D concentration is the most useful laboratory measurement of the body's vitamin D.** 1,25-dihydroxyvitamin D is the active form of vitamin D, but it has a shorter half-life and circulates in smaller amounts (pmol/L concentrations compared with nmol/L for 25-hydroxyvitamin D).

The main roles of vitamin D are maintaining calcium homeostasis and increasing the plasma concentration of calcium ions (**Figure 8.7**). There are three key mechanisms through which vitamin D, or more accurately 1,25 dihydroxyvitamin D, exerts its influence:

- increased uptake of calcium from the gut
- increased resorption of calcium from the kidney
- increased bone resorption to release calcium

There is increasing evidence that vitamin D has effects outside its classic roles in calcium

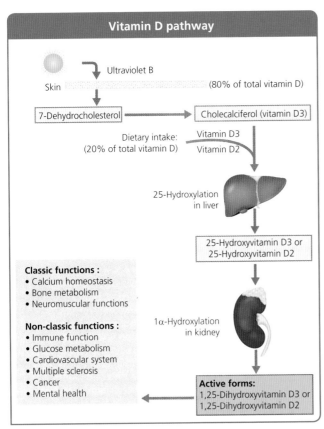

Figure 8.6 Vitamin D pathway.

Vitamin D pathway

Skin

Ultraviolet B

(80% of total vitamin D)

7-Dehydrocholesterol → Cholecalciferol (vitamin D3)

Dietary intake:
(20% of total vitamin D)
Vitamin D3
Vitamin D2

25-Hydroxylation
in liver

25-Hydroxyvitamin D3 or
25-Hydroxyvitamin D2

Classic functions :
• Calcium homeostasis
• Bone metabolism
• Neuromuscular functions

Non-classic functions :
• Immune function
• Glucose metabolism
• Cardiovascular system
• Multiple sclerosis
• Cancer
• Mental health

1α-Hydroxylation
in kidney

Active forms:
1,25-Dihydroxyvitamin D3 or
1,25-Dihydroxyvitamin D2

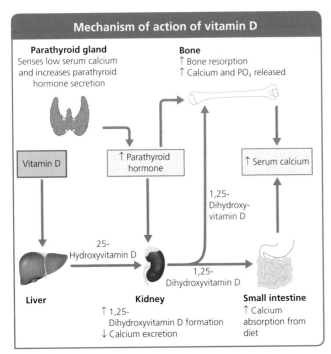

Figure 8.7 Mechanism of action of vitamin D.

Mechanism of action of vitamin D

Parathyroid gland
Senses low serum calcium
and increases parathyroid
hormone secretion

Bone
↑ Bone resorption
↑ Calcium and PO₄ released

Vitamin D

↑ Parathyroid
hormone

↑ Serum calcium

1,25-
Dihydroxy-
vitamin D

25-
Hydroxyvitamin D

1,25-
Dihydroxyvitamin D

Liver

Kidney
↑ 1,25-
Dihydroxyvitamin D formation
↓ Calcium excretion

Small intestine
↑ Calcium
absorption from
diet

homeostasis and bone metabolism. Roles in cell growth, neuromuscular and immune function, and reduction of inflammation have been suggested.

Vitamin D deficiency is linked with increased risk of numerous conditions, including diabetes, cancer, infections, cardiovascular disease and neurological disorders. Exact mechanisms are not proven but it is suggested that the interaction of 1,25-dihydroxyvitamin D with the vitamin D receptor on cells, e.g. malignant cells triggers an intracellular cascade which can result in cell apoptosis, increased immune function by activation of T cells, or slow cell growth. These are only a few mechanisms and research is continually evolving in this area.

Vitamin D deficiency

This arises in various ways, as listed in Table 8.6. Endogenous vitamin D is produced by the action of sunlight of wavelength 290–310 nm, equivalent to ultraviolet B wavelength, on the skin. In the UK, no sunlight of this wavelength is available between October and March, so body stores are used. With the increasing use of sunscreen products that block ultraviolet B light, exposure of the skin to adequate sunlight in the summer months is frequently insufficient for the accumulation of adequate stores.

Vitamin D deficiency affects bone mineralisation, which in children results in rickets, and in adults, osteomalacia. In children, the effect of rickets on bone mineralisation leads to soft, deformed bones. If the condition is not corrected by calcium and vitamin D supplementation, failure of adequate growth results. In adults, as the bones are formed, the effect is demineralisation of existing bones and increased fracture risk.

Rickets is caused by vitamin D deficiency and was epidemic in the 19th century. The condition presents with growth retardation, muscle weakness and skeletal deformities. It can be treated with sunlight, because ultraviolet B radiation is absorbed by 7-dehydrocholesterol in the skin to form cholecalciferol (vitamin D3). This is then hydroxylated in the liver and kidney to form 1,25-dihydroxyvitamin D3, the biologically active form.

Causes of vitamin D deficiency	
Cause	Groups at risk
Decreased dietary intake	Vegans, because vitamin D is absent from food of plant origin
Inadequate exposure to sunlight of the correct wavelength	People living in areas where ultraviolet B light is seasonally limited
	Women and children of Asian and African ethnic origin living in sunlight-poor areas
	Elderly and housebound people
	People who use sunscreen all year round
Glucocorticoids	People on long-term high-dose glucocorticoid therapy; these drugs inhibit intestinal vitamin D and calcium absorption
Decreased 1-α-hydroxylation of 25-hydroxyvitamin D	People with renal disease, which leads to inadequate formation of active 1,25-dihydroxyvitamin D
Decreased formation of 25-hydroxyvitamin D	People with liver disease, which results in decreased precursor formation
Fat malabsorption	People with coeliac disease, Crohn's disease, gastrointestinal tract surgery, pancreatic insufficiency, cystic fibrosis and short gut syndrome
Hereditary vitamin D-resistant rickets	People with end organ sensitivity to active vitamin D
Storage in fat tissue	People with obesity; they store fat-soluble vitamin D in adipose tissue, resulting in reduced amounts available for adequate functions

Table 8.6 Predominant causes of 1, 25-dihydroxyvitamin D deficiency.

Vitamin D excess

Vitamin D excess is normally well tolerated, but it presents with nausea, vomiting and muscle weakness due to hypercalcaemia. Excess vitamin D is not possible from excessive exposure to sunlight, because a photo-degradation pathway converts vitamin D to its inactive forms. Excess is generally from high intake of oral supplements. Long-term excess intake can result in increased calcium absorption, increased bone resorption, and calcium deposition in soft tissues (e.g. the arteries, heart, liver, kidney and pancreas).

Vitamin E

Vitamin E encompasses eight fat-soluble compounds that have vitamin E activity:

- four are tocopherols (α, β, Υ and δ)
- four are tocotrienols (α, β, Υ and δ)

The most active form of vitamin E is the natural isomer of α-tocopherol (**Figure 8.8**), which accounts for 90% of the vitamin E in humans. Vitamin E is present in vegetable oils, nuts and green vegetables.

Vitamin E is soluble in dietary fat and is absorbed through the gastrointestinal tract. It is transported to the tissues, mainly the liver, in chylomicrons and circulates in the blood in lipoproteins, specifically very-low-density lipoproteins. Vitamin E is a fat-soluble vitamin, so it is stored in adipose tissue.

The main function of vitamin E is as an antioxidant protecting vitamins A and C, red blood cells and essential fatty acids from destruction by free radicals. Because it is fat-soluble, it is incorporated into cell membranes to protect them from oxidative damage.

Vitamin E deficiency

This deficiency is rare and generally seen only in premature infants because of a deficiency in the mother. In adults and children, vitamin E deficiency is secondary to severe fat malabsorption or lipoprotein deficiency. Severe vitamin E deficiency leads to neuromuscular abnormalities and myopathies. Deficiency will lead to anaemia because of oxidative damage to red blood cells.

Vitamin E excess

Vitamin E is the least toxic of all the fat-soluble vitamins and has few adverse effects. However, hypervitaminosis E is able to counteract vitamin K, leading to vitamin K deficiency, which will potentiate anticoagulant therapy.

Vitamin K

This is a group of two forms of vitamin K: vitamin K1 (phytomenadione or phylloquinone) and vitamin K2 (menatetrenone or menaquinone). They are structurally similar and both fat-soluble.

Vitamin K1 and vitamin K2 are required for post-translational modification of proteins in the clotting cascade pathway (**Figure 8.9**). Vitamin K is a coenzyme and is required for the γ-carboxylation of the first 10 amino terminal glutamate residues of factor II (prothrombin). The carboxylation of prothrombin facilitates the binding of calcium. Calcium is necessary for conversion of prothrombin to thrombin in the final common pathway of the clotting cascade.

Vitamin K is also required for the γ-carboxylation of factors VII, IX and X to form sites with a high affinity for calcium.

A similar mechanism of carboxylation occurs in other proteins outside the clotting pathway, including:

- osteocalcin and matrix Gla protein, two extracellular matrix proteins in bone
- nephrocalcin in the renal cortex
- cell growth–regulating, growth arrest–specific gene 6 protein, which functions

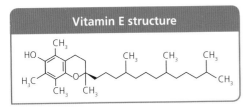

Vitamin E structure

Figure 8.8 Structure of vitamin E.

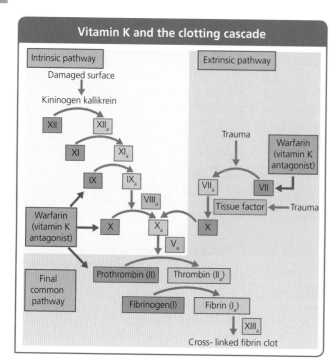

Figure 8.9 Role of vitamin K in the clotting cascade.

as a growth factor to stimulate cell proliferation or prevent apoptosis

> **Vitamin K status is assessed by prothrombin time, a measurement of the time required for blood to clot.** A prolonged clotting time suggests vitamin K deficiency, although prothrombin time does not detect mild deficiencies.

The predominant dietary form of vitamin K is K1, which is in leafy green vegetables, egg yolk and liver. Vitamin K2 encompasses several subtypes, which differ in the length of their isoprenoid chains (**Figure 8.10**). Vitamin K2 is the main storage form and is produced by conversion of vitamin K1 by gut bacteria. Circulating vitamin K is normally K1, whereas hepatic stores are K2.

Vitamin K deficiency

True deficiency of vitamin K is rare, because most of the body's vitamin K is synthesised by the bacteria in the gastrointestinal tract. However, any factor that affects the bacteria in the gastrointestinal tract, such as long-term antibiotic therapy, will lead to a decreased level of bacteria. In addition, newborn babies have sterile gastrointestinal tracts, so are unable to initially make vitamin K. Deficiency results in inhibition of the clotting cascade, leading to an increased tendency to bleed and bruise easily.

Vitamin K excess

Toxicity from naturally occurring vitamin K is rare, even at very high doses.

Water-soluble vitamins

The water-soluble vitamins are the B family of vitamins and vitamin C. They tend to be rapidly absorbed through the gastrointestinal tract and are not stored in large quantities in the body. Because of their solubility, these vitamins are easily destroyed or washed out during food preparation and cooking. Eight of the water-soluble vitamins are known as the vitamin B complex group. **Table 8.7** summarises the key functions of the B family of vitamins.

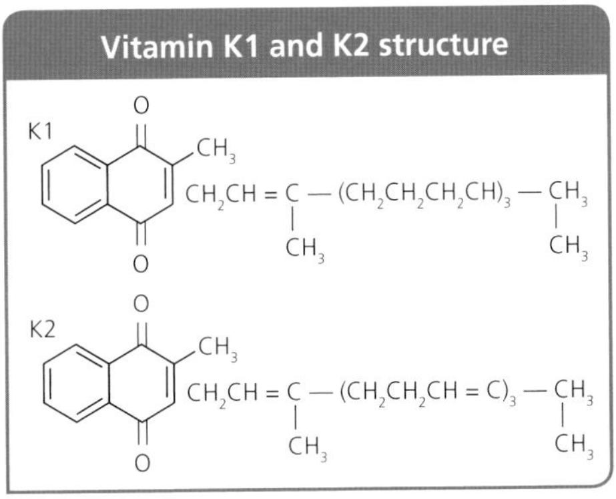

Figure 8.10 Structure of vitamin K1 and vitamin K2.

Vitamin B1 (thiamin)

The physiologically active form is thiamin pyrophosphate, whose key functions are listed in **Table 8.7** and shown in **Figure 8.11**. The body has about 1 month's store of vitamin B1. Deficiency is rare, because cereals and grain products are enriched with the B vitamins B1, B2, B3 and folate, as well as iron. Low-calorie diets and diets high in processed carbohydrates confer a risk of deficiency, and people who frequently consume an excessive amount of alcohol are at increased risk. This is due to reduced absorption and ingestion of vitamin B1, reduced storage by the liver and the inhibition of intestinal vitamin B1 transport by alcohol.

> **Wernicke's encephalopathy and Korsakoff's psychosis are related neurological diseases resulting from localised brain atrophy caused by vitamin B1 deficiency.** They are both associated with alcohol dependence.
>
> ■ Wernicke's encephalopathy has an acute presentation, with the symptoms of ataxia, ophthalmoplegia and confusion
>
> ■ Korsakoff's psychosis results from chronic deficiency, and presents with anterograde and retrograde amnesia and other cognitive dysfunctions
>
> Both diseases are treated with vitamin B1 infusion, although much of the pathology is irreversible by the time it becomes clinically evident.

Symptoms of vitamin B1 deficiency include muscle weakness, mental confusion, oedema, impaired growth and the disease beriberi. Beriberi occurs in two forms: 'dry' and 'wet'.

■ Dry beriberi specifically causes muscle wasting and peripheral neuropathy
■ Wet beriberi specifically causes oedema and heart failure

Beriberi generally affects people in poorer regions of South East Asia, who eat rice with the husk removed (the husk contains the vitamins).

Vitamin B2 (riboflavin)

Riboflavin deficiency is rare in countries in which milk is a regular part of the diet. Features of deficiency include angular stomatitis (inflammation at the sides of the mouth), cheilosis (fissures at the corners of the mouth), glossitis (soreness and inflammation of the tongue) and cataracts. Riboflavin is not toxic in excess, because absorption from the gastrointestinal tract is readily saturated, with excess rapidly excreted in the urine.

> **Riboflavin is destroyed by ultraviolet light.** This is why milk, a rich source of riboflavin, is generally transported in opaque plastic containers or glass, which will stop most ultraviolet light.

Vitamin B3 (niacin)

Vitamin B3 is known as niacin; however, this term often refers to both nicotinic acid and nicotinamide. Nicotinic acid is the precursor of nicotinamide. Nicotinamide is a constituent of the oxidised forms of nicotinamide adenine dinucleotide (NAD^+) and nicotinamide adenine dinucleotide phosphate ($NADP^+$), which are reduced to NADH and NADPH, respectively. Niacin is also made from tryptophan. However, this is an inefficient mechanism and requires thiamin, riboflavin and pyridoxine as cofactors (vitamins B1, B2 and B6, respectively).

Deficiency of niacin, a condition known as pellagra, is described as the three D's:

The vitamin B family		
Vitamin	Sources	Key functions (physiologically active form)
Vitamin B1 (thiamin)	Wheatgerm, oatmeal, yeast, liver and legumes	Cofactor in conversion of pyruvate to acetyl coenzyme A Conversion of 2-oxoglutarate to succinyl coenzyme A Cofactor in pentose phosphate pathway Metabolism of branched chain amino acids
Vitamin B2 (riboflavin)	Milk, eggs and offal	Constituent of two flavoproteins (flavin mononucleotide and flavin adenine dinucleotide) that act as electron carriers
Vitamin B3 (niacin)	Wholegrain cereals, meat and fish	Formation of NAD^+ and $NADP^+$
Vitamin B5 (pantothenic acid)	Liver, meat, cereals, milk, egg yolk and fresh vegetables	Used in synthesis of coenzyme A, which is required for transfer of acyl groups Component of fatty acid synthase
Vitamin B6	Wholegrain wheat and corn, meat, fish and poultry	Pyridoxal phosphate is a cofactor for >60 enzymes involved in: amino acid metabolism haem synthesis glycogen phosphorylate tryptophan conversion
Vitamin B7 (biotin)	Offal, milk and eggs	Cofactor responsible for transfer of carbon dioxide in reactions catalysed by carboxylase enzymes, including: acetyl coenzyme A carboxylase propionyl coenzyme A carboxylase pyruvate carboxylase Coenzyme in 1-carbon transfer reactions
Vitamin B9 (Folate)	Green vegetables, liver and wholegrain cereals	Synthesis of amino acids (e.g. methionine and glycine) Synthesis of purines, AMP and GMP Synthesis of thymidine
Vitamin B12 (cobalamin)	Only animal-derived foods (e.g. meat, offal, fish, eggs and milk)	Carrier of methyl groups and acts as coenzyme for two enzymes: Deoxyadenosylcobalamin required for methylmalonyl coenzyme A mutase (involved in breakdown of odd-numbered fatty acids) Methylcobalamin required for homocysteine methyltransferase (synthesises methionine)

AMP, adenosine monophophate; GMP, guanosine monophosphate; NAD^+, nicotinamide adenine dinucleotide (oxidised form); $NADP^+$, nicotinamide adenine dinucleotide phosphate (oxidised form).

Table 8.7 The B family of vitamins and their key functions

dermatitis, diarrhoea and dementia. Pellagra ultimately may lead to death. Dietary and endogenous niacin are both important, because pellagra can develop in deficiency of either. Dietary deficiency of niacin is rare, but decreased formation from tryptophan occurs with existing riboflavin (vitamin B2) or vitamin B6 deficiency.

Toxicity, as with all water-soluble vitamins, is rare. If it does occur, it results in vasodilation and flushing.

> **Premenopausal women are more at risk of borderline niacin deficiency.** This is because their high levels of oestrogen decrease the rate of tryptophan metabolism.

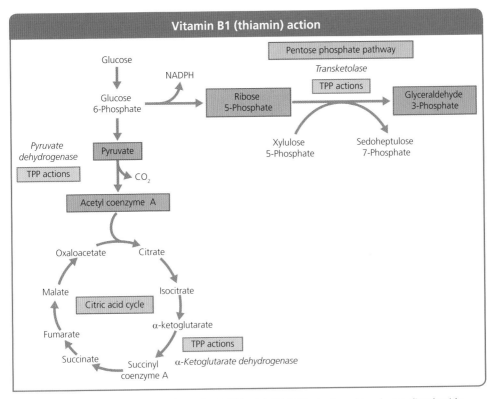

Figure 8.11 Mechanism of action of vitamin B1 (thiamin). NADPH, nicotinamide adenine dinucleotide phosphate (reduced form); TPP, thiamin pyrophosphate.

Vitamin B6

Vitamin B6 exists in three forms: pyridoxine, pyridoxal and pyridoxamine (**Figure 8.12**). The 5′ phosphates of the three forms also have B6 activity. The predominant active form of the vitamin is pyridoxal phosphate, which is produced from all three forms of B6.

Severe vitamin B6 deficiency results in dermatological and neurological changes. Mild deficiency reduces the activity of the enzymes for which pyridoxal phosphate acts as a cofactor. This results in abnormal amino acid metabolism, hypochromic microcytic anaemia and secondary pellagra. Deficiency occurs as a result of the use of certain drugs affecting vitamin B6 metabolism, for example penicillamine and isoniazid, the latter of which is used to treat tuberculosis. These drugs form a complex with vitamin B6, and thus prevent its activity or displace pyridoxal phosphate from the active binding sites.

Vitamin B9 (Folate)

Folate, present in leafy green vegetables, cereals, grains, nuts and meat, is a natural form of vitamin B9. Folic acid is the synthetic form, and is in fortified food and supplements. Folic acid is more bioavailable than folate, but they have the same biologic effects.

Folate is absorbed in the duodenum and jejunum, and stored in the liver. The amount stored is small relative to daily requirements, so deficiency occurs within 2–3 months.

The role of folate is linked to that of vitamin B12 (**Figure 8.13**). Therefore even if the diet provides adequate folate, a deficiency in vitamin B12 will cause secondary folate deficiency.

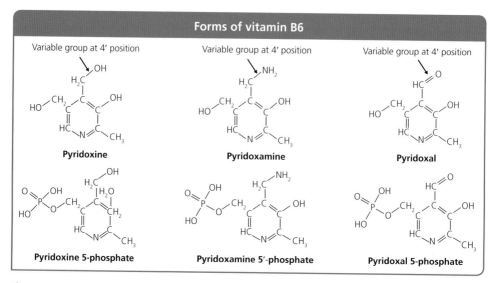

Figure 8.12 Various forms of vitamin B6.

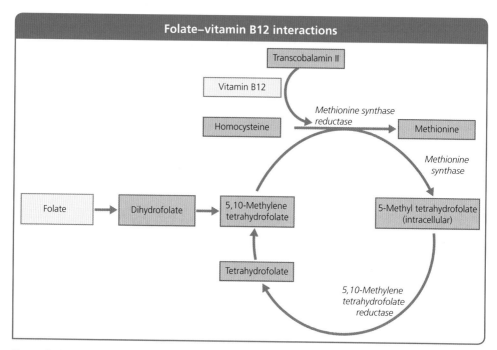

Figure 8.13 Interactions between folate and vitamin B12. A deficiency of either folate or vitamin B12 will have similar results namely an increase in homocysteine, a risk factor for cardiovascular disease. However, increasing folate concentrations has the potential to mask a B12 deficiency and enhance the symptoms of vitamin B12 deficiency.

Folate deficiency

The following cause folate deficiency.

- Dietary deficiency: the elderly, people with alcohol dependence and those with poor nutritional intake are at increased risk

- Malabsorption: resulting from coeliac disease or gastrointestinal tract surgery, for example
- Inability to sustain folate demand during periods of increased requirement caused by:

- rapid cell growth (e.g. during pregnancy, infancy or adolescence)
- cell growth in cancer
- inflammatory states
- recovery from illness
- haemolytic anaemias
- Use of certain drugs
  - anticonvulsants, such as phenytoin and phenobarbital (phenobarbitone), which impair folate absorption
  - dihydrofolate reductase inhibitors, for example methotrexate
  - antimalarial drugs
- Vitamin B12 deficiency, because folate deficiency may be secondary to this (see **Figure 8.13**)

Folate deficiency is treated by supplementation; this is particularly important during pregnancy, because folate is required for DNA, RNA and cell synthesis and production. Inadequate folate especially during early embryo development reduces the risk of neural tube defects predominantly spina bifida.

> **Development of the neural tube during embryogenesis depends on folate.** All pregnant women are advised to take folate supplements to reduce the risk of neural tube defects such as spina bifida and anencephaly. The critical period for supplementation is just after conception, during very early development.

Vitamin B12 (cobalamin)

This vitamin has two active forms: deoxyadenosylcobalamin and methylcobalamin. Both forms have cobalt as the central atom. However, they have different functions (see **Table 8.7**):

- deoxyadenosylcobalamin is used to break down fatty acids
- methylcobalamin is used to synthesise methionine

Although vitamin B12 is water-soluble, the body stores a large proportion, 60% of which is in the liver and 30% in muscles. The absorption and transport of vitamin B12 occurs in several steps.

1. Release of vitamin B12 from protein by gastric acid in the gastrointestinal tract
2. Binding of vitamin B12 to a glycoprotein carrier, intrinsic factor, which is produced by the parietal cells
3. Binding of the B12–intrinsic factor complex to mucosal cell receptors in the terminal ileum
4. Absorption of vitamin B12 by the into the portal circulation enables B12 to bind to transcobalamin II which transports B12.
5. The transcobalamin II-B12 complex is then endocytosed into the cells which require B12, where free B12 is released into the cytoplasm

Dietary deficiency is rare, because the body contains sufficient stores of vitamin B12 to last a couple of years. However, vegetarians are at risk of dietary deficiency, because animal products are the predominant source of vitamin B12. Deficiency occurs more often as a result of impaired absorption, intrinsic factor deficiency or disease of the terminal ileum, such as Crohn's disease. Intrinsic factor deficiency develops in pernicious anaemia, an autoimmune condition in which the body produces antibodies to intrinsic factor.

The effects of vitamin B12 deficiency result in two main sequalae linked to the vitamin's two main functions (see **Table 8.7**).

- Accumulation of abnormal odd-numbered fatty acids, which are incorporated into the cell membranes of nerves, resulting in neurological symptoms and neural degeneration
- Secondary folate deficiency, because vitamin B12 is necessary for the processing of folate; megaloblastic anaemia then results from decreased nucleotide synthesis, because folate is blocked as methyl tetrahydrofolate (see **Figure 8.13**)

Vitamin B7 (biotin)

Biotin is widely distributed in foods, and deficiency is rare because gut bacteria also produce biotin in excess of daily requirements. When biotin deficiency does occur, it is mild. It occurs in patients receiving parenteral nutrition (see page 229) and people who consume large amount of raw eggs. Egg white contains a glycoprotein called avidin, which binds biotin, thus preventing its absorption. Symptoms of deficiency include scaly dermatitis and hair loss.

Some metabolic disorders result from reduced activity of biotin-dependent carboxylases. One such disorder is deficiency of the enzyme holocarboxylase synthetase. This enzyme is required for the effective use of biotin, because it activates the other specific carboxylase enzymes by transferring biotin to them. Biotin is harmless in excess.

Vitamin B5 (pantothenic acid)

This vitamin is in most food, with high amounts in wholegrain cereals, eggs, meat and avocados. Structurally, pantothenic acid exists as a D isomer and an L isomer, but only the former is biological active.

Pantothenic acid has a role in the synthesis of coenzyme A, which acts as an acyl group carrier to form acetyl coenzyme A (see page ???).[8] Coenzyme A is vital for many functions and essential for metabolism and other key biological processes.

- In energy metabolism, coenzyme A enables pyruvate to enter the citric acid cycle[9] as acetyl-coenzyme A
- As acetyl coenzyme A in the citric acid cycle, it is used to convert α-ketoglutarate to succinyl coenzyme A
- It is used in the biosynthesis of fatty acids, cholesterol and acetylcholine
- Coenzyme A forms the acyl carrier protein, which is required alongside it in fatty acid synthesis
- It is used in acetylation and acylation

Pantothenic acid is converted to free pantothenic acid to enable absorption. In food, pantothenic acid is in the form of the coenzyme A of acyl carrier protein. Hydrolysis of coenzyme A and acyl carrier protein produces 4'-phosphopantetheine, which is dephosphorylated into pantetheine. A gut enzyme, pantetheinase, then hydrolyses the molecule further into free pantothenic acid. Free pantothenic acid is absorbed through a sodium-dependent active transport system.

Deficiency of pantothenic acid is rare. It produces symptoms similar to those of other vitamin B deficiencies. Consistent with its identified functions, low levels of pantothenic acid lead to impaired energy production, with symptoms of fatigue, lethargy and apathy. Impairment of acetylcholine synthesis can occur, which causes neurological symptoms.

Pantothenic acid is water-soluble, so excess is unlikely as the kidneys will excrete surplus to requirements.

Vitamin C (L-ascorbic acid)

Vitamin C is in citrus fruit, tomatoes, berries and green vegetables. Being labile, it is destroyed by heat, light, oxygen, metal ions and alkaline conditions. Vitamin C:

- scavenges antioxidants and free radicals
- is used in the post-translational reduction of proline to form hydroxyproline in collagen synthesis
- aids intestinal absorption of non-haem iron
- acts as a cofactor in enzymatic reactions

Vitamin C excess

The claim that megadoses of vitamin C prevent or cure illness is unfounded. There is no proof that excess vitamin C intake confers the benefits suggested. High intake may be harmful, leading to the formation of kidney stones and diarrhoea.

Vitamin C deficiency

Deficiency of vitamin C leads to scurvy. Scurvy first presents with symptoms of lethargy and malaise. The more advanced symptoms then develop; these are linked to decreased collagen synthesis, poor connective tissue formation and impaired wound healing. Stores of vitamin C are equivalent to 6 months' requirement. However, scurvy can occur even in high-income countries in the elderly, smokers and people with alcohol dependence. Smokers lose more vitamin C from tissues and require more to counteract the damage that smoking causes. Treatment involves oral replacement of vitamin C with symptoms resolving in days to weeks.

> **Vitamin C is required for the synthesis of collagen.** Vitamin C deficiency (scurvy) presents with malaise and lethargy, followed by spongy bleeding gums. In previous centuries, it caused many deaths among sailors because fresh fruit and vegetables could not be stored on long sea voyages.

Minerals and trace elements

In simple terms, living organisms comprise just 11 elements: carbon, hydrogen, oxygen, nitrogen and seven major minerals. The major minerals are obtained from a healthy diet containing meat, cereals, fish, vegetables, nuts, fruit and dairy products. The body also requires trace minerals, more correctly referred to as trace elements.

Minerals

Minerals are inorganic substances required by the body, in small amounts, for a range of functions (**Table 8.8**). The term mineral is a misnomer, because all the major minerals are actually elements. They are used to form bones and teeth, as constituents of body fluids and tissues, for normal nerve and muscle function and as components of enzyme systems.

The seven major minerals are:

- calcium, phosphorus and magnesium (predominantly in the skeleton)
- sodium, potassium and chloride (the main electrolytes)
- sulphur (used in amino acids and therefore proteins)

With the exception of sulphur, dietary guidelines have been published for the above minerals; the recommended nutritional intake is > 100 mg/day. Sodium potassium and calcium have been discussed in Chapter 7.

Trace elements

Trace elements are essential, because the body is unable to make them in sufficient amounts. They are called 'trace', because the recommended intake is < 100 mg/day. There is debate about which substances qualify as essential trace elements (**Table 8.9**). Iron, zinc, copper, selenium, manganese, chromium, molybdenum, cobalt and iodine are well accepted trace elements. Other elements that have physiological roles but have not been proved to be essential trace elements are nickel, vanadium, silicon, lithium and fluoride. Iron has been discussed in Chapter 6 (see page 165).

Zinc

Zinc is in most foods but meat, nuts and lentils are its key sources. Zinc is absorbed in the duodenum and jejunum with 20–40% efficiency. Therefore although the dietary requirement is 2–3 mg/day, the recommended intake is 10 mg/day. Zinc absorption is regulated by metallothionein. Metallothionein is a metalloprotein that binds copper and other divalent cations.

Zinc absorption is impaired in pancreatic disease and pancreatic insufficiency, because pancreatic enzymes are necessary for release of dietary zinc. Zinc, copper and iron have similar absorption components and compete for absorption. Zinc is excreted mainly through the gut, with only 10% excreted through the kidneys.

The functions of zinc (**Table 8.10**) are attributed to its ability to form tight bonds with particular amino acids, especially histidine and cysteine. When zinc binds four amino acids, it acts as a structural motif maintaining protein structure, nuclear stability and histone structure.

Minerals: sources and functions		
Mineral	Source	Major functions
Calcium	Milk, leafy green vegetables	Strengthens bones and teeth Muscle contraction Energy conversion Blood clotting
Phosphorous	Milk. Meat, fish, poultry, beans	Strengths bones and teeth Energy conversion Muscle and nerve function Acid base balance
Magnesium	Nuts, leafy greens, milk	Minor constituent of bones and teeth Cofactor for >300 numerous reactions and enzymes Regulate nerve and muscle contraction
Sodium	Salt, meat, fish, dairy products	Controls water balance and blood pressure Regulates nerve impulses and muscle contractions
Potassium	Fruit, meat, vegetables, fish, poultry, milk	Helps control water balance Muscle contractions and cardiac function Regulates nerve impulses
Chloride	Table salt, vegetables, seaweed	Controls water balance Key component of stomach acid Acid base regulation
Sulphur	Meat, fish, egg yolk and milk, vegetables	Formation of collagen Component of amino acids (cysteine, cysteine, methionine and taurine) Present in keratin (skin, hair and nails) Cell respiration – used in redox reactions

Table 8.8 Summary of main functions of minerals

Zinc binding enables the creation of zinc finger proteins, which are small protein motifs in which zinc stabilises the protein folding. Zinc fingers function to interact with DNA, RNA or proteins to alter the binding and configuration of the molecule.

Zinc deficiency

Deficiency of zinc results from inadequate dietary intake, increased zinc loss or increased zinc requirement. A rare cause is acrodermatitis enteropathica, an autosomal recessive disorder causing malabsorption in the small intestine.

Zinc excess

Excess zinc ingestion affects copper and iron absorption; it induces synthesis of metallothionein which binds copper, preventing its absorption. Excess zinc has been linked to changes in lipoprotein levels resulting in increased low density lipoprotein and decreased high density lipoprotein. Therefore, it is potentially atherogenic. Zinc poisoning is serious and treatment involves supporting breathing and zinc removal.

Copper

Dietary copper is absorbed in the stomach and duodenum, and then transported, bound to albumin, to the liver. The amount of dietary copper absorbed varies from 30% to 70%. The reasons for this variability are unclear, but zinc is known to reduce copper absorption by increasing synthesis and competitive binding to metallothionein.

Once absorbed, copper is incorporated into caeruloplasmin, a glycoprotein synthesised by the liver. Caeruloplasmin transports copper to the tissues, where it is incorporated into proteins and metalloenzymes for the development and maintenance of bone and other connective tissues, for the formation of red blood cells and the for metabolism of glucose and cholesterol. Caeruloplasmin bound copper accounts for 80–90% of copper entering the circulation. Once absorbed, the main function of copper is as a component of metalloenzymes. Metalloenzymes contain a metal ion bound within its structure to catalyse the reaction. The most common metalloenzyme that requires copper is cytochrome oxidase.

Copper is excreted in the bile, not through the kidneys. Therefore the presence of copper in urine is abnormal and suggests renal damage or the use of copper-chelating agents, such as penicillamine.

Dietary sources of trace elements

Trace element	Source	Key function(s)
Iron	Liver, meat, green vegetables, cereals	Oxygen transport Transport of electrons
Zinc	Seafood, meat, nuts	Co-factor for over 100 enzymes
Copper	Offal	Synthesis of copper-containing enzymes
Selenium	Meat, green vegetables	Co-factor of glutathione peroxidase
Manganese	Vegetables, whole grains	Co-factor for pyruvate carboxylase, superoxide dismutase, glycosyl transferase
Chromium	Beef, liver, eggs	Glucose tolerance
Molybdenum	Legumes (beans, peas, lentils), liver, nuts	Purine breakdown, constituent of xanthine oxidase
Cobalt	Foods of animal origin	Constituent of Vitamin B12 as cobalamin
Iodine	Supplemented salt	Synthesis of thyroid hormones
Nickel	Nuts, dried peas	Suggested role in iron absorption. Present in DNA and RNA - role in synthesis
Vanadium	Shellfish, green beans	Oxidizing agent, lipid metabolism
Silicon	Green vegetables	Cartilage matrix calcification in proteoglycan, glycosaminoglycan formation
Lithium	Grains and vegetables	Mood stabilizer, interaction with neurotransmitters
Fluoride	Drinking water (5–6% global population), toothpaste and dental products	Increases teeth hardness and prevention of dental caries

Table 8.9 Dietary sources of trace elements

Zinc functions

Role	Details
Cofactor	Present in > 250 proteins, including enzymes such as: – angiotensin-converting enzyme – alkaline phosphatase – carbonic anhydrase – DNA and RNA polymerases – copper–zinc superoxide dismutase – metallothionein
Zinc fingers	Gene transcription
Wound healing	Suggests a role for topical zinc in enhancing re-epithelialisation and decreasing inflammation and bacterial growth

Table 8.10 The many functions and interactions of zinc

Copper deficiency

Copper deficiency is rare, because the liver contains adequate copper stores. Deficiency is seen in malnourished children (who have inadequate copper stores) and adults on long-term supported nutrition. Symptoms of deficiency include neutropenia, skeletal fragility and, in cases of prolonged deficiency, microcytic hypochromic anaemia.

Menkes disease is a rare X-linked recessive disorder of copper absorption. Patients with this condition have excessive renal excretion of copper. Boys have progressive developmental delay, intellectual disability, abnormal bone structure and loss of pigment from their hair. Female carriers are rarely affected. Even with copper replacement therapy, patients with Menkes disease have a high mortality, with a life expectancy of only 3 years.

Copper excess

Excess copper is toxic, but dietary overload is a rare cause of copper toxicity. Wilson's disease is a rare autosomal recessive disorder in which the liver fails to excrete copper in the bile, and incorporation of copper into caeruloplasmin is also impaired. These effects lead to deposition of copper in the liver, basal ganglia of the brain, kidneys and eyes (see page 205). Treatment is chelation of the copper and excretion in the urine.

Selenium

Selenium is essential to the activity of the enzyme glutathione peroxidase. Glutathione peroxidase reduces lipid hydrogen peroxides to their corresponding alcohols and reduces free hydrogen peroxide to water. The overall role of glutathione peroxidase is to protect cells from oxidative damage.

Selenium is also a cofactor in several thyroid hormone deiodinases. These include iodothyronine deiodinase, which catalyses the conversion of thyroxine to tri-iodothyronine.

Selenium deficiency results in reduced activity of these enzymes. About half of dietary selenium is absorbed, so deficiency in health is rare and generally occurs in patients on long-term nutritional support, or those with malabsorption disorders such as Crohn's or ceoliac disease.

Excess selenium is toxic. It leads to loss of hair and nails, dermatitis, irritability, and in severe cases, neurological damage.

Manganese

Manganese is a component of certain enzymes, for example pyruvate carboxylase (see Chapter 4) and superoxide dismutase. It also activates other classes of enzymes, such as hydrolases, kinases and decarboxylases. These groups of enzymes are pivotal to carbohydrate metabolism, so manganese deficiency can impair metabolism.

Most of the body's store of manganese is in bone. The remainder is in the liver and kidneys.

Chromium

There has been some debate about whether or not chromium is an essential element. Chromium has been ascribed a role in potentiating the action of insulin through the action of chromodulin. Chromodulin, a low-molecular-weight chromium-binding substance, transports chromium and interacts with the insulin receptor.

Chromium supplements have been suggested to reduce insulin levels and improve blood glucose metabolism, especially in people with obesity or type 2 diabetes. However, the evidence to support this theory is uncertain.

Molybdenum

Molybdenum is concentrated in the liver and kidneys, with lower concentrations in the vertebrae. Molybdenum combines with molybdopterin to form molybdenum cofactor. Molybdenum cofactor is essential for the activity of numerous enzymes, of which the main one is xanthine oxidase.

Xanthine oxidase is used in purine breakdown, as described in Chapter 2 (see page 54). The activity of xanthine oxidase is directly proportional to the amount of molybdenum in the body but only up to a certain point, after which the molybdenum becomes inhibitory.

Additional enzymes that depend on molybdenum are sulphite oxidase and aldehyde oxidase.

- Sulphite oxidase is present in the mitochondria, where it oxidises sulphite to sulphate; the electrons produced by this reaction are transferred through cytochrome c to the electron transport chain (see page 113).
- Aldehyde oxidase catalyses the oxidation of aldehydes into carboxylic acids; aldehyde oxidase also helps metabolise numerous drugs through oxidation in the liver and subsequent hepatic clearance

Cobalt

Cobalt is an essential constituent of vitamin B12 (cobalamin). Vitamin B12 acts as the source of cobalt reserves in the body.

The function of cobalt is essentially the same as that of vitamin B12 (see **Table 8.7**), and cobalt deficiency impairs these functions. Excess cobalt is known to decrease fertility in men, and when taken in excess leads to overproduction of red blood cells and damage to the heart muscles.

Iodine

Iodine is essential for synthesis of the thyroid hormones thyroxine and tri-iodothyronine (**Figure 8.14**). Iodine also has a nutritional association with selenium (see page 226).

> **Iodine deficiency causes thyroid gland hyperplasia.** An enlarged thyroid gland (goitre) develops because increased thyroid-stimulating hormone is secreted by the anterior pituitary gland to try to increase thyroid hormone levels. Goitre effects are more evident in lower income countries, because iodine is added to table salt in higher income countries.

Adults living in iodine-deficient parts of the world may develop hypothyroidism. This condition is characterised by tiredness, goitre, depression, weight gain and low body temperature. Hypothyroidism is also the result of auto-immune disease, as a consequence of treatment for hyperthyroidism; post thyroid surgery, pituitary disorders and from medications including lithium. Treatment is the replacement of thyroxine.

The babies of mothers who were iodine-deficient during pregnancy are at risk of congenital hypothyroidism either because

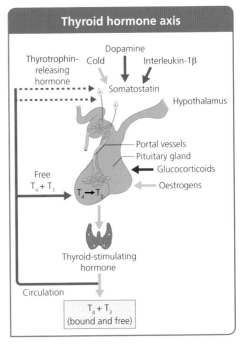

Thyroid hormone axis

Figure 8.14 The thyroid hormone axis. T_3, tri-iodothyronine; T_4, thyroxine; TRH, thyrotrophin-releasing hormone; TSH, thyroid-stimulating hormone.

the thyroid gland did not develop or lack of iodine for hormone synthesis. Congenital hypothyroidism requires lifelong thyroxine therapy. It is essential that this starts in the first few weeks of life. Without early diagnosis and treatment, the condition causes intellectual disability and growth retardation.

Excess iodine is rare but results from taking too many supplements or from areas where a high seafood and seaweed diet is ingested. It can result in the symptoms of hyperthyroidism. Symptoms include increased heart rate, temperature, tremors and anxiety, insomnia and weight loss. Treatment is either blocking the production of thyroid hormones by propylthiouracil or carbimazole or destruction of the gland by radioactive iodine.

Nutrition and disease

Nutritional status is the condition of the body resulting from the intake, absorption and utilisation of food. Assessment of nutritional status is key to diagnosis and appropriate treatment, especially in demanding clinical situations where adequate nutrition is vital to recovery and life. It is also necessary to determine whether patients' needs are being met and to identify those who are likely to be at increased risk of morbidity and mortality without nutritional support.

All patients who are admitted to hospital or residential care should undergo nutritional assessment. This is necessary because poor nutrition is linked to increased duration of hospital stay, slower recovery and higher mortality.

Several tools are available to assess nutritional status; some are more complex than others. The assessment tools that include biochemical, haematological, anthropometric and clinical information have economic and practical implications when used routinely. This is because test results take time, anthropometric measurements require equipment and clinical information is not always available.

In the UK, the Malnutrition Universal Screening Tool is often used for screening in the National Health Service. This tool uses body mass index, unplanned weight loss and acute illness to calculate the patient's overall risk of malnutrition.

Malnutrition is associated with many complications (**Table 8.11**). Therefore it is essential that patients who are undernourished, or at risk of becoming undernourished, are identified and provided with nutritional support.

Nutritional support

Nutritional support provides adequate food appropriate for the patient's needs and is supplemented (enriched) as required. If a patient is unable to tolerate eating, swallowing or chewing, then further support will be provided by either an enteral or a parenteral route.

■ In enteral nutrition, food is delivered into the stomach or small bowel through a tube
■ In parenteral nutrition, the patient is fed intravenously, thus bypassing the processes of eating and digestion

The provision of any type of nutritional support is matched to the patient's nutrient requirements and basal metabolic rate, as well as any additional needs identified from their current metabolic state. Numerous formulae are used to calculating the patient's requirements. However, some are impractical in an acute clinical setting, because a patient may be in a hyper- or hypometabolic state, fluid balance is difficult and determination of body composition is restricted. For simplicity, energy requirement can be calculated from body weight, with an assumption of 25–35 kcal/kg/24 h. Other calculations and formulae are available, but most institutions will have a preferred formula.

Table 8.12 details the basic composition and requirements for nutrients when a patient requires nutritional support.

Enteral feeding

This type of feeding is required when the patient has prolonged difficulty with swallowing, has upper gastrointestinal tract obstruction or is unable to eat. It is also be used as a transition feeding method between parenteral nutrition and normal nutrition.

Enteral feeding delivers nutrients into the gastrointestinal tract. These nutrients then stimulate normal digestion and absorption processes, so that they reach the bloodstream through the gut. Thus enteral feeding helps maintain gut integrity.

Complications associated with malnutrition	
Effect of malnutrition	Complication(s)
Decreased muscle strength	Fatigue, inactivity and increased risk of falls
Inactivity	Pressure sores and increased risk of thromboembolism
Impaired wound healing	Increased recovery times, duration of hospital stay and risk of further infections
Impaired immune response	Increased infection rates
Impaired thermoregulation	Hypothermia
Decreased respiratory muscle strength	Increased incidence of chest infection

Table 8.11 Effects of malnutrition on many physiological processes

Basic nutrients required in nutritional support		
Component	Healthy adult	Hospitalised adult
Protein	0.75 g/kg/24 h	1 g/kg/24 h Increased to 1.5 g/kg/24 h in cases of sepsis or trauma
Fluid	Fluid 30–35 mL/kg/24 h	Extra 2–2.5 mL/kg/24 h for every 1°C temperature rise above 37°C
Sodium	About 1 mmol/kg/24 h	In pyrexia, additional 15 mmol sodium per 100 mL additional fluid With large gastrointestinal, loss of 130–150 mmol/L
Potassium	1 mmol/kg/24 h	Increased up to 7 mmol/kg/24 h when refeeding is a risk

Table 8.12 Components to consider when balancing nutritional support

The composition of the feeds depends on the individual patient. The standard feed contains protein, vitamins and trace elements, as well as adequate electrolytes.

Parenteral feeding

Parenteral nutrition is often referred to as TPN, which stands for total parenteral nutrition. TPN is used only when neither oral nor enteral support are an option. This type of feeding is required when patients do not have a functioning gastrointestinal tract, or if there is bowel obstruction, short bowel syndrome, prolonged diarrhoea or a high-output fistula. Other conditions, for example severe Crohn's disease, may also require TPN.

Parenteral nutrition contains carbohydrate, fat, protein, vitamins, minerals, trace elements, electrolytes and water; these are usually provided in one bag of solution.

■ Carbohydrate is provided as glucose
■ Fat is an efficient source of calories and provides essential fatty acids

■ Protein, provided as nitrogen, is a mixture of amino acids, including essential amino acids
■ Fat-soluble and water-soluble vitamins are provided
■ The various trace elements include iron, zinc, copper, manganese, chromium, selenium and molybdenum

The nutritional solution is light-protected to prevent degradation of vitamins A and E.

Nutrition is essential before and after surgery and injury. Good nutrition aids healing:

■ Protein is necessary for tissue repair and the generation of scar tissue
■ Carbohydrates are needed to maintain energy and prevent protein (muscle) catabolism
■ Lipids are required for the absorption of fat-soluble vitamins, the generation of energy and the functioning of the immune system

Monitoring

Monitoring of nutritional support is essential. Routine daily laboratory tests are required to monitor renal and liver function and the concentration of electrolytes, glucose, calcium, albumin, magnesium and phosphate. Trace elements and vitamins are measured at baseline and then at suitable weekly or fortnightly intervals, depending on the duration of feeding and the patient's risk of deficiency.

Biochemical disturbances

Parenteral nutrition has many potential metabolic complications, but these are prevented with adequate monitoring. **Table 8.13** summarises the key biochemical complications associated with parenteral nutrition support.

Refeeding syndrome

Refeeding syndrome encompasses the metabolic processes that occur when malnourished patients are started on nutritional support. During periods of prolonged starvation, metabolic pathways switch from using glucose as the major energy source to using ketones. This results in a decreased basal metabolic rate and decreased insulin production.

Once carbohydrates are reintroduced, metabolism switches back to using glucose, and these metabolic pathways require phosphate to make the intermediates and products of the glycolytic pathway (see page 103). The increased demand for phosphate can result in hypophosphataemia. In addition, insulin is released, which causes potassium and magnesium to move into the cells.

Refeeding syndrome is avoided by following the advice in **Table 8.13**.

Obesity

Obesity is the other end of the nutritional spectrum, and develops when energy intake is surplus to energy requirements and expenditure; the extra is deposited or stored as fat tissue. The condition is commonly defined as a body mass index (calculated by dividing a person's weight by the square of their height in metres) of $> 30 \, \text{kg/m}^2$.

Excess body fat has negative effects on health, including reduced life expectancy and increased risk of other diseases. These diseases include coronary heart disease, type 2 diabetes, cancer and osteoarthritis, and are associated with increased mortality.

Parenteral nutrition complications		
Disturbance	Mechanism	Treatment
Glucose	Hyperglycaemic occurs particularly in cases of sepsis and in glucose-intolerant patients	Treated using intravenous insulin to maintain strict glycaemic control
	Hypoglycaemia occurs after abrupt cessation, both with and without insulin	Use of lipids in the mix prevents this complication, and feeds should not be stopped abruptly
Electrolytes	Hyperkalaemia may occur in patients with renal failure or metabolic acidosis	Insulin
	Hypokalaemia occurs when potassium lost in excess is not replaced	Potassium replacement
	Hyperchloraemic metabolic acidosis occurs with excessive gastrointestinal or renal bicarbonate loss	Acetate or lactate to correct acidosis
	Mild hyponatraemia resulting from: increased antidiuretic hormone secretion during stress of acute illness decreased ability to maintain fluid balance with high osmolar load	Sodium and water, unless secondary to ascites or odema, in which case fluid restriction is necessary
	Hypernatraemia resulting from sodium excess or water deficiency	Fluids
Calcium and magnesium	Hypercalcaemia is rarely due to excess vitamin D and immobility in cases of long-term nutrition	Adjust concentrations and reduce vitamin D
	Hypocalcaemia resulting from inadequate calcium, magnesium or both	Replace calcium and magnesium
	Hypomagnesaemia secondary to gastrointestinal loss or use of diuretics	Replace or stop diuretics
Phosphate	Hypophosphataemia occurs at start of feeding because of refeeding syndrome (see page 229)	Start feeds slowly in 'at-risk' patients, and if refeeding occurs, increase provision of potassium, phosphate, magnesium and thiamin

Table 8.13 Metabolic complications of parenteral nutrition

Obesity is recognised as a global issue and a major public health concern, because of the increasing demands that obesity places on health service providers.

Many theories have been proposed regarding the causes of the positive energy balance that is driving the increasing prevalence of obesity worldwide. The following factors have all been considered:

- dietary intake
- physical activity
- age and gender
- genetics
- psychological issues
- socioeconomic status

Dietary intake

Diets and access to food have changed greatly over the past few decades. Processed food with a high fat content is more easily available. Conversely, a variety of low-calorie, low-fat food products are being marketed. According to one theory, decreased energy expenditure may underlie the positive energy balance resulting in obesity. However, the results of nutritional studies suggest a positive fat balance rather than a positive energy balance.

A diet high in carbohydrates produces satiety through the action of hormones, including insulin, noradrenaline (norepinephrine) and gastric inhibitory polypeptide. A carbohydrate-rich diet also results in storage of glucose and inhibition of fat oxidation. In health, the processes of carbohydrate metabolism are well regulated to ensure glucose homeostasis.

However, fat metabolism does not have the same degree of autoregulation, because the body has a great capacity to store fat. Excess fat intake will be stored unless an equivalent amount of the energy it represents is used. Fat is stored very efficiently, using minimal energy in the process. A diet high in fat does not provide the satiety of a carbohydrate-rich diet, with a small portion of fat providing the same amount of energy as that of a larger portion of carbohydrate, because the energy content of fat per gram is higher. These factors are thought to explain the positive fat energy balance underlying the increased rate of obesity.

Physical activity

If energy input equals energy output, then a system is in balance.

- Increased energy requirements or output result in weight loss
- Increasing energy input produce weight gain

Lifestyles have become increasingly sedentary.

> The UK Royal College of Physicians 2013 report *Action on Obesity* estimates the current cost of obesity to be £5 billion per year. The authors of the report also state that this figure will double by 2050.

Age and gender

Several periods have been identified as critical in the development of obesity: early infancy, 5–7 years, adolescence and during pregnancy. This is because of the hormonal changes during these key developmental stages.

An overweight child is more likely to become an overweight adult. However, an overweight adult was not always an overweight child. This seeming discrepancy is related to the positive energy balance during adulthood. During adulthood, basal metabolic rate decreases, and if energy intake is not reduced accordingly, this will lead to a positive energy balance. In women, the loss of oestrogen activity that occurs at menopause may lead to increased central deposition of fat. However, both men and women lose weight when >70 years due to a combination of many factors (e.g. reduced appetite, change of taste and effect of taking a greater amount of medications).

Genetics

A parent's weight is related to that of their children; however, no single genetic defect is responsible for this relationship. Factors such as environment, nutrition, psychology and social environment all have a role. It is estimated that 40–70% of cases are the result of heritable factors, and that environmental factors have a 30% contribution to the number of cases.

> **Prader–Willi syndrome is a rare genetic disorder associated with an insatiable appetite and obesity.** The condition presents in infancy with poor muscle tone. This is followed by behavioural problems, which usually manifest in early childhood. Hyperphagia (overeating) begins between the ages of 2 and 8 years and carries on into adulthood. It commonly leads to the endocrine consequences of obesity, such as hypogonadism, infertility and an increased risk of diabetes.

Psychological issues

Overeating has been attributed to depression, anxiety and emotional disturbances. With increasing weight gain, additional depression and low self-esteem a cycle is created, especially if eating is the response to these feelings. When the cycle continues, it is difficult to distinguish cause and effect under these circumstances.

Stress has been linked to weight gain because of the actions of the stress response hormone, cortisol. Cortisol stimulates fat and carbohydrate metabolism and counteracts the effects of insulin. Anorexia and bulimia nervosa are associated with poor body image, self-esteem and public pressure. There are many links between psychological issues and poor control of energy balance. Depression, stress, emotional events (e.g. death) can all influence eating patterns which lead to weight gain or weight loss. Anorexia and bulimia are generally initiated from a psychological issue.

Socioeconomic status

The World Health Organization now state that obesity is affecting all ages and socioeconomic groups, worldwide. Originally there was a link to socioeconomic status, with a healthy diet and access to leisure facilities perceived as prohibitively expensive. Other contributory factors are the increased use of bottle-feeding (nutrient-enriched formula leading to increased fat deposition linked to obesity in childhood), poorer self-esteem (especially in women) and propogated parental attitudes in groups with low socioeconomic status. With an increased sedentary lifestyle, reliance on transport, increase in availability of processed high fat food, the socioeconomic trend for obesity is across all social groups, especially evident in children.

Health risks of obesity

As weight increases, so do the risks of mortality and morbidity. Cardiovascular disease, hypertension and type 2 diabetes are strongly associated with obesity. Obesity has many medical consequences (**Table 8.14**), which place additional burdens on health service providers.

Consequences of obesity

Category	Consequences
Endocrine effects	Infertility and menstrual dysfunction
	Increased incidence of oestrogen-dependent cancers, including those of the breast and prostate
Metabolic effects	Cardiovascular disease (coronary heart disease and stroke)
	Hypertension
	Type 2 diabetes
	Hyperlipidaemia
	Increased risk of gallstones
	Increased risk of blood-clotting abnormalities
Physical effects	Joint disorders and back pain
	Arthritis
	Oedema
	Breathlessness
	Physical inactivity
	Sweating
	Varicose veins
	Sleep apnoea
Surgical complications	Increased risk for complications during anaesthesia
	Chest infections
	Poor wound healing
	Deep vein thrombosis
Psychological and social effects	Low self-esteem
	Depression
	Tiredness
	Discrimination
	Agoraphobia

Table 8.14 Health consequences of obesity

Orlistat is a pancreatic lipase inhibitor that decreases fat digestion and absorption. Lipase breaks triglycerides into absorbable free fatty acids. The results of clinical trials have shown that orlistat, in conjunction with a reduced-calorie diet, improves weight loss compared with diet and exercise alone. An adverse effect of this drug is steatorrhea (oily loose stools), which are a consequence of the reduced absorption of fats.

The treatment or reversal of weight gain requires a negative energy balance. This can be achieved by decreasing food intake, increasing exercise, gaining advice from healthcare professionals, medication or surgical intervention.

Answers to starter questions

1. Thiamin (vitamin B1)-dependent enzymes are present in all cells, but deficiencies of thiamin present in the nervous system due to the reliance on thamine for oxidative phosphorylation atrophy in some areas of the nervous system. Thiamin pyrophosphate is a co-factor of four key enzymes, whose activity is reduced in thiamine deficiency: pyruvate dehydrogenase and α-ketoglutarate dehydrogenase – causing reduced acetyl CoA and ATP formation and therefore acetylcholine, branched chain amino acid α-ketoacid dehydrogenase and transketolase, which results in decreased activity of the pentose phosphate pathway. The result is a decrease in NADPH, which is required for fatty acid synthesis of the myelin. Myelin is required for functioning of the nervous system and loss of myelin results in impairment of signal conduction along the nerves, leading to peripheral neuropathy.

    In addition, neurotransmitter production is dependent upon thiamin.

2. In a fed state, the main fuel to provide blood glucose is exogenous carbohydrate. In a fasting state the glucose originates from liver and muscle glycogen stores (though only the muscle uses its own stores). These stores are generally only adequate for 12–24 hours, after which gluconeogenesis will proceed; using protein and fat to produce glucose.

3. Fat content in food provides texture and taste. The fat affects how volatile compounds are released in the mouth and how flavours are perceived. Some flavours stick to fat prolonging the taste and others are enhanced by the presence of fat. The perception of fat in a meal uses several senses, taste, smell, sound and sight.

4. Hunger in the physical sense is related to contractions of the stomach muscles, often known as hunger pangs. The hormone ghrelin is believed to trigger the contraction of the muscles and its release is triggered by a low glucose.

5. In cholestasis the flow of bile is impaired in the bile ducts of the liver, pancreas or biliary tract. This can be caused by hepatic or extra-hepatic blockages. As bile normally binds bilirubin, this now escapes into the blood stream and manifests as jaundice as it appears yellow as it deposits under the skin. Meanwhile, vitamin K – essential for healthy blood clotting – is a fat-soluble vitamin and hence requires bile for absorption. Cholestatic disease results in reduced absorption of vitamin K and hence decreased activation of vitamin K dependent enzymes involved in the clotting cascade. In addition vitamin K is required for inhibitors of coagulation, protein C and S.

6. Metabolic syndrome is a term for a combination of diabetes, hypertension and obesity. Individually, these increase the risk of heart disease but in combination the effect is magnified. Characteristically, people with metabolic syndrome will have high triglyceride levels, high blood pressure, insulin resistance, increased risk of deep vein thrombosis and a large waist circumference. Asian and African-Caribbean populations are particularly susceptible.

7. The basal metabolic rate is the number of calories required to keep the body functioning at rest. It is relative to body mass, age, weight and height. Gender also plays a role as men need more calories than women. The formula for men is:

$$66.47 + [13.7*weight(kg)] + [5*size(cm)] - [6.8*age(years)]$$

    For women it is:

$$655.1 + [9.6*weight(kg)] + [1.8*size(cm)] - [4.7*age(years)]$$

Answers *continued*

8. In general, vitamin supplements are unnecessary, as a varied healthy diet should satisfy all requirements. However, there are certain groups of people where supplementation is advised, such as: folic acid in pregnancy to reduce the risk of neural tube defects, vitamin D supplements in pregnancy and during breastfeeding and for children 6 months to 5 years and in the over 65 years old.

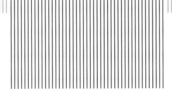

Chapter 9
Self-assessment

SBA Questions

Nucleic acids

1 A 24-year-old man has mild jaundice (bilirubin 45 µmol/L) and no significant past medical history. Liver function tests are unremarkable. Gilbert's syndrome is suspected.
What single laboratory test result will support a diagnosis of Gilbert's syndrome?

A Decreased TA repeats in the TATA box promoter sequence of UGT1A1
B Decreased unconjugated bilirubin
C Increased serum conjugated bilirubin
D Increased serum haptoglobin
E Increased TA repeats in the TATA box promoter sequence of UGT1A1

2. A 42-year-old man presents with a painful swollen big toe and is suspected to have gout. Determining the concentration of which single substance in the blood is most likely to support this diagnosis?

A Allantoic acid
B Rasbicurase
C Urea
D Uric acid
E Xanthine

3. A 46-year-old man had chemotherapy 48 hours ago for acute myeloid leukaemia with nausea, vomiting, lethargy and oliguria. Routine blood tests are sent to the biochemistry laboratory.
What single set of blood results would you expect to see?

A High calcium, high potassium, high phosphate, high uric acid
B High calcium, low potassium, low phosphate, high uric acid
C Low calcium, high potassium, high phosphate, high uric acid
D Low calcium, low potassium, low phosphate, high uric acid
E Low calcium, low potassium, low phosphate, low uric acid

4. A 23-year-old woman has ulcerative colitis. She has suffered several relapses in the last few months and is started on azathioprine.
What is the single most useful test to perform before starting her on therapy?

A Faecal calprotectin
B Serum CRP
C Serum renal profile
D Serum 6-thioguanine nucleotide
E Whole blood thiopurine methyltransferase activity

5. A 42-year-old pregnant woman consents to antenatal screening for Down's syndrome. A nuchal translucency scan and blood testing is performed at 12 weeks and the results indicate she has a high risk.
What single test would confirm her baby has Down's syndrome?

A Karyotyping fetal DNA
B Mitochondrial DNA analysis of maternal DNA
C PCR analysis using fetal DNA
D Restriction fragment length polymorphism analysis using fetal DNA
E Single nucleotide polymorphism analysis using fetal DNA

6. A 17-year-old man is given high dose IV methotrexate therapy following surgical resection of an oestosarcoma. 14 hours post therapy he develops acute kidney injury, oliguria and neutropenia.
What is the single most effective therapy to give?

A Haemodialysis
B Hydrocortisone

C IV saline 0.9%
D IV sodium bicarbonate
E Leucovorin

7. A 5-year-old girl's parents say she is very sensitive to light and her skin blisters and burns easily after slight sun exposure. She has many freckles over her face, neck, hands and arms. On examination she is found to have a basal cell carcinoma on her face.
What single process is most likely to be defective in this patient?

A Repair of DNA double strand breaks
B Repair of nucleotide mismatch errors during DNA replication
C Removal of methylated guanine bases from DNA
D Removal of pyrimidine dimers from DNA
E Removal of uracil from DNA

8. A 4 year-old-boy has poor language skills and developmental delay. He has a waddling gait and hypertrophy of the calf and his parents report that he falls frequently. Genetic analysis revealed a mutation in the promoter region of the dystrophin gene.
What is the single most likely effect of this mutation?

A Defective end capping of the mRNA for dystrophin
B Defective initiation of transcription of the dystrophin gene
C Defective splicing of the mRNA for dystrophin
D Extended transcription of the dystrophin gene
E Premature termination of translation of the dystrophin protein

9. A 2-month-old girl has failure to thrive and pneumonia. She has suffered previously with respiratory tract infections and recurrent candidiasis. Blood tests reveal she has low T, B and NK lymphocytes.
What single enzyme defect is most likely in this patient?

A Adenine deaminase
B Adenine phosphoribosyltransferase
C Hypoxanthine-guanine phosphoribosyl-transferase
D Ribonucleotide reductase
E Thymidylate synthase

Proteins

1. A 74-year-old woman has progressive lethargy. Physical examination reveals significant weight loss and anaemia. The most likely diagnosis is multiple myeloma.

What investigation will best support this diagnosis?

A Albumin concentration
B β_2-microglobulin concentration
C Blood film
D Full blood count
E Serum and urine protein electrophoresis

2. A 55-year old man has poorly controlled type 2 diabetes.
What single test would confirm long term poor glycaemic control?

A Carbohydrate deficient transferrin
B Fructosamine
C Glucose
D Glycated albumin
E Glycated haemoglobin

3. A 40-year-old man has a history of recurrent chest infections and laboured breathing on exertion. He smokes 20 cigarettes a day. He is concerned there is a genetic basis for his symptoms.
What is the single best test to investigate this possibility?

A Albumin
B Alpha-1-antitrypsin
C Caeruloplasmin
D Ferritin
E Haptoglobin

4. A 5-year-old girl with phenylketonuria (PKU) has frequent high phenylalanine concentrations.
What single foodstuff should be excluded from her diet?

A Bananas
B Butter
C Corn starch
D Diet carbonated drinks
E Salt

5. A 40-year-old woman has weight loss, abdominal pain and altered bowel movements.
What single investigation would best support a diagnosis of coeliac disease?

A Anti-gliadin antibody
B Caeruloplasmin
C Faecal elastase
D IgA tissue transglutaminase
E Urine protein

6. A 3-week-old male neonate has failure to thrive and is encephalopathic. His ammonia concentration is 400 µmol/L.
Which single disorder can be excluded before further tests are performed?

A Galactosemia
B MCAD deficiency
C Phenylketonuria

D Propionic acidaemia

E Tyrosinemia type 1

7. An 18-year-old man has a clear fluid running from his ear (rhinorrhoea) following a head trauma. It is suspected that it is cerebral spinal fluid secondary to a fractured skull.
What single test should be performed to confirm this?

A Albumin

B Alpha-1-anti trypsin

C Alpha-2 macroglobulin

D Protein S100

E Tau protein (β_2 transferrin)

8. A-19 year-old woman claims to have taken an overdose of acetaminophen (paracetamol) tablets 8 hours previously. Her blood acetaminophen concentration is 142 mg/L on admission.
What is the single most appropriate management?

A Activated charcoal

B Methionine

C N-acetylcysteine

D Naloxone

E Penicillamine

9. A 14-year-old female has a fractured tibia following a minor fall. She has a past medical history of fractures, including two previous fractured arms and several fingers. She has attended the emergency department three times for a dislocated shoulder. On examination her sclera are noted to blue.
What single protein is she most likely to be deficient in?

A Collagen I

B Collagen III

C Elastin

D Fibrillin I

E Keratin

Carbohydrates

1. A 62-year-old man with type 2 diabetes mellitus has a fever, shortness of breath and a cough productive of green sputum. His blood glucose is 45.0 mmol/L and serum sodium 129 mmol/L. He is on metformin normally. His urine osmolality is 350 mOsmol/kg and urinary sodium 30 mmol/L. He appears dehydrated.
What is the single most likely cause of his hyponatraemia?

A Congestive heart failure

B Furosemide

C Osmotic diuresis

D SIADH

E Spurious result

2. A 15-year-old girl has recurrent hypoglycaemic episodes. Samples are taken while she is hypoglycaemic for further investigations.
What single investigation will best help identify the cause of hypoglycaemia?

A Cortisol

B Growth hormone

C Insulin and c-peptide

D Oral glucose tolerance test

E Sulphonylurea screen

3. A 45-year-old man has polyuria and polydipsia. A glucose tolerance test is performed and the baseline fasting sample had a serum glucose of 5.2 mmol/L. 2 hours after he had taken the glucose load, the second glucose sample was 13.8 mmol/L.
What single interpretation best describes this man's ability to handle the glucose load?

A Diabetic response to glucose load

B Impaired fasting glycaemia

C Impaired glycaemic control

D Normal response

E Post-prandial hypoglycaemia

4. A 52-year-old man has diabetic ketoacidosis. His serum glucose is 47 mmol/L and β-hydroxybutyrate concentration 7 mmol/L. His breathing is deep and laboured. An arterial blood gas analysis was performed.
What is the single most likely set of blood gas analysis results for this patient?

A pH 7.2, pCO_2 2.7 kPa, BE -12.6

B pH 7.2, pCO_2 8.0 kPa, BE +2.4

C pH 7.4, pCO_2 5.4 kPa, BE -1.2

D pH 7.45, pCO_2 5.6, Std bicarb 28 mmol/L

E pH 7.5, pCO_2 6.9 kPa, Std bicarb 38 mmol/L

5. A 40-year-old man has joint pains and lethargy. He works on a building site and is struggling with his work. He has also noticed his hard hat isn't fitting his head securely. His oral glucose tolerance test results are:

Time	Glucose mmol/L	Growth Hormone µg/L (<1.0)	IGF1 nmol/L (9–28)
0	7.9	7.1	56
30	8.9	6.5	
60	12.6	6.1	
90	14.8	6.9	
120	13.5	6.5	

What is the single most appropriate interpretation of these results?

A Acromegaly

B   Diabetes
C   Diabetes and acromegaly
D   Impaired fasting glycaemia
E   Impaired glucose tolerance

6. A 40-year-old woman has bloods taken for glycated haemoglobin (HbA1c); the result is 75 mmol/mol. She has no past medical history and is well.
Which single interpretation best describes this result?

A   Diagnoses diabetes without further tests
B   High risk of diabetes, suggests lifestyle changes
C   Impaired glucose tolerance
D   Suggestive of diabetes, repeat sample required
E   Within normal reference range

7. A 66-year-old woman with diabetes has routine blood tests analysed in the laboratory and an arterial blood gas sample taken. The glucose concentration in both samples is 19 mmol/L. The potassium concentration is 5.9 mmol/L in the laboratory and 5.6 mmol/L on the arterial blood gas.
What single reason best describes the difference in potassium level?

A   Blood gas analyser is not working correctly
B   Delayed analysis of the blood gas sample
C   Laboratory assay is running with a positive bias
D   Serum sample in the laboratory is contaminated with potassium
E   Serum sample is a clotted sample and potassium is released from platelets

8. A 28-year-old woman has a glucose tolerance test performed because she often feels unwell after a large carbohydrate load and thinks she may be diabetic. The fasting glucose concentration is 5.2 mmol/L and 2 hours post glucose load the serum glucose concentration is 2.4 mmol/L.
What is the single best interpretation of these results?

A   Diabetic response
B   Impaired fasting glycaemia
C   Normal response
D   Reactive hypoglycaemia
E   Sample mix up with the baseline 2.4 mmol/L

9. A premature neonate is born to a diabetic mother and is hypoglycaemic, with a plasma glucose concentration of 1.8 mmol/L.
What is the single most likely cause of the hypoglycaemia?

A   Addison's disease
B   Neonate has type I diabetes

C   Glycogen storage disorder
D   Increased circulating insulin
E   Insulinoma

10. A 48-year-old man was diagnosed as a type 2 diabetic 6 months ago. His glycated haemoglobin (HbA1c) is now 85 mmol/mol (target control 48–59 mmol/mol). He has been compliant with diet and exercise recommendations. He is started on sulphonylurea treatment.
What is the single most likely result of this treatment?

A   Decreased secretion of insulin from pancreas
B   Decreased absorption of carbohydrate from the GI tract
C   Increased production of glucose from the liver
D   Increased secretion of insulin from the pancreas
E   Increased absorption of carbohydrate from the GI tract

Fats

1. A 59-year-old women has her atorvastatin dose increased from 40mg to 80mg to treat her hypercholesterolaemia. She complains of muscle pain and weakness.
What single biochemical test will indicate that the atorvastatin has caused muscle damage?

A   Alanine aminotransferase
B   Aspartate aminotransferase
C   Creatine kinase
D   Haptoglobin
E   Lactate dehydrogenase

2. A 35 year-old man has been unwell for 6 weeks and has bilateral pitting oedema of the lower limbs. Urine analysis reveals severe proteinuria. He is considered to have nephrotic syndrome. A lipid profile (cholesterol, triglyceride and HDL) is requested.
What single abnormality would you expect to see on the lipid profile?

A   High HDL cholesterol
B   High total cholesterol
C   Low LDL cholesterol
D   Low total cholesterol
E   Low triglyceride

3. A 22-year-old man's brother is recently diagnosed with familial hypercholesterolaemia. A lipid profile is performed.
Which single set of results will confirm the diagnosis of familial hypercholesterolaemia?

A   Total cholesterol >6.7 mmol/L, LDL cholesterol >4.0 mmol/L

B Total cholesterol >7.0 mmol/L, LDL cholesterol >4.0 mmol/L, HDL cholesterol <2.0 mmol/L

C Total cholesterol >7.5 mmol/L, LDL cholesterol >4.9 mmol/L

D Total cholesterol >7.5 mmol/L, LDL cholesterol >4.9 mmol/L, HDL cholesterol >2.0 mmol/L

E Total cholesterol >9.0 mmol/L, LDL cholesterol >3.0 mmol/L, HDL cholesterol >2.0 mmol/L

4. A 45-year-old woman has an infected foot ulcer. Routine biochemistry blood tests reveal that she has a significantly increased triglyceride concentration.
Which single reason is responsible for increased fatty acid concentrations in type 2 diabetes?

   A Decreased cholesteryl ester transfer protein activity
   B Decreased hepatic flux of free fatty acids
   C Hyperglycaemia
   D Increased hormone sensitive lipase activity
   E Increased lipoprotein lipase activity

5. A 54-year-old man has a history of lethargy, weight gain and constipation. Blood results requested 1 week earlier reveal cholesterol 14.9 mmol/L and triglyceride 2.9 mmol/L.
What single laboratory investigation will best support a secondary cause for the lipid abnormality?

   A Alcohol measurement
   B Glucose measurement
   C Liver function tests
   D Urea and electrolytes
   E Thyroid function tests (TSH and free T4)

6. A 45-year-old obese woman (BMI 34 Kg/m²) with a history of alcohol excess is referred for an endoscopy following frequent complaints of epigastric pain. Endoscopy reveals a duodenal ulcer. Hospital blood tests reveal a significantly elevated triglyceride concentration.
What is the single most appropriate treatment?

   A Ezetimibe
   B Fibrate
   C Insulin
   D Lifestyle advice (abstain from alcohol and weight loss)
   E Statin

7. A 54-year-old man with poorly controlled type 2 diabetes has routine blood tests that reveal serum triglyceride 40 mmol/L and sodium 125 mmol/L. His plasma glucose is 10.3 mmol/L.

What is the single most likely cause of the hyponatraemia?

   A Addison's disease
   B Drug-induced
   C Hyporeninaemia hypoaldosteronism (type 4 renal tubular acidosis)
   D Inadequate sodium intake
   E Pseudohyponatraemia

8. A 15-year-old boy with an enlarged liver and spleen, and a brownish pigmentation of his skin is suspected to have type 1 Gaucher's disease (lysosomal storage disorder). His eyes also contain yellow spots called pingueculae.
What is the single most appropriate blood test to perform?

   A Cholesterol
   B Glucocerebrosidase enzyme activity
   C Lipoprotein lipase enzyme activity
   D Platelets
   E Triglycerides

9. A 20-year-old woman with orange hyperplastic orange-yellow tonsils, corneal opacity and thrombocytopenia has a high density lipoprotein concentration of HDL=0.2 mmol/L.
What is the single most likely diagnosis?

   A Chronic kidney disease
   B Familial hypercholesterolaemia
   C Familial combined hyperlipidaemia
   D Hypothyroidism
   E Tangier disease

Haemoglobin

1. A 16-year-old woman is feeling tired and is jaundiced. The doctor suspects she has intravascular haemolysis.
Which single panel of biochemistry tests will confirm this?

   A Albumin, potassium, ALT, calcium
   B LDH, haptoglobin, albumin, bilirubin
   C LDH, haptoglobin, ALT, reticulocytes
   D Reticulocytes, ALT, calcium, potassium
   E Sodium, potassium, LDH, haemoglobin

2. 65-year-old man complains that his skin is becoming deep yellow in colour. He has had weight loss but no pain and has noticed that his stools are pale. Physical examination revealed only deep icterus. There is no history of drug therapy. A urine dipstick test is performed for bilirubin and urobilinogen.
What is the single most likely set of results for the urine dipstick?

   A Bilirubin absent and urobilinogen present
   B Bilirubin and urobilinogen both absent
   C Bilirubin and urobilinogen present

D   Bilirubin present and urobilinogen absent
E   Bilirubin, urobilinogen and haemoglobin
    present

3. A 30-year-old man is jaundiced and with no
    previous medical history of note. Routine
    blood tests show glucose 18 mmol/L and biliru-
    bin 60 μmol/L.
    What single test will confirm a diagnosis hae-
    mochromatosis?

    A   Ferritin
    B   HFE genotyping
    C   Iron
    D   Total iron binding capacity
    E   Transferrin

4. A 19-year-old woman has abdominal pain.
    She recently started the oral contraceptive pill
    and has a family history of acute intermittent
    porphyria.
    What single investigation will establish a diag-
    nosis of an acute attack of acute intermittent
    porphyria?

    A   Blood lead
    B   Faecal coproporphyrinogen
    C   Serum biliverdin
    D   Serum iron
    E   Urine porphobilinogen

5. A 17-year-old woman complains of tiredness.
    Thyroid function tests, vitamin B12 and folate,
    full blood count and iron studies are request-
    ed. Results show she has iron deficiency
    anaemia.
    What single set of iron study results would be
    expected?

    A   High transferrin, high iron, low ferritin
    B   High transferrin, low iron, low ferritin
    C   Low transferrin, high iron, high ferritin
    D   Low transferrin, high iron, low ferritin
    E   Low transferrin, low iron, low ferritin

6. A 14-month-old infant born outside of the
    UK has pallor with slight scleral icterus and an
    enlarged abdomen. There is no previous medi-
    cal history. The baby is suspected to have beta
    thalassemia.
    What single laboratory test would be used to
    confirm that this is the case?

    A   Alpha fetoprotein
    B   Full blood count
    C   Haemoglobin electrophoresis
    D   Iron studies
    E   Peripheral blood smear

7. A 35-year-old man with cystic fibrosis has
    abnormal clotting results. His prothrombin
    time and activated partial thromboplastin time
    are 18 seconds and 41 seconds.

What is the single most likely cause of this
abnormality?

A   Disseminated intravascular coagulopathy
B   Dysfibrinogenaemia
C   Heparin
D   Low fibrinogen
E   Vitamin K deficiency

8. A 5-year-old boy is rescued from a house fire
    and is having difficulty breathing. Blood gas
    results show hypoxia (PaO_2 8KPa) and carbon
    monoxide poisoning (CO=30%, reference
    range in non-smoker <5%).
    What is the single most likely cause of the
    hypoxia?

    A   Carbon monoxide impaired oxygen delivery
        and utilisation at a cellular level
    B   Carbon monoxide enhanced oxygen con-
        sumption
    C   Carbon monoxide altered the oxidation
        state of iron so oxygen delivery to the tissue
        is impaired
    D   Carbon monoxide decreased 2,3-bispho-
        phoglycerate, reducing oxygen delivery to
        the tissues
    E   Metabolic alkalosis reduced oxygen delivery
        to the tissues

9. A 40-year-old woman has mild jaundice. She
    has a yellow discolouration to her sclera and
    blood tests reveal a total bilirubin concentra-
    tion of 60 μmol/L and a direct (unconjugated)
    bilirubin of 50 μmol/L. Other liver function
    tests are unremarkable.
    What is the single most likely cause of these
    results?

    A   Gallstones
    B   Gilbert's syndrome
    C   Hepatitis
    D   Intravascular haemolysis
    E   Pancreatic cancer

Body fluid homeostasis

1. A 73-year-old man is drowsy and unwell. He is
    known to have COPD (chronic obstructive pulmo-
    nary disease) but also appears to be septic. Blood
    gases reveal elevated hydrogen ions, elevated
    $Paco_2$ and low PaO_2, bicarbonate and pH.
    What is the single most likely diagnosis?

    A   Metabolic acidosis
    B   Mixed metabolic and respiratory acidosis
    C   Respiratory acidosis
    D   Respiratory acidosis with metabolic com-
        pensation
    E   Respiratory alkalosis with metabolic com-
        pensation

2. A 20-year-old man is hypotensive (BP: 105/60 mmHg) and tachycardic (105 bpm). Blood tests reveal mild hyponatraemia (Na: 130 mmol/L), hyperkalaemia (K$^+$: 6.3 mmol/L), hypoglycaemia (glucose: 2.2 mmol/L) and pre-renal uraemia (urea: 10 mmol/L).
What is the single most appropriate next test to perform?

   A Plasma ACTH
   B Plasma renin
   C Serum cortisol
   D Serum osmolality
   E Urine sodium

3. A 30-year-old man has a broken ankle. Routine blood results are unremarkable apart from a low serum potassium and bicarbonate (with a normal anion gap).
What is the single most likely diagnosis?

   A Aspirin overdose
   B Chronic kidney disease
   C Diabetic ketoacidosis
   D Ischaemic limb
   E Proximal renal tubular acidosis

4. A 25-year-old woman has a persistently low serum potassium concentration of 2.6 mmol/L. She has a history of anorexia nervosa and complains of muscle weakness and polyuria.
What is the single most appropriate next test to perform?

   A Plasma aldosterone
   B Plasma renin
   C Serum magnesium
   D Serum osmolality
   E Urine potassium

5. A 45-year-old man has polyuria and abdominal pain. He is also low in mood. Blood tests reveal hypercalcaemia. His adjusted calcium is 3.4 mmol/L.
What is the single most appropriate next test to perform?

   A Plasma parathyroid hormone
   B Plasma phosphate
   C Serum 25-hydroxyvitamin D
   D Serum magnesium
   E Urine calcium

6. A 52-year-old woman has been vomiting for 2 days following food poisoning. Blood gas analysis results revealed pH: 7.62, Paco$_2$: 7.1 KPa, PaO$_2$: 14.2 KPa and base excess: +20.2.
What is the single most likely diagnosis?

   A Compensated metabolic acidosis
   B Metabolic acidosis
   C Metabolic alkalosis

   D Partially compensated metabolic alkalosis
   E Respiratory alkalosis

7. A 70-year-old man is discovered lying on the floor at home by his son following a stroke. He is unable to swallow. Clinical assessment revealed he was dehydrated with pulse rate: 110 bpm and BP: 95/65 mmHg with lax skin. Biochemical results were sodium: 169 mmol/L, potassium: 3.9 mmol/L, urea: 23.5 mmol/L, creatinine: 162 µmol/L, glucose: 7.1 mmol/L.
What is the single most appropriate intravenous fluid to give for treatment?

   A Dextrose 5%
   B Hartmann's solution
   C Potassium chloride 0.3% and sodium chloride 0.9%
   D Sodium chloride 0.9%
   E Sodium chloride 0.45%

8. A 19-year-old woman with chronic kidney disease stage 4 has a potassium concentration of 7.2 mmol/L.
What is the single most appropriate treatment?

   A Intravenous Calcium gluconate
   B Oral Calcium resonium
   C Haemodialysis
   D Intravenous Insulin and dextrose
   E Salbutamol nebulizer

9. A 35-year-old woman has abdominal pain and is hyperventilating (respiratory rate 30 breaths per minute). Blood gas results show she has a respiratory alkalosis and routine blood tests show a phosphate result of 0.32 mmol/L.
What is the single most likely cause of the phosphate result?

   A Dietary phosphate deficiency
   B Drug-induced hypophosphataemia
   C Fanconi syndrome
   D Refeeding syndrome
   E Respiratory alkalosis promoting cellular uptake of phosphate

10. A 15-year-old girl has urea and electrolytes and a bone profile measured after an appendectomy. Results reveal marked hyperkalaemia and hypocalcaemia (K$^+$: 8.5mmol/L and adjusted calcium: 1.50mmol/L). All other results are unremarkable.
What is the single most likely cause of these results?

   A Acute kidney injury
   B Delayed sample centrifugation
   C Haemolysis
   D Potassium-ethylenediamine tetraacetic acid contamination
   E Potassium-sparing diuretics

11. A 25-year-old East Asian man with thyrotoxicosis and profound muscle weakness has urea and electrolytes measured which reveal marked hypokalaemia (K$^+$ 1.9 mmol/L). What is the single most likely cause?

A Bartter's syndrome
B Gittelman's syndrome
C Hypokalaemic periodic paralysis
D Liddle's syndrome
E Vomiting

Nutrition

1. A 32-year-old African man has dehydration and hypercalcaemia (adjusted calcium: 3.20 mmol/L). He has no significant drug or medical history. Initial investigations reveal an appropriately suppressed PTH concentration and an adequate 25-hydroxyvitamin D concentration (55 nmol/L).
What is the single most appropriate next investigation?

A Blood ionised calcium
B Serum 1,25-hydroxyvitamin D
C Serum magnesium
D Serum thyroid function test
E Serum vitamin A

2. An 85-year-old woman has a fractured neck of femur and is unable to stand up. The Malnutrition Universal Screening Tool (MUST) is used to assess her nutritional status.
What single measurement is required in this assessment?

A Head circumference
B Length of ulna
C Metatarsal length
D Mid lower arm circumference
E Recent planned weight loss

3. A 23-year-old woman is unable to get pregnant despite trying for 12 months. Her BMI is 16.5 kg/m^2.
Which single biochemical result would you most likely see?

A Low LH, FSH and oestradiol
B Low serum cortisol
C Raised creatinine
D Raised free T4 and free T3 concentrations
E Raised potassium

4. A 58-year-old man is unconscious following a fall. He is well-built and has chronic kidney disease. His serum phosphate is 2.85 mmol/L with abnormal renal function.
What is the single most likely cause of the hyperphosphataemia?

A Hyperparathyroidism
B Hyperthyroidism
C Metabolic alkalosis
D Respiratory acidosis
E Rhabdomolysis

5. A 25-year-old woman has weakness, increasing occurrence of pins and needles and is generally feeling down. She has a low serum potassium (3.0 mmol/L) and a low serum magnesium (0.41 mmol/L).
What single differential diagnosis can be excluded?

A Diarrhoea
B Furosemide use
C Gitelman syndrome
D Hypoaldosteronism
E Laxative abuse

6. An 84-year-old women is in intensive care and having daily assessments for nutritional support. Trace metal analysis has identified a low serum zinc of 3.4 μmol/L.
What is the single most likely cause of the low zinc level?

A Acute inflammation and tissue damage
B Increased dietary intake and acute inflammation
C Reduced dietary intake and acute inflammation
D Tissue damage and hypoalbuminaemia
E Tissue damage and reduced dietary intake

7. A 35-year-old woman has active coeliac disease. At her gastroenterology outpatient review she has a full blood and physical assessment.
What is the single most likely finding?

A Hypercalcaemia
B Iron excess
C Sodium deficiency
D Vitamin C deficiency
E Weight loss

8. A 16-year-old girl swims for her local team and regularly exercises for 2–3 hours a day. She has not had a menstrual period for the last 4 months. Prior to this her periods were regular; she has recently lost weight. Upon examination she is underweight for her height and she has purpuric lesions on her body and arms. Full blood count reveals low platelets and neutrophil count with a macrocytic anaemia.
What is the single most likely deficiency?

A Folic acid
B Iron
C Magnesium
D Niacin
E Zinc

9. A 78-year-old woman has pins and needles in her arms and legs and generally feeling weak. Examination shows weakness of the extensor and flexor muscles of the lower extremities with exaggerated knee reflexes.
What single vitamin deficiency is most likely to be causing her symptoms?

A Niacin
B Vitamin B1
C Vitamin B2
D Vitamin B6
E Vitamin B12

10. A 14-year-old girl has very heavy periods and when examined says her gums bleed when she cleans her teeth. Her mother says that when she had a tooth extracted recently it wouldn't stop bleeding. Blood tests show platelets 300 x10⁹/L, prothrombin time 11 s and activated partial thromboplastin time 47 s.
What is the single most likely diagnosis?

A Factor VII deficiency
B Factor X deficiency
C Haemophilia
D Vitamin K deficiency
E Von Willebrand disease

SBA answers

Nucleic acids

1. E
An increase in the number of TA repeats in the TATA box promoter sequence of UGT1A1 is responsible for Gilbert's syndrome. The conjugation reaction that converts bilirubin to bilirubin glucuronide (water soluble) is defective. The conjugation process is catalysed by the enzyme UDP-glucuronyltransferase. The mutation observed in Gilbert's syndrome causes a reduced level of expression of the UDP-glucuronyltransferase.

2. D
Uric acid is measured as a first line biochemical screen for gout. The clinical manifestations of gout result from uric acid crystals forming in the joint. The definitive diagnosis of gout is based upon microscopy analysis on the joint fluid and the presence of urate crystals.

3. C
Presentation and history of the patient is suggestive of tumour lysis syndrome. Tumour lysis syndrome is caused by the rapid death of cancer cells following chemotherapy and the release of large amounts of intracellular contents into the circulation. This results in hyperkalaemia and hyperphosphataemia. Hyperphosphataemia causes precipitation of calcium phosphate and subsequent hypocalcaemia. The breakdown of large amounts of cellular DNA causes hyperuricaemia. Tumor lysis syndrome is often associated with haematological malignancies such as the acute leukaemias, where large numbers of cells are affected.

4. E
Azathioprine is metabolised either to the active 6-thioguanine nucleotide by hypoxanthine-guanine phosphoribosyltransferase or to inactive methylated metabolites by thiopurine methyltransferase (TPMT). TPMT activity varies between individuals and patients with low or no TPMT activity are at risk of toxicity due to increased conversion of azathioprine to its active metabolite. Measurement of TPMT activity is performed before starting azathioprine treatment to identify patients with low TPMT activity, who require a lower dose to prevent myelosuppression. Azazthioprine treatment is not suitable for patients with TPMT deficiency.

5. A
Down's syndrome is caused by an additional copy of chromosome 21 (trisomy 21). Pre-natal diagnosis involves karyotyping DNA extracted from fetal cells. Up to 12 weeks gestation fetal DNA is extracted from chorionic villi cells sampled from the placenta, after 12 weeks gestation fetal cells are sampled from the amniotic fluid via amniocentesis.

6. E
Methotrexate competes with dihydrofolate for the active site of dihydrofolate reductase, preventing the formation of the essential metabolite tetrahydrofolate. Leucovorin (folate) inhibits this effect and in methotrexate toxicity high dose leucovorin rescue therapy is required immediately to rapidly restore tetrahydrofolate levels. Haemodialysis is sometimes used in cases of toxicity to remove circulating methotrexate, but it has no effect on intracellular levels. Hydration with IV fluids and urine alkalinisation

with sodium bicarbonate are used as preventative therapy during methotrexate treatment to prevent renal damage.

7. D

The clinical presentation of the patient with excessive freckling, sunlight sensitivity and presence of cancer at a young age, suggests she is suffering from xeroderma pigmentosum. This disorder is caused by a defect in DNA nucleotide excision repair proteins, which remove pyrimidine dimers from ultra-violet damaged DNA.

8. B

Global developmental delay, abnormal gait and calf hypertrophy is the typical presentation of Duchenne muscular dystrophy, a recessive, x-linked inherited disorder. Duchenne muscular dystrophy is caused by mutations in the gene encoding for the muscle protein dystrophin. Mutations in the promoter region of a gene alter the binding of RNA polymerase to the promoter site. This leads to inhibited or reduced transcription of the gene.

9. A

The clinical presentation of pneumonia, recurrent infections and lymphocytopenia (low lymphocyte count) is suggestive of severe combined immunodeficiency (SCID). SCID is a recessive genetic disordered caused by mutations in numerous genes involved in the immune response. Adenosine deaminase deficiency is found in 15–20% of SCID cases and causes a reduction in lymphocyte proliferation due to reduced dNTP production.

Proteins

1. E

Serum and urine protein electrophoresis will identify an excess of intact immunoglobulin(s) in serum and urine. It would also identify if κ and or λ light chains were being excreted. Not all forms of myeloma produce both intact immunoglobulins and immunoglobulin light chains.

2. E

Glycated haemoglobin provides an assessment of glycaemic control over an 8–12 week period. Fructosamine and glycated albumin are useful when there is an increased turnover of red blood cells and where an assessment of short term glycaemic control is required (e.g. pregnancy, advanced liver disease).

3. B

Alpha-1-antitrypsin is a serine protease inhibitor. It protects the lower airways from damage caused by the enzyme elastase. Elastase breaks down the protein elastin. The normal alpha-1 antitrypsin allele is called the M allele. Over 100 allelic variants exist. The most severely deficient variant is the Z allele. Clinical manifestations of severe deficiency of AAT typically involve the lung and liver disease

4. D

Diet carbonated drinks. The artificial sweetener aspartame (e.g. NutraSweet) is added to many medications, diet foods and carbonated drinks. This additive contains phenylalanine.

5. D

The antigen against which anti-endomysial antibodies are directed is a tissue transglutaminase (tTG). Anti-tTG antibodies are highly sensitive and specific for the diagnosis of coeliac disease in most reports. Anti-gliadin antibody tests are not recommended due to their low positive predictive value in a general population.

6. A

This is a disorder of carbohydrate metabolism and hyperammonaemia is not observed as part of the pathogenesis of the disease. Galactosemia can result from deficiencies of three different enzymes: galactose-1-phosphate uridyl transferase; galactokinase and uridine diphosphate galactose 4-epimerase.

7. E

Tau proteins are abundant in neurons of the central nervous system and are less common elsewhere. The detection of tau protein will confirm if there has been a leak of cerebral spinal fluid from the skull.

8. C

Acetaminophen is metabolised in the liver to the toxic metabolite N-acetyl-p-benzoquinone imine. NAPQI is normally detoxified by glutathione but in an overdose the cellular glutathione stores are rapidly depleted leading to liver damage. N-acetylcysteine is a precursor to glutathione and replenishes the cellular glutathione stores, preventing liver damage. Methionine is also a precursor to glutathione but must first be converted to cysteine so it is not as effective as N-acetylcysteine. Charcoal is only useful if given within one hour of acetaminophen ingestion to inhibit its absorption.

9. A

The clinical presentation with blue sclera, fragile bones and loose ligaments, is suggestive of osteogenesis imperfecta. This is an inherited disorder of collagen type I where a person has either too little collagen type I or the collagen type I is of a poor quality due to a genetic mutation. Collagen type I is the major protein in mineralised connective tissues such as bones and teeth and is also a component of ligaments and tendons.

Carbohydrates

1. C

Osmotic diuresis is the most likely cause of the hyponatraemia in this man. This is confirmed by the increased urinary sodium. While the kidney can reabsorb 99.9% of sodium in health, the re-absorptive capacity of the kidney is reduced in the presence of hyperglycaemia as the glomerular filtration rate is increased and thus the kidneys re-absorptive efficiency is reduced. The renal threshold for glucose is 10 mmol/L. If for every 16mmol/L of glucose metabolised, serum sodium increases by 6mmol/L, then the sodium is approx 144mmol/L reflecting the dehydration of this patient.

2. C

Measurement of insulin and c-peptide will help identify whether excess endogenous insulin is being produced inappropriately by the body (insulin and c-peptide increased) or whether insulin is being administered exogenously (insulin increased, c-peptide low). Cortisol and growth hormone deficiency are both rarer causes of hypoglycaemia.

3. A

Based on the World Health Organisation (WHO) criteria you would classify this patient as having a diabetic response to a glucose load. If fasting glucose is ≥ 7.0 mmol/L and or 120 minute glucose is ≥ 11.1 mmol/L the WHO classifies this patient as diabetic

4. A

At the time of presentation he has a metabolic acidosis due to the elevated β-hydroxbutyrate (ketoacidosis). The compensation for a metabolic acidosis is a respiratory alkalosis, hence deep breathing to remove the CO_2, known as Kussmaul breathing.

5. C

The baseline glucose and the two hour sample are diagnostic of diabetes. The growth hormone excess and failure to suppress with the glucose load is consistent with acromegaly. Suppression of growth hormone would have ruled out acromegaly. The musculoskeletal clinical features are as a result of soft tissue and bony overgrowth resulting in enlargements of hands, feet, expansion of the skull and protrusion of the jaw. Diabetes is a systemic complication along with hypertension, heart failure and renal failure.

6. D

Although HbA1c of 48 mmol/mol is recommended as the cut-off point for screening for diabetes, if the patient is non-symptomatic then a repeat would be required. If the repeat was < 48 mmol/mol then the patient is at high risk of diabetes and the test should be repeated within six months. In symptomatic adults with relatively slow onset of symptoms a single result ≥ 48 mmol/mol is sufficient for the diagnosis of diabetes.

7. E

The blood sample analysed within the laboratory is collected into a serum tube which contains a clot activator. This causes the sample to clot, thereby releasing potassium from the platelets. An arterial sample analysed on the blood gas analyser contains lithium heparin to prevent clotting, so the potassium will be lower by 0.2-0.3 mmol/L. If there is a greater discrepancy then review of the platelet concentration is important as if this is higher than the reference range 150-400 × 10^9/L then this can further contribute to raise the serum potassium in a clotted sample.

8. D

Reactive hypoglycaemia or postprandial hypoglycaemia can occur when excess insulin is released in response to a glucose load. The patient does not have diabetes. This can occur in people who have had stomach surgery or who may have hereditary fructose. Although the samples could have been swapped, this would be eliminated by ensuring the time of sampling was written on the tubes.

9. D

After birth, a neonate of a diabetic mother will still have insulin circulating without the high glucose concentrations from the mother, hence will become hypoglycaemic. The glucose concentrations require monitoring until the insulin clears the infants system. If hypoglycaemic persists after this time, then investigation of metabolic causes would be required.

10. D

Sulphonyurea therapy is used to increase the released of insulin from the beta cells in the pancreas. The use of this treatment relies on the fact that the beta cells are still producing insulin, therefore sulphonylureas are not used in treatment of type 1 diabetes, where due to the lack of insulin production, they are ineffective. Treatment occasionally results in hypoglycaemia due to the increase in insulin production especially in dose adjustment or during periods of fasting.

Fats

1. C

Statins can induce muscle myopathy, the exact mechanism of which is unclear. It is recommended that creatine kinase is measured before starting statin therapy. This is because CK is present at high concentrations in muscle and therefore is a good indicator of muscle damage.

2. B

As a response to hypoproteinemia the liver tries to compensate by increasing the synthesis of proteins. This includes lipoproteins. An increase in the latter can cause the hypercholesterolaemia.

3. E

The Simon Broom criteria states that total cholesterol should be > 7.5 mmol/L and LDL cholesterol > 4.9 mmol/L to fulfil the criteria for definite diagnosis of familial hypercholesterolemia in an adult.

4. D

The absolute or relative lack of insulin and its action in diabetes means that hormone sensitive lipase activity is not suppressed when adequate energy reserves are available. Insulin inhibits hormone sensitive lipase and catecholamines and ACTH stimulates lipoprotein lipase activity. Lipoprotein lipase hydrolyse triglycerides into glycerol and fatty acids.

5. E

Hypothyroidism frequently causes hypercholesterolemia. This is because there is decreased removal of low density lipoprotein from circulation. Treatment of hypothyroidism with thyroxine replacement frequently corrects the hypercholesterolemia in the absence of a coexisting pathology.

6. D

Alcohol promotes triglyceride synthesis and obesity promotes insulin resistance, thus increased lipoprotein lipase activity and fatty acid metabolism.

7. E

Sodium concentration is measured in the aqueous portion of plasma using indirect ion selective electrode measurement. A low serum sodium concentration can occur when increased concentrations of triglyceride or protein are present as they displace a portion of the aqueous portion (so called electrolyte exclusion principle) and thus also exclude electrolyte that is present. This generates an artifactually low sodium result.

8. B

Gaucher's disease is due to a defect in a gene that encodes for the enzyme glucocerebro-sidase. Measurement of glucocerebrosidase enzyme activity would confirm the diagnosis. Enzyme activity is reduced and as a consequence glucocerebrosides accumulate.

9. E

Tangier disease is a very rare inherited disorder characterised by significantly reduced high-density lipoprotein concentrations, large yellow-orange tonsils and enlarged liver, spleen and lymph nodes. It is caused by mutations in the ATP-binding cassette transporter A1 gene (ABCA1 gene).

Haemoglobin

1. C

LDH and ALT are present at high concentrations within the red blood cell and should increase in the presence of haemolysis. Reticulocyte count should also increase to compensate for a decrease in the number of red blood cells. Reticulocytes are precursors to red blood cells. Haptoglobin should fall as it binds haemoglobin when it is released into circulation when red blood cells are broken down. This is a detoxification mechanism.

2. D

Detection of bilirubin in the urine signifies that conjugation of bilirubin is occurring (bilirubin monoconjugates and diconjugates are water soluble; therefore they can be excreted in the urine).

3. A

Blood ferritin concentrations increase when the body's iron stores increase. Ferritin does not rise until iron stores are high. A ferritin concentration greater than 300 µg/L in men and 200 µg/L in women supports a diagnosis of hemochromatosis. However, ferritin levels can also be increased by many common disorders other than hemochromatosis (e.g. inflammation, renal failure, liver disease). HFE genotyping will only detect the two most common mutations found in haemochromatosis and only a minority of people carrying a mutation develop clinical symptoms.

4. E

Acute intermittent porphyria results from a defect in an enzyme called hydroxymethylbilane synthase. The consequence of this defect is the accumulation of porphobilinogen, which is the substrate the HMBS acts on to form hydroxymethylbilane.

5. B

The presenting feature of iron deficiency is a hypochromic microcytic anaemia (low mean cell volume) and is classically associated with low serum iron and ferritin and high transferrin. The former representing depleted iron stores and the latter a response by the body to maximise iron binding capacity.

6. C
Thalassaemia is screened for at birth using a type of electrophoresis called isoelectric focussing. This is used with genetic techniques to classify the type of haemoglobinopathy.

7. E
Cystic fibrosis is characterised by deficiency of fat soluble vitamins A, D, E and K as the exocrine pancreas is dysfunctional and fat absorption is impaired. Vitamin K is an essential cofactor in the blood coagulation cascade and deficiency results in abnormal PT and APTT times.

8. A
Carbon monoxide (CO) toxicity causes impaired oxygen delivery and utilization at the cellular level. It affects several different sites within the body but has its most profound impact on the organs with the highest oxygen requirement (e.g. brain, heart). CO reversibly binds haemoglobin, resulting in relative functional anaemia.

9. B
In the absence of other clinical features and otherwise normal liver function tests Gilbert's syndrome is the most likely diagnosis. This genetic disorder affects 5% of the population and is a benign condition exacerbated by infection and fasting.

Body fluid homeostasis

1. B
Increased hydrogen ions indicate an acidaemia. Increased pCO_2 indicate a respiratory component and low bicarbonate a metabolic component.

2. A
This case demonstrates a classic presentation of hypoadrenalism (Addison's disease) where patients present with postural hypotension and with a lack of mineralocorticoids (i.e. aldosterone) and glucocorticoids (i.e. cortisol). This means water and electrolyte (typically increased sodium excretion and potassium retention) and glucose homeostasis (i.e. hypoglycaemia) are disturbed.

3. E
Proximal renal tubular acidosis results from a defect in the reabsorption of bicarbonate at the proximal tubule. It presents with a normal anion gap hyperchloraemic metabolic acidosis. The loss of bicarbonate is compensated for by an increase in chloride reabsorption.

4. C
Magnesium is a cofactor for the Na-K-ATPase pump that maintains intra- and extracellular potassium stores within tight limits. Low serum magnesium concentrations can lead to low serum potassium concentrations as it is lost from intracellular stores.

5. A
Parathyroid hormone will establish whether the hypercalcaemia is due to a parathyroid or non-parathyroid cause.

6. D
Vomiting causes a metabolic alkalosis. The body's compensation to this is to maintain the balance of bicarbonate and carbon dioxide at a ratio of 20:1. In order to do this the respiratory centre in the brain reduces the rate of respiration to reduce the elimination of carbon dioxide (respiratory compensation). This results in an increase in the concentration of carbon dioxide. An acid base disorder can only be called fully compensated if the pH is back within the normal range.

7. A
This patient requires water as the clinical and biochemical (increased sodium and urea concentration) picture supports dehydration. Intravenous dextrose will correct the water deficit as dextrose is metabolised to water and carbon dioxide.

8. A
Hyperkalaemia is a life threatening electrolyte abnormality that can result in cardiac arrhythmias. Calcium gluconate is given first to stabilise the myocardium, followed by insulin and dextrose which promotes the movement of potassium into the cell thus lowering the plasma potassium concentration.

9. E
Respiratory alkalosis (low pCO_2) reduces intracellular hydrogen ion concentration and thus increases pH. This promotes the activation of the glycolytic enzyme phosphofructokinase, the rate limiting step of glycolysis. This process requires phosphate for the generation of ATP, and therefore leads to a reduction in extracellular phosphate concentration and an increase in intracellular phosphate. This essentially is the result of a cellular shift of phosphate.

10. E
The most likely explanation for the results is potassium-ethylenediaminetetraacetic acid (K-EDTA) contamination. This is because there was no significant drug history and all other biochemical tests were normal. Contamination is often observed due to the preservative

present in the blood bottle used for a full blood count which uses K-EDTA as a preservative. This happens when the full blood count sample is collected first and the needle or venflon used to collect the blood gets contaminated.

11. C

Thyrotoxic periodic paralysis is a rare genetic caused by mutations in genes that code for certain ion channels that transport sodium and potassium across cell membranes. It present with attacks of muscle weakness in the presence of thyrotoxicosis. Hypokalaemia is usually present during attacks. It can be life threatening if the low potassium concentrations cause cardiac arrhythmias.

Nutrition

1. B

The suppressed PTH indicates a non-parathyroid cause of hypercalcaemia and a normal 25-hydroxyvitamin D excludes iatrogenic vitamin D toxicity. The next appropriate investigation is a 1,25 dihydroxyvitamin D to determine if there is extra-renal hydroxylation of 25-hydroxy vitamin D. In health, conversion of 25-hydroxy vitamin D to 1,25 dihydroxyvitamin D occurs under the physiologic control of PTH, FGF23 and serum phosphate concentration. Sarcoidosis and other granulomatous diseases such as tuberculosis are the most common causes of extra-renal hydroxylation which is independent of PTH.

2. B

If a patient is unable to stand, as in this case with a fractured neck of femur, then height can be estimated from measurement of the ulna. Head circumference is not a requirement for the MUST screening tool. BMI can be estimated from the mid upper arm circumference not the lower arm, but this only provides an indication of BMI. Unplanned weight loss and nutritional intake can be determined from clinical history.

3. A

Typically you would expect hypokalaemia not hyperkalaemia due to vomiting and or misuse of diuretics and laxatives. The BMI is typical of anorexia nervosa which results in hypothalamic dysfunction. She has been unable to get pregnant as she has secondary amenorrhoea and a typical pattern seen in anorexia or excessive extreme exercising with hypothalamic hypogonadism; similar hypothalamic dysfunction results in decreased production of thyroid hormones not increased. Raised cortisol is typical with increased production and decreased

metabolic clearance typical of anorexia. Low creatinine is expected due to the low muscle mass.

4. E

Metabolic alkalosis is not a cause of hyperphosphataemia. Phosphate is an intracellular anion and causes of high circulating levels are related to redistribution from cells, decreased renal excretion or increased intake. Rhabdomyolysis involves cell damage and increased release of phosphate from the cells, particularly muscle cells as seen in this case, following a fall. In chronic kidney disease phosphate filtration and excretion is reduced, however the reabsorption of phosphate is then decreased by the increased secretion of parathyroid hormone (PTH) and FGF23. Eventually the maximum level of suppression is reached and hyperphosphataemia occurs. PTH is phosphaturic and results in phosphate excretion, hence hypoparathyroidism will result in decreased excretion leading to increased concentrations.

5. D

Mineralcorticoid excess rather than deficiency is a cause of hypomagnesaemia via renal excretion. Magnesium can be lost through the gut (diarrhoea, laxative abuse) and via the kidneys (furosemide a loop diuretic, Gitelman syndrome leading to reduced absorption of magnesium from distal convoluted tubule).

6. C

They all affect serum zinc measurement; dietary intake can result in fluctuations and zinc will fall with a decrease in albumin as approximately 80% is protein bound. Zinc will also decrease in the acute phase response as albumin is a negative acute phase responder. Tissue damage results in a raised serum zinc concentration, as zinc is released into the blood from damaged cells.

7. E

Typically coeliac disease will result in weight loss when active due to inability to absorb carbohydrates and fats. This in turn make fat soluble vitamin deficiency likely (A,D,E and K). Iron malabsorption can lead to iron deficiency anaemia and malabsorption of folate and B12 can lead to megaloblastic anaemia.

8. A

Macrocytic anaemia results from either B12 or folate deficiency. Folate deficiency results from inadequate intake, malabsorption or increased demand. In this case the platelet count is also low as is the white cell count. This is because the bone marrow is not producing adequate amounts of cells due to the folate deficiency. With regards to the weight loss it is difficult to know which is cause and which effect −extreme exercise leads to weight loss particularly if the energy intake does not account for the increase in activity. Her periods have stopped due to the excessive physical activity (secondary amenorrhea) where the training schedule interrupts the normal pulsatile nature of gonadotrophin releasing hormone which influences the secretion of leutinizing hormone (LH) and follicle stimulating hormone (FSH).

9. E

Deficiency in vitamin B12 results from absorption difficulties or inadequate intake. Absorption requires intrinsic factor and stomach acid for efficient absorption. In the elderly, nutrition plays a role (decreased intake and dietary changes) as does inflammation of gut, pernicious anaemia and the interference from medications.

10.E

Von Willibrand disease characteristically has a normal prothrombin time but prolonged activated partial thromboplastin time. An increased bleeding tendency, often in the form of easy bruising, bleeding gums and nosebleeds, is characteristic. The disease is due to a deficiency of Von Willebrand factor or if the protein has reduced functionality. The role of Von Willebrand factor is to promote platelet aggregation and to transport factor VIII, also involved in the clotting cascade.

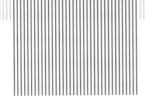

Index

Note: Page numbers in **bold** or *italic* refer to tables or figures, respectively.